The Fascinating Body

How It Works

Sheldon Margulies, M.D.

SCARECROWEDUCATION
Lanham, Maryland • Toronto • Oxford
2004

Published in the United States of America
by ScarecrowEducation
An imprint of The Rowman & Littlefield Publishing Group, Inc.
4501 Forbes Boulevard, Suite 200, Lanham, Maryland 20706
www.scaroweducation.com

PO Box 317
Oxford
OX2 9RU, UK

British Library Cataloguing in Publication Information Available

Library of Congress Cataloging-in-Publication Data

Margulies, Sheldon.
    The fascinating body : how it works / Sheldon Margulies.
        p. cm.
    Includes index.
    ISBN 1-57886-076-8 (pbk. : alk. paper)
    1. Body, Human—Juvenile literature. 2. Human physiology—Juvenile
literature. I. Title.
QP37 .M348 2004
612—dc22

                                                    2003018883

⊗ ™ The paper used in this publication meets the minimum requirements of
American National Standard for Information Sciences—Permanence of
Paper for Printed Library Materials, ANSI/NISO Z39.48-1992.
Manufactured in the United States of America.

To my wife and children, and to teachers everywhere

CONTENTS

INTRODUCTION

There are always two issues in teaching: what to teach and how to teach it. For twelve years, I taught clinical neurology to third- and fourth-year medical students—after they had already studied neuroanatomy, neurophysiology, neuropathology, neurochemistry, and neuropharmacology. It was shocking how little third-year medical students knew about the brain and the nervous system. It finally got to the point where in my introductory talk, I would tell the students that I knew for a fact that the *only* thing they knew about the brain was that it was in the skull. Their response would be smiles of acknowledgment and sighs of relief.

My take on why such bright kids knew so little after so much teaching was that they were taught too much material. They were taught about the twigs on the trees without ever being taught to see the forest. For this reason, *The Fascinating Body* does not contain a lot of microscopic detail or sophisticated chemistry, not because they aren't important, but because they are unnecessary for a day-to-day understanding of how the body works.

That takes care of how to teach; now the harder problem: what to teach about the human body. It seems to me that by the end of high school people ought to know something about the body they expect to occupy for the next 60 to 80 years. Also, it's inevitable that someday your parents will get sick, you'll get sick, or your kids will get sick, and you'll want to talk with the doctors and nurses. If you can't understand more than "He okay. She not okay," you'll never be able to make an informed decision about your own healthcare. And if you ever expect to *avoid* doctors, you might want to rely on something more than cautionary premonitions of your mother and grandmother.

This book lays out in a straightforward fashion what I think any high school graduate should know about the human body, things a person can use in everyday life, things so common that if you haven't asked them before now, you ought to be asking yourself why not. Most of us float through life as passive observers, looking without seeing. We don't ask why things are the way they are, or why things happen the way they do. This is not a new problem. Man has been looking at his world forever, but it was the 14th century before the first artist, Giotto, began to understand perspective—that images recede to one or two vanishing points on the horizon. What have we been looking at for the past million years?

All of us can become good observers, but what separates the great observers from the good observers is that the great ones know what to look for. They're not just looking at something, they're looking *for* something. The trick is knowing what to look for. The greatest observer of all time, of course, was Sherlock Holmes. Holmes was modeled after Dr. Joseph Bell, a Scottish surgeon who practiced medicine in the latter part of the 19th century. One of Bell's students was Arthur Conan Doyle, who went on to create Sherlock Holmes. From careful observation of details like calluses, debris clinging to a coat, speech inflections, and scratches on shoes, Bell would draw remarkably accurate conclusions about his patients. At almost the same time, there lived another equally observant doctor by the name of William Osler. His students once paraded a naked man before him and asked Osler what was wrong with him. The man felt fine and had no symptoms of any kind. Dr. Osler recognized immediately that the patient had been born with his heart inverted, positioned on the right side of his chest and facing the wrong way, a condition called situs invertus. How did Osler know this? Because he saw that the man's right testicle hung lower than the left one when normally the left one hangs lower than the right. The inverted testicles tipped Osler off to the diagnosis of situs invertus. Now *that's* observant. I want you to be that observant.

And if you *are* a good observer of your world, you'll see more than science. You'll see people's physical traits and behavior and begin to understand and even appreciate the differences between us, and with a little space warp, you'll see the world through other people's eyes. In other words, this book is not meant just to teach you science, though I'm sure it will, but also to make you more observant of everything around you.

Currently, human biology is taught by introducing the biochemical foundations of life, such as proteins, DNA, carbohydrates, and lipids. In logical progression, the student is then introduced to the cell, how cells interact to form tissues, how tissues work together to form organs, how organs carry out vital functions of the body, and eventually how all this fits together into some observable activity such as exercise. *The Fascinating Body* reverses that teaching process by beginning with everyday events and then seeking out the anatomic and physiologic bases for those observations. The format is question and answer. Each question concerns some everyday observation or notion about the body and is followed by an answer that includes only enough anatomy and physiology to answer the question.

I think you'll learn a great deal from this book; not enough to put "M.D." after your name, but when you finish you *will* be a step ahead of the public, and what you learn here you will carry with you for the rest of your life. Hopefully, this book will motivate some readers to pursue a career in medicine or an allied field. At the very least this book will jump-start your understanding of the human body. Before you know it, you will begin relating what you've learned in this book to a variety of other fields, which will further expand your knowledge into still other fields. It won't be long before you experience that thrilling rite of passage—when someone facing a hard choice turns to you and asks for *your* opinion about what to do next, and you give it.

1

~~~~~~~~~~~~~~~

ORGAN SYSTEMS

Like any machine, the body works through the coordination of its many organs—the lungs, heart, liver, intestines, brain, and so on. An organ "system" is a particular set of organs that cooperate among themselves to carry out some important function. A good example is the gastro-intestinal system, whose job it is to digest food. The gastrointestinal system extends from the mouth to the rear end and includes the salivary glands, mouth, esophagus, stomach, liver, gall bladder, pancreas, and the small and large intestines.

Each organ in turn is made up of tissues—groups of similar cells acting together to carry out the function of that particular organ. For example, the lungs contain vascular tissue, hematologic tissue, immunologic tissue, and neurologic tissue. All tissues are made of cells, which are living, walled-off sacks of fluid capable of taking in nutrients to make structures vital to the cell's survival.

There are 14 organ systems in the human body, each with one or more specialized function. The functions of the skin are to protect the underlying tissues and help control the temperature of the body. The immunologic system protects the body from infection. The eyes inform the brain of visual events in the environment. The ears inform the brain of auditory events and help maintain our sense of balance. The respiratory system takes in oxygen, exhales carbon dioxide, and helps regulate the acidity of the bloodstream. The cardiac system pumps blood around the body. The gastrointestinal system digests food and supplies the body with nutrients to run the machinery of the body. The endocrine system squirts chemicals into the bloodstream to control the function of distant organs. The vascular system is the blood's highway system. The urologic system rids the body of waste products and helps regulate the acidity and chemical balance of the blood. The genital system controls reproduction. The hematologic system delivers oxygen, nutrients, metabolic waste products, and hormones to their proper destinations. The bones and joints provide the framework necessary for us to stand and move about without collapsing under the force of gravity. The neurologic system deciphers signals from the environment, decides what to do about them, and sends instructions to the body to carry out its decisions.

When illnesses disrupt the function of organ systems, each organ system reacts with specific symptoms and signs. Symptoms are things a person complains about, such as fatigue, dizziness, double vision, and trouble thinking. Signs are abnormal physical findings a doctor discovers during a physical examination, such as swollen glands, a rapid heart rate, an enlarged liver, or a lump in a breast. There are only a limited number of ways in which an illness can disrupt an organ system. It can do it with inflammation, infection, cancerous destruction, chemical disruption, genetic mistakes, mechanical force (compression, twisting, swelling), and trauma. These mechanisms are explained more as we explore each organ system. Each chapter from chapter 2 to chapter 15 answers a series of questions relating to one of the organ systems.

2

~~~~~~~~~~~~~~~~~~~

SKIN

Because beauty is only skin deep, the skin assumes major importance.

Why, for example, does hair turn gray?

We don't know why, only how. Each shaft of hair, or follicle, is formed by a little cluster of cells in the skin, or epidermis. These cells are slowly added to the base of the hair shaft, packing the cells in front of them and pushing the hair shaft upward. In their ascent, the cells die and are replaced by a protein called keratin. The hair-forming cells also add pigment to the hair shaft, but at the age of 45 or so they inexplicably stop making the pigment and the hair turns a colorless gray.

How does electrolysis work?

Electrolysis uses electricity or heat to destroy the cells at the base of the hair follicle. Since electrolysis destroys only one follicle at a time, dermatologists have begun to use lasers to destroy larger numbers of hair follicle cells.

Why don't eyebrows grow as long as a beard?

Each hair follicle is programmed to live only a certain length of time. When that time is up, the hair follicle dies and falls out. The hair on our head lives longer than the hair elsewhere on our body, so it grows the longest.

Why does hair fall out in cancer victims?

Hair falls out because of the drugs used to treat the cancer. Chemotherapy drugs act on any rapidly growing cells, such as cancer cells and hair follicle cells. Once the chemotherapy stops, hair follicles generally recover and the hair grows back.

What is acne?

To help hair follicles slide upward to pores at the skin surface, sebaceous glands secrete oil, called sebum, onto each growing hair follicle (see figure 1). Carried onto the skin surface, sebum also lubricates the skin and helps protect it from bacteria. During teenage years, in response to rising levels of the male sex hormone testosterone in boys *and* girls, sebaceous glands secrete excessive amounts of sebum, which mixes with dead hair cells and clogs the pores, causing collections of oil called whiteheads and blackheads. Whiteheads are located under the skin. If they break through to the skin surface, air turns the oil black and forms blackheads. Pimples develop when whiteheads and blackheads get infected.

How does the drug Accutane work to lessen acne?

Accutane works by slowing the production of sebum and inhibiting the bacteria that infect clogged pores.

Is it okay to pop pimples?

Yes, so long as the bacteria in a pimple are popped onto the surface of the skin. Squeezing pimples that are still deep in the skin can squeeze bacteria into the deeper layers of the skin, where they may form a nasty infection.

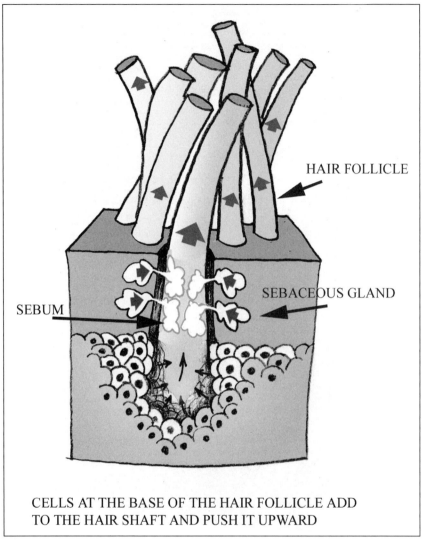

CELLS AT THE BASE OF THE HAIR FOLLICLE ADD
TO THE HAIR SHAFT AND PUSH IT UPWARD

Figure 1

Bacteria squeezed downward into the skin can also gain entry into the bloodstream through small blood vessels. Bacteria in the bloodstream can be very dangerous if they lodge in an internal organ and start a deep-seated infection. For example, in the triangle of death, the area across the face, veins normally carry blood directly into the brain, so squeezing pimples on the face can squirt bacteria directly into the brain (see figure 2). It's best not to squeeze any pimple until it's ready to pop onto the skin surface. First, moisten the head of the pimple to soften it and be sure to squeeze gently from the sides of the pimple, preferably with a sterile gauze pad.

Why does armpit sweat smell so bad?

Armpit and groin sweat are slightly thicker than skin sweat. Armpit sweat smells, in part, because of bacteria flourishing in the thick, moist secretions. As bad as this sweat smells, one scientific study showed that when a man's sweat is dabbed onto the upper lips of women, within a few hours the women report feeling more upbeat and relaxed.

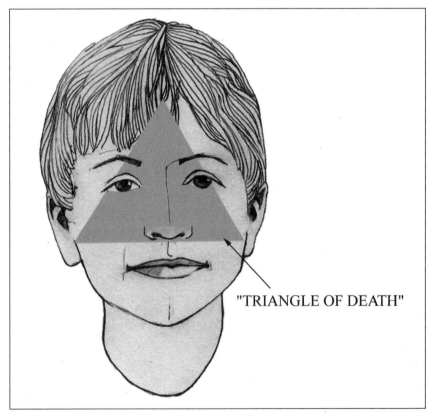

"TRIANGLE OF DEATH"

Figure 2

What's the difference between a callus and a corn?

A callus is a painless thickening of skin from continual rubbing or pressure. A corn is a painful thickening of the skin due to continual rubbing or pressure—painful because the thickened skin is being pushed inward.

What's a keloid?

After a cut, a developing scar knows when to stop growing, but in some people the scar keeps growing beyond the edges of the cut into a thick, raised rope called a keloid. Scar tissue can form anywhere in the body in response to any kind of injury, which is good and bad—good because scar tissue is durable and tough; bad because it has no other useful properties. Scar tissue does not function like the underlying tissue, and too much scar tissue can interfere with the function of the underlying organ.

What's so bad about sun bathing?

Over many years, ultraviolet light in sunshine damages the DNA in skin cells, turning them cancerous. To protect itself, skin releases melanin, a chemical that absorbs ultraviolet rays. Melanin gives skin its brown color, and as man migrated out of Africa the diminished sunshine led to less melanin production and hence lighter skin. Unfortunately, the DNA in melanin-producing cells is particularly vulnerable to cancer-causing ultraviolet light. The cancer that develops in pigmented cells is called a malignant melanoma, a highly dangerous cancer because of its tendency to spread rapidly (metastasize) to distant areas of the body. The risk of melanoma is quite significant. In the United States, there are now more new cases of melanoma per year than new cases of HIV infection. Sunscreens provide pretty good protection against ultraviolet rays and should be used generously.

What's a mole, and why are they sometimes removed?

Moles are pigmented areas of the skin. Melanomas often form in moles, especially atypical moles. For this reason, some people prefer to have atypical moles removed before they have a chance to become malignant.

Atypical moles are those that have irregular shapes and indistinct borders, contain two or more shades of brown, have a bumpy surface, and are larger than the diameter of a pencil eraser.

The real tip-off to a developing melanoma, though, is a change in a mole, even if the mole is typical (small, flat, smooth surfaced, sharp edged, symmetrically shaped). So, if a new mole develops; if an existing mole begins to become raised or larger in diameter or changes shape or color; or if a dark-looking "pimple" develops, especially one that bleeds and doesn't go away, it's best to see a dermatologist, as you don't have a great deal of time to remove a melanoma before it metastasizes.

How do they make tattoos, and what's the risk?

Tattooing involves puncturing the skin with a needle dipped in ink that permanently stains the deeper layers of the skin. The major risk of tattooing is that the needle or the ink may be contaminated with a serious infection like HIV, hepatitis, or syphilis—three diseases that are transmitted when tiny amounts of infected blood are passed from one person to another. It's vital that the needles be sterilized at high temperature between clients and that fresh, sterile ink be used on every new client. First, you have to ask the owner of the tattoo parlor if he does this, and then you have to be able to trust the answer.

What are wrinkles?

Skin is a lot thicker than it looks. Underneath the surface is an elaborate array of elastic fibers that keep the skin taught and collagen fibers that provide a scaffolding for fat cells, blood vessels, sweat glands, oil glands, and hair follicles. Aging causes a loss of all these supporting structures, permitting the surface of the skin to sag and wrinkle. Besides aging, smoking is the worst destroyer of collagen and elastic fibers in the skin. Repeated scientific studies have proven what is obvious on the street: smokers get wrinkles early on and get lots of them. Also, the loss of subcutaneous tissue in the face hollows out the temples and sinks in the cheeks, giving older smokers a characteristic gaunt, wrinkly appearance. To top it off, tobacco smoke also contributes to baldness by damaging delicate hair follicles in the scalp.

3

IMMUNOLOGIC SYSTEM

The immunologic, or immune, system is a collection of lymphoid tissue—white blood cells—strategically placed around the body in the bone marrow, lymph nodes (glands), bloodstream, tonsils, adenoids, appendix, lining of the intestines, liver, and spleen (see figure 3).

The purpose of the immunologic system is to keep bacteria, viruses, and fungi from invading the body. These critters are everywhere, and anytime the immune system is shut out (e.g., by cutting off the blood supply to an organ) or shut down (e.g., by anticancer drugs or the HIV virus), infection is soon to follow.

What's the difference between a bacterium and a virus?

A bacterium is an actively growing cell that takes in nutrients, digests them to make new molecules, and excretes waste products. The instructions governing a bacterium's activities are contained in its DNA. A virus, in contrast, is simply a tiny compact sack of DNA. If a cell from the body were the size of a car, a virus would be the size of an ant. A virus infects its victim by injecting its DNA into a cell and substituting its DNA for the cell's. The viral DNA now controls what the cell makes, which will include more viruses (see figure 4).

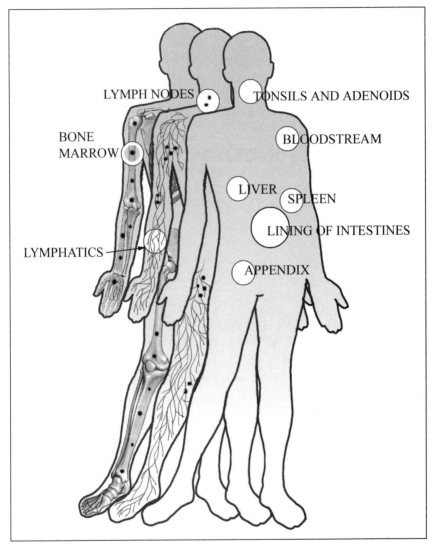

Figure 3

What is inflammation?

Inflammation is a mass attack by white blood cells. The site of inflammation is in its name: arthritis (inflammation in a joint), conjunctivitis (inflammation in the white of the eye), hepatitis (inflammation of the liver), gastritis (inflammation in the stomach), and arteritis (inflammation of arteries).

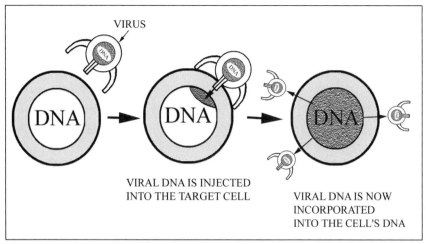

VIRUS

DNA

DNA

DNA

VIRAL DNA IS INJECTED
INTO THE TARGET CELL

VIRAL DNA IS NOW
INCORPORATED
INTO THE CELL'S DNA

Figure 4

There are three reasons for an inflammatory attack. First, the immune system may be attacking something it considers foreign to the body, usually a protein. To the immune system, a foreign substance, called an antigen, could pose a threat to the body, so inflammation is a protective weapon against foreign antigens. Any protein foreign to the body can trigger an inflammatory response, whether it's an infectious agent (bacterium, virus, fungus, protozoa, parasite), a bit of pollen, a transplanted organ, or a splinter of wood. The second reason for an inflammatory attack is that immune surveillance may have turned on itself and attacked something home grown in our own body. The resulting inflammation can persist for months and years and damage the targeted organ system. Two good examples of such autoimmune diseases are systemic lupus erythematosus ("lupus" for short), which attacks our arteries, and rheumatoid arthritis, which attacks the joints. Third, an inflammatory attack may be in response to tissue damage that releases special chemicals that attract white blood cells to repair the damaged tissue.

How does the immune system recognize a protein as foreign?

Proteins and antigens entering the body, and those already in the body, are continually being checked for citizenship by nubbins of lymphoid tissue. The adenoids, for example, located in the back of the throat up behind the soft palate (the thing that flaps up and down in the back of your throat), check the air passing by and the snot dripping down the back of your throat. Food entering the mouth brushes by more lymphoid tissue in the tonsils attached to the side walls of the pharynx—at the very back of the throat.

The adenoids and tonsils are loaded with white blood cells checking for unfamiliar proteins. Once one is detected, white cells in the adenoids and tonsils alert other white blood cells to prepare an immediate two-pronged defense: some white blood cells manufacture antibodies against the foreigner, while other white blood cells seek out and destroy the foreign invader (see figure 5). The wonderful thing about white blood cells is that they remember what the foreign antigen looks like. In fact, they stay primed to respond even faster the next time the protein tries to reenter the body. This is why old folks only contracted measles, mumps, and chicken pox once in their lives. (Now, with vaccines, kids don't even contract these diseases once.)

When a foreign protein does try to reenter the body, antibodies specific to that protein quickly attach to it, and the antigen–antibody complex is taken up by lymph nodes scattered throughout the body. Inside the lymph node, white blood cells swarm around the antigen, causing the lymph node to enlarge. The next time you get an upper respiratory infection, feel for enlarged, tender lymph nodes along each side of the trachea

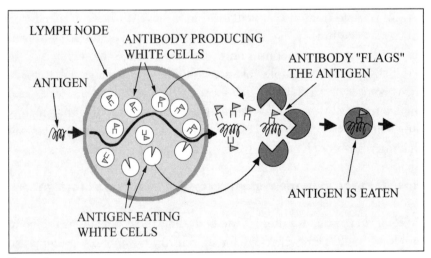

Figure 5

(wind pipe) in the neck. Doctors also check for enlarged lymph nodes in the armpits and groin.

If the tonsils and adenoids are so important for warning against potentially dangerous proteins in the food and air, why are the tonsils and adenoids sometimes surgically removed?

When the tonsils become repeatedly infected, or when the adenoids become large enough to obstruct airflow through the nose, they are sometimes removed. Kids who have tonsils and adenoids removed do lose the benefit of an early warning system, but other lymphatic tissue, called Peyer's patches, densely lining the gut wall suffices to protect against foreign proteins that make it past the nose and mouth into the intestines. Other white blood cells also lie in wait in the lungs.

Are the lymph nodes connected to one another?

Yes, through a system of channels called lymphatics, an entire circulation separate from the blood circulation. Arteries carrying blood from the heart divide into smaller and smaller arteries, until finally blood reaches tiny capillaries where oxygen and glucose being carried by the blood are released into the body's tissues. All capillaries, except those in the brain, continually leak lots of protein and fluid from the bloodstream into the spaces between cells, collectively called the interstitial space. Most of the proteins and fluids reenter the capillaries, but some remain in the interstitial space. Proteins in the interstitial space soak up water, so if they are not returned to the bloodstream, the extremities and organs will swell up with edema fluid. Accordingly, in every part of the body except the brain is a network of tiny canals, the lymphatics, which reabsorbs interstitial fluid and carries it to the nearest lymph node for analysis by white blood cells. If the proteins check out as native to the body, they are then transported through the lymphatics to large veins in the upper chest carrying blood back to the heart. If the proteins are not native, a new antibody is made specifically directed against each foreign protein.

Women who have had a breast removed for cancer sometimes run into problems with swelling in the arm (lymphedema) if the surgeon, in examining for spread of the cancer, has had to remove a lot of lymph nodes in the axilla (armpit). Postsurgical scarring in the axillary lymphatics backs up lymph and edema into the arm.

Why are there two kinds of immunologic defense—antibodies and white blood cells?

Antibodies are easy to produce, can be dumped into the bloodstream for widespread distribution, and can attach themselves to a wide variety of foreign antigens. In doing so, antibodies can neutralize viruses or poisonous toxins such as rattlesnake poison or tetanus toxin. Antibodies are not enough, though. For example, by attaching themselves to foreign antigens sticking out from the surface of bacteria and viruses, antibodies don't actually kill the invaders; they only flag them to be devoured and disassembled by white blood cells (in some circumstances the antibody flag attracts special complement proteins that punch a hole in the bacteria). The other problem with relying solely on antibodies is that some infections such as tuberculosis, syphilis, and viruses grow inside cells, out of reach of antibodies. Only white blood cells can reach those infectious agents.

What's a vaccine?

A vaccine is a way of mobilizing the body's immune system before an infectious agent has a chance to gain a foothold in the body. A small part of the infectious agent, or even the whole infectious agent after it's been killed or disabled in some way, is purposefully introduced into the body for the immune system to analyze. Forewarned is forearmed, so the next time the infectious agent tries to enter the body, the immune system will be waiting for it.

The idea of introducing a mild form of a disease to prevent a more severe form stemmed from milkmaid's complexion. For a thousand years or more it was noted that some milkmaids (women who milked cows) had beautiful complexions, unlike everyone else, whose faces were scarred by smallpox infections. Eventually, it was realized that milkmaids who contracted cowpox, a mild cousin of smallpox, never contracted the face-scarring smallpox. Figuring that the reason the milkmaids did not contract smallpox was because they had contracted cowpox, the next logical step was to purposely infect a person with cowpox in order to prevent a later infection with smallpox. In 1796, Edward Jenner did just this and then later, rather boldly, injected his volunteer patient with smallpox to prove he was now protected.

If we have vaccines, why do we still have infections?

An antibody to a virus is only effective against that particular virus, until the virus switches masks. Many viruses repeatedly change their outward appearance, the best examples being the common cold virus and the HIV virus, which causes AIDS.

Many bacteria are coated with a layer of carbohydrates that make the proteins in the bacterial walls less antigenic (irritating) to the immune system, meaning they are less likely to elicit an antibody response.

What's the difference between infection and inflammation?

An infection is an invasion of an organ system by an infectious agent—a bacterium, virus, or fungus. An infection usually, but not always, elicits an inflammatory response. For example, no inflammatory response occurs when the infection develops in tissue deprived of a blood supply, because white blood cells have no way of reaching the infection. Nor does an inflammatory response occur when the white blood cells have been disabled, for example, by cancer chemotherapy drugs.

What is pus?

Pus is the remnants of an inflammatory attack, usually one directed against bacteria or fungi. When bacteria first invade the body, white blood cells circulating in the bloodstream immediately depart capillaries adjacent to the bacteria to seek the bacteria out. Sometimes, the white blood cells encircle the bacteria with a dense wall of white cells before moving in for the kill. This is quite common when the bacteria are able to hide out in a foreign body, such as a splinter or piece of dirt, which because it has no blood supply is able to harbor bacteria beyond the reach of white blood cells. When the white cells are finished destroying the bacteria and any other tissue in the region, all that's left is a walled-off pocket of gooey yellow pus, called an abscess, filled with dead bacteria, white cells, and destroyed tissue.

The problem with pus is that it has no blood supply, so like the splinter, white blood cells have no way of reaching any bacteria still alive in the pus. Even antibiotics have great difficulty reaching the bacteria and often won't cure an abscess. One way or another the pus has to go or else the bacteria will continue to multiply. If those bacteria get into the bloodstream, a dangerous situation called sepsis, the bacteria can travel anywhere in the body and cause an infection—in the brain, lungs, liver, you name it.

For a long time, pus was thought to be beneficial—a sign that the wound was healing. No one thought of cleaning away "laudable pus" until Ambrose Pare discovered that cleansing pus from wounds improved soldiers' chances of survival. Later, around the time of the Civil War, Joseph Lister considered the possibility that germs, which had recently been proposed by Louis Pasteur as the cause of wine and milk spoilage, might also be the cause of wound infections. Looking around for something to kill germs, Lister learned that carbolic acid was being introduced as a way to prevent sewage from rotting. Gambling that germs were the cause of wound infections, and that carbolic acid might have a beneficial effect on such germs, Lister applied carbolic acid to the wounds of two separate accident victims with broken bones sticking out of their skin—a perfect setup for infection. Both patients recovered without infection, and yet, despite similar successes over the next several decades, many reputable surgeons remained skeptical of Lister's antiseptic approach.

Sometimes when a person coughs, he coughs up clear fluid, sometimes white mucus, and when he has a chest cold, globs of yellow or green mucus. Why the different colors?

The clear stuff is just plain mucus. The white phlegm is mucus mixed with white blood cells. The yellow and green goop is mucus mixed with white blood cells and bacteria—pus.

White phlegm typically occurs when something in the air irritates the bronchial mucosa. (Mucosa is that soft, warm, moist, pink lining of the mouth, nose, bronchial tubes, intestines, and just about every other hollow structure that comes in contact with the air but needs to stay moist.) White blood cells arriving to attack the irritant release chemicals that stimulate the bronchial tubes to make more mucus, which is released into the bronchial tubes. The usual irritant is cigarette smoke, which is why many if not most smokers have a chronic cough, as they try to clear their bronchial tubes of inflamed mucus, a condition called chronic bronchitis. Heavy smokers walk around hacking out pus. Bacteria love bronchial mucus because it's nutritious and, again, out of reach of white blood cells. So long as the infected mucus stays confined to the bronchial tubes, the pus won't do too much immediate damage, but if it gets into the lungs, the bacteria will cause pneumonia.

How do you get rid of pus?

When pus forms in an open wound, the wound has to be soaked in water and the pus scraped away. For abscesses deep in the body, antibiotics typically fail and the only way to cure the abscess is to cut it open and drain out the pus. For abscesses right under the skin, such as a pimple, surgery can be avoided by simply soaking the abscessed area in water. Soaking softens the skin over the abscess, allowing the pus to break through and drain out onto the skin.

Open wounds are not to be fooled with. They need to be thoroughly cleaned, especially to remove any foreign bodies, such as dirt or splinters. If a wound is gaping and fresh, it needs to be sutured closed to reduce the chance of bacterial infection, but only after ensuring that no foreign material is in the wound. Surgeons to this day routinely leave drains in a wound to prevent blood and lymph from accumulating and becoming infected.

What's gangrene?

Gangrene is an infection of necrotic (dead) tissue—dead usually because it's lost its blood supply. A good example is a necrotic foot that's lost its blood supply because of atherosclerotic arteries. Frostbite (skin frozen to death) can also result in tissue necrosis. Bacteria love to infect necrotic tissue, because there's no fear of white blood cells reaching them there. Gangrenous tissue is incurable and has to be amputated.

Three highly dangerous bacteria infect only necrotic tissue because they cannot grow in the presence of oxygen, and without a blood supply necrotic tissue has virtually no oxygen in it. Bacteria that don't need oxygen to grow—and that in fact are *inhibited* by oxygen—are called anerobic bacteria. (Bacteria that do need oxygen to grow are called aerobic bacteria.) Anerobic bacteria are extremely dangerous because they make deadly poisons. One of the most deadly anerobic bacteria is Clostridium tetani, which makes a potent nerve toxin that causes every muscle in the body to contract. The victim's body becomes totally rigid, including the jaw muscles, hence the name lockjaw. (The scientific name tetanus is derived from the Greek for "to stretch," because massive muscular contractions associated with tetanus would arch the body into such extreme hyperextension that only the heels and the back of head would touch the bed.) Tetanus patients have to be placed on a ventilator to help them breathe because, with every muscle contracting, the chest and diaphragm cannot expand and contract to draw air into the lungs. Eventually, the toxin is destroyed and the nerves return to normal functioning.

Another anerobic bacteria, a cousin of *Clostridium tetani*, is *Clostridium perfringens*. When *Clostridium perfringens* contaminates necrotic wounds, it makes vicious proteins that rapidly destroy tissue, turning muscles to soup within hours. Bubbles of carbon dioxide and hydrogen gas produced by the rapidly growing *Clostridium perfringens* give this infection its wartime tag: gas gangrene.

The third anerobic bacterium is *Clostridium botulinum*. If even minuscule amounts of botulinus toxin from a contaminated wound reach the bloodstream, widespread paralysis ensues, including the respiratory muscles. Unless victims of botulism are put on a ventilator, they too will die of respiratory paralysis. If they are placed on a ventilator, however, the body will eventually restore the affected muscles to full power.

Botox is a dilute form of botulinus toxin, and when injected in small amounts it will paralyze muscles in the area of injection that, for various neurologic reasons, involuntarily contract. For example, Botox relaxes wrinkles by paralyzing the tiny muscles forming the edges of the wrinkle. The effects of Botox last four to six months, until the affected muscles recover.

Because *Clostridium tetani*, *Clostridium perfringens*, and *Clostridium botulinum* live in the soil, wounds contaminated by dirt must be thoroughly cleaned and all tissue in the wound that's lost its blood supply must be snipped away to prevent infection by these anerobic bacteria.

Puncture wounds can also be contaminated by clostridium. When a dirty nail punctures the thick skin of the sole, the hole seals up without any bleeding. The reason the sole does not bleed is that it is composed of a thick layer of capillary-free skin cells (which is why a sliver in the sole of your foot can be dug out without much bleeding). The relatively bloodless sole provides an ideal anerobic environment for *Clostridium tetani* or *Clostridium perfringens*. Since *Clostridium tetani* (but not *Clostridium perfringens*) can be prevented with a vaccine, and since we don't go to the doctor for every puncture wound, it's a good idea to get a routine tetanus shot every 5 to 10 years.

Have you ever seen inflammation? How would you recognize it?

Inflammation causes four things to happen: the skin overlying the inflammation gets *red* as blood vessels dilate and leak to deliver white blood cells; all that extra blood causes the skin to get *hot*; fluid and white blood cells pouring out of the leaking capillaries cause the inflamed tissue to become *swollen* with edema (fluid) and *tender* to the touch because of irritating chemicals released by the damaged tissue and white cells. So, a warm, swollen, red, tender elbow is inflamed.

A paronychia is a pretty common example of inflammation. A paronychia is an infection at the edge of a nail in and around the cuticle, causing the adjacent skin to swell and turn red, warm, and very tender. In the foot, similar inflammation occurs along the edge of the great toe when the edge of the toenail grows into the skin, which is called an ingrown toenail. The best place to see dilated capillaries is in the conjunctiva (the white of the eye) when the eyes are bloodshot.

Why do you put ice on a sprained ankle?

Ice is applied to a sprain to reduce edema formation. Edema slows the healing process because inflammatory white blood cells have to swim through all the edema to reach the injury site. Cold constricts blood vessels (which is why your hands turn white in the cold), so less fluid leaks out of the blood vessels. Compression by an ace bandage is also helpful in reducing edema because it forces fluid into other parts of the limb. Elevation of the ankle is another simple technique to drain edema from the injury site, because it allows the extra fluid to simply flow downhill into the calf and thigh.

Why do you get a fever when you get an infection?

Because white blood cells devouring bacteria release chemicals into the bloodstream, chemicals that reset the brain's thermostat to a higher temperature. Suddenly, our body's temperature, which was fine a moment ago, feels too cold and we have to get under some covers to warm up. If the brain's thermostat is really raised, muscles shiver to generate lots of heat. Total body, bed-shaking shivers are known as rigors. This explains *how* we get a fever, but it doesn't explain why we get a fever with an infection. It's unclear if a fever helps white blood cells fight infections, or whether the fever is just one of those things that happens when white blood cells fight infection. A fever can be deadly. If the temperature gets above 106 degrees, the brain begins to seize, or even cook! That's why febrile children, who can quickly run a fever of 105, should be quickly cooled off in a tepid bath.

How does the body rid itself of heat when it has a fever?

Normally, blood vessels in the skin dilate to carry hot blood to the skin surface in order to radiate heat into the air. That's why you look flushed (red) when you get hot. Also, of course, we sweat, sometimes with drenching pajama-changing sweats, and the evaporating sweat cools the skin.

Frequently, patients with a high fever due to infection feel too sick to drink. Between sweating, moisture evaporating from the mouth, and not drinking, fever can make a person dry, or dehydrated. Fluids are desperately needed to maintain the flow of blood because blood is 50% water. Without fluids, the blood pressure will begin to drop as the river of blood dries up. Normally, the body responds to low blood pressure by diverting blood from the skin to the vital internal organs, but that creates a problem because the best way to get rid of body heat is to direct blood to the skin, where the heat can be radiated into the air. If blood flow to the skin is shut off, heat can't escape through the skin, and body temperature will continue to rise. That's why you need to drink plenty of fluids when you have a fever—to allow the body the luxury of supplying blood to the skin, where all that heat can be radiated into the air. Heat radiates from the skin more efficiently if the skin is in contact with water rather than air—another reason febrile children are placed in tepid baths.

What are some of the chemicals released by damaged tissue and white blood cells?

Scores of chemicals are released, among them the prostaglandins, so named because they were first discovered in the prostate gland. Chemically, they are fat molecules, and there are lots of different ones throughout the body, each of which has some important effect on a particular organ in the body. The prostaglandins released from damaged tissue contribute to the fever, swelling, and pain of inflammation. Other prostaglandins stimulate the production of the stomach's mucous lining. Each of these two branches of prostaglandins is synthesized with the help of an enzyme called cylcooxygenase (COX): COX-1 for the mucous prostaglandins and COX-2 for the inflammatory prostaglandins. (An enzyme is a protein that helps assemble or disassemble other molecules.)

Can't prostaglandins be blocked so you don't suffer pain when injured?

So far, the best way to block the prostaglandins is to block their synthesis by inhibiting COX-2 with anti-inflammatory drugs such as aspirin, Motrin, Naprosyn, Alleve, Celebrex, Vioxx, and Bextra. Unfortunately, all but Celebrex, Vioxx, and Bextra also block COX-1, the mucus-producing enzyme. Without its mucous lining, the stomach is exposed to its own digestive enzymes and acids. That's why aspirin, Motrin, Naprosyn, Alleve, and others can cause stomach ulcers (an ulcer is an open sore). Since Celebrex, Vioxx, and Bextra don't interfere with COX-1, the mucous lining of the stomach is maintained, greatly reducing the incidence of stomach ulceration from these anti-inflammatory drugs.

Why do you take antihistamines for allergic skin reactions and poison ivy?

Poison ivy, mosquito bites, and allergic reactions to foods and drugs trigger the release of histamine and other inflammatory chemicals such as leukotrienes and cytokines, all of which cause blood vessels to dilate and leak fluid. The dilating blood vessels turn the skin red, and the leaking fluid collects under the skin as bumps in the skin or blebs of fluid, called hives. The itching is from histamine irritating itch nerve fibers in the skin. Antihistamines such as Benadryl counteract the irritating effect of histamine.

Is Tylenol an anti-inflammatory drug?

No. Even though Tylenol inhibits the production of prostaglandins, it's unclear why Tylenol doesn't stop inflammation. Tylenol does, however, stop the pain of inflammation by acting on pain centers in the brain. (Drugs that stop pain are called analgesics.) Tylenol also lowers body temperature, primarily by blocking the temperature-raising effect of prostaglandins and other chemicals on the brain.

Why shouldn't febrile children be given aspirin?

For reasons not entirely understood, in febrile children aspirin precipitates a dangerous waterlogging of the brain called Reye's syndrome (pronounced "rize"). Since there's only so much room inside the skull, a swollen brain quickly raises intracranial pressure. If steps are not taken to lower the intracranial pressure, the raised pressure can do serious damage to the brain.

What anti-inflammatory medicine do they inject into joints?

Corticosteroids. Examples of corticosteroids include prednisone and cortisone. Corticosteroids are superpotent anti-inflammatory agents because they block almost the entire inflammatory response, including the synthesis of prostaglandins and other inflammatory chemicals. Like aspirin and Motrin, corticosteroids interfere with the production of the mucous lining of the stomach, risking the development of stomach ulcers.

Why can't white blood cells get rid of the HIV virus (the virus that causes AIDS)?

Because the HIV virus is already living comfortably inside white blood cells. HIV is able to penetrate white blood cells, take over their DNA, hang out, and eventually kill the host cells. Only a few other infectious agents, such as leprosy and tuberculosis, have the audacity to live and prosper inside white blood cells. As the HIV virus kills off more and more white blood cells, the body loses its ability to defend itself against infections from bacteria, fungi, and other viruses. Consequently, patients with HIV infection end up suffering difficult-to-treat infections.

What's an antibiotic?

An antibiotic is a drug that kills a bacterium, fungus, or virus. With the exception of herpes simplex virus, which is inhibited by the antibiotic acyclovir and its offshoots, viruses are resistant to antibiotics.

Why are antibiotics often given by vein?

By delivering antibiotics through a needle inserted into a vein—intravenous, or IV, injection—much higher concentrations of antibiotics can be delivered into the bloodstream, and therefore more antibiotics can be delivered to where they are needed. An IV is also handy for delivering any medication that's needed in a hurry. A slower method is to inject the medication into a muscle—intramuscular, or IM, injection. Still slower is a subcutaneous injection, between the skin and muscle, and slowest of all is taking a substance by mouth.

Why do antibiotics kill bacteria but not your body's own cells?

Antibiotics selectively damage vital bacterial functions that animal cells don't utilize. For example, penicillin interrupts the way bacteria synthesize their cell walls but not the way animal cells synthesize their cell walls.

What is tuberculosis?

Tuberculosis is a bacterium that causes a dangerous and highly contagious form of pneumonia. In Charles Dickens's day, the cause of tuberculosis was unknown, but because tuberculosis literally consumed the lungs it was called consumption. Even after the cause of tuberculosis was discovered, there was still no cure, so the government would remove people with tuberculosis from their homes and isolate them on large estates called sanitoriums. Finally, in 1949, Dr. Henry Waxman discovered a chemical made from the fungus *streptomyces* that killed tuberculosis. This chemical, which he named *streptomycin*, freed thousands of patients from sanitoriums.

Unfortunately, tuberculosis is still a highly dangerous pneumonia because it is so very resistant to antibiotics. Nearly one-third of the world's population is infected with tuberculosis, albeit mostly in a quiescent stage akin to bacterial hibernation. Nevertheless, tuberculosis remains the world's leading cause of death from infectious agents. The reason the tuberculosis bacterium is so resistant to antibiotics is that it has a fatty coat that antibiotics cannot penetrate and white blood cells cannot consume. The fatty coat gives tuberculosis its subclassification name, mycobacterium.

Tuberculosis loves oxygen, so much so that it primarily affects the *upper* lungs, where there's more air and less blood (gravity pulls blood into the lower lungs). How would you take advantage of this liking for oxygen to slow down the onslaught of tuberculosis in the lungs? You could remove the upper lungs, but the lower lungs would just expand and elevate to fill up the vacant space. You need something that is well aerated, that is rigid, and that can be sterilized to be placed inside the chest wall around the upper lungs to compress them. Exactly—ping-pong balls. By inserting sterile ping-pong balls into the upper chest cavity to compress the upper lungs, surgeons used to deny the tuberculosis bacteria their favorite feeding grounds.

What's a fungus?

A fungus looks like a plant but doesn't contain chlorophyll—which means two things. One, it can't use sunlight as an energy source, so it must get its nutrients from some other dead or living substance. Two, if it doesn't have chlorophyll, it doesn't need sunlight, meaning fungi can live in dark, moist places, such as a forest or between your toes as athlete's foot. Yeast, mushrooms, and molds are all fungi. All that fuzzy stuff growing on stale bread and oranges is mold, but not all molds make food inedible. Blue cheese gets its flavor from the blue mold growing inside it.

Why should a fungus make streptomycin?

In competing with bacteria for food and living space, a fungus armed with an antibiotic that kills a wide range of bacteria, such as streptomycin, is at a distinct advantage. The problem is that only a rare fungus makes an antibiotic. The real reason a few fungi make antibiotics is still unknown.

What other fungus or mold makes an antibiotic?

Penicillin mold—the green fuzzy mold that commonly grows on stale oranges. Penicillin mold triggered the antibiotic revolution. In 1928, Dr. Alexander Fleming was doing a routine experiment of growing staphylococcus bacteria on a plate of agar (agar is like gelatin). In a few spots a mold had accidentally landed on the culture plate and grew into a small round colony. Fleming noticed that all around the mold colony was a rim of clear agar in which no staphylococci were growing. He puzzled over why there were no bacteria growing in that clear halo around the mold colonies. Was there something being released into the agar by the mold preventing the bacteria from growing? If so, what was it?

How would you go about answering these questions?

Fleming grew another plate of staphylococcus bacteria. He then scraped out some of the agar from the clear halo around the mold colony and placed it on the plate of bacteria. When Fleming came back a few hours later, there were clear spots where he had placed the agar, indicating that the bacteria had been killed. Fleming surmised that the mold had made something that seeped into the agar.

How would you go about proving that theory, and how would you find the magic molecule and prove that it killed bacteria?

Fleming scooped up the mold and grew it in a nutritious, clear liquid. The liquid quickly turned yellow from whatever the mold was making. Fleming took some of the yellow liquid and dripped it onto another plate of staphylococcus bacteria. Holes again developed in the plate where he dripped the solution. Fleming named this magic molecule after the mold that it came from: penicillin. Unfortunately, he did not know how to manufacture penicillin in mass quantities for general use. That discovery was made ten years later, by Dr. Howard Florey, an Australian chemist who became so revered by his countrymen that his face adorns the Australian $50 bill (he also received the Nobel Prize).

4

EYES

The eyes are an extension of the brain. During fetal development, the eyes form as little out-pouches from the developing brain and remain connected to the brain by means of the optic nerve behind each eyeball.

We all know that the eyes detect light, but what is light?

Light is one form of energy, a combination of electricity and magnetism called electromagnetic radiation. The electrical part of electromagnetic radiation vibrates back and forth—the more energy, the faster the vibration. How fast the electrical wave vibrates determines the color you see. Slow vibration (low energy) is red, a little faster vibration is orange, then yellow, green, and finally blue (the fastest vibration, or highest energy). When a blacksmith places a cold rod of steel in a hot fire, energy from the fire is transferred into the rod. Slowly, the energy in the rod rises high enough to send out electromagnetic radiation, which you see as a glowing red-hot rod. Red is the lowest frequency of light. If the blacksmith's rod gets any hotter, it should begin to turn yellow, green, and blue. This doesn't happen, because some parts of the rod still emit red light even though the fire is continuing to heat the rod hotter and hotter. The continuing red light combines with the other colors and eventually all the colors of the rainbow are seen simultaneously as a white light, and the rod becomes white hot.

Can electromagnetic radiation vibrate faster than visible light?

Sure. Electromagnetic energy vibrating slightly faster than visible light is called ultraviolet light (which bees and butterflies can see), and faster still are X-rays. These high-energy waves pack quite a wallop. X-rays have so much energy, they pass right through your skin, but they are not strong enough to pass through bones. That's why an X-ray shows the bones but not the skin or any other soft tissue, such as the liver, kidneys, or stomach.

How about electromagnetic radiation vibrating *slower* than visible light?

Not a problem. Electromagnetic radiation vibrating at very low frequency is what carries radio and TV signals. At a little faster frequency are radar waves and faster still are microwaves—the same ones a microwave oven uses to heat up food. A little faster than microwaves is invisible infrared radiation, which is just below the frequency for visible light. Infrared light is used by restaurants to keep food hot after it is cooked, and a pulse of infrared light shot from the remote controls your TV. So visible light, infrared light, ultraviolet light, microwaves, TV signals, radio signals, radar, and X-rays are all forms of electromagnetic radiation. The only difference is how fast the electromagnetic energy vibrates.

If it takes more energy to generate a blue light than a red light, why are heat lamps red, not blue?

Even though blue light contains more energy, infrared light is warmer. If you passed sunlight through a prism to break up light into a rainbow, and then placed a thermometer in each of the colors, as William Herschel did around 1800, you'd find that red light is warmer than blue light. When Herschel moved the thermometer into the dark zone just beyond the red light zone, he found that the temperature was even higher in the infrared zone than in the red zone.

Infrared light heats our skin by transferring its energy to the skin. High-energy blue and ultraviolet light penetrate deeper into the skin and damage it. The resulting inflammatory response is felt as sunburn. Infrared detectors are found in night goggles and in the pits of pit vipers, making them very good at hunting mice underground or at night.

How many of you have ever been woken up by your parents' flipping on the lights in your room? Your first reaction is to squint to reduce the amount of light entering your eyes. The lights are too bright, yet they're the same lights you have on during the evening and they're not too bright then. What gives? Why are the lights too bright when you first wake up? And, conversely, why does it take time for your eyes to adjust to sudden darkness, for example, when you first enter a movie theater?

When light enters the eye, it passes straight through to the back wall of the eye—the retina. Embedded in the retina are thousands and thousands of cells called rods and cones. They are called rods and cones because that's what they are shaped like. When struck by a ray of light, rods and cones send an electrical signal to the brain (see figure 6).

It turns out that rods and cones have different functions. Rods detect the intensity of light, and cones detect the color of light. Rods are 10,000 times more sensitive to light than cones; because of this we use rods at night, not during the day. The chemical in rods that detects light is called rhodopsin. Daylight breaks down rhodopsin, but during the night the rhodopsin in rods is reassembled. In the morning, then, the rising sun gradually inactivates rhodopsin, and the cones take over for daylight vision. If the transition from darkness to brightness is rapid, however— such as when someone flips on the lights when you're asleep—it takes a few minutes for the rhodopsin to be inactivated. During those few minutes, the bright light dazzles the light-sensitive rods. Everything looks too bright and you have to squint (see figure 7).

During the day, when rhodopsin is inactivated by sunlight, any sudden darkness, such as when you walk into a darkened movie theater, will catch the rods without sufficient rhodopsin to see in dim light. Even though the pupils dilate when you walk into a dark room, it takes a few minutes for the rods to build up enough rhodopsin for you to see an empty

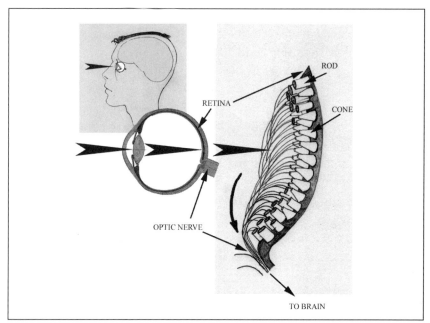

RETINA

ROD

CONE

OPTIC NERVE

TO BRAIN

Figure 6

seat, and another 10 to 15 minutes to reach maximal acclimation to the dark.

Why don't we use rods for daytime vision?

There are two reasons. The first is that rods, while fine for seeing in dim light, don't see as much fine detail as cones do because of what happens to the light impulse after it reaches the rods and cones. When a ray of light strikes a rod or cone, the signal is converted into an electrical signal, which then stimulates a nerve cell in the retina. This nerve cell, called a ganglion cell, sends the electrical signal along its axon to the brain, telling the brain exactly which part of the retina was stimulated.

In the center of our vision, each cone in the retina has its own ganglion cell, so the brain can see things in our central vision with the utmost clarity. For rods, however, one ganglion nerve cell may connect to twenty to thousands of rods, which means a rod ganglion cell services a wider area than a cone ganglion cell (see figure 8). Here's the trade-off: a

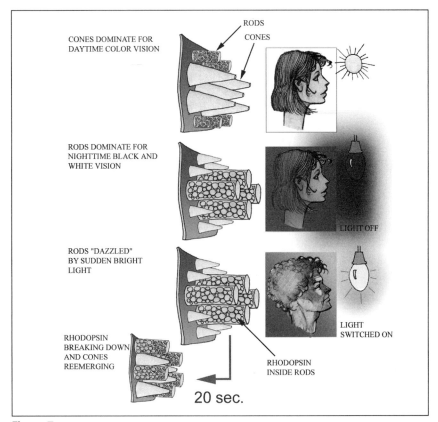

Figure 7

ganglion nerve cell servicing many light-sensitive rods is much more likely to be stimulated by low-level light than a ganglion nerve cell servicing a single cone, which is great for night vision, but the ganglion cell does not know which of the 100 or more rods actually received the light on the retina. Without knowing exactly which rod cell sent the electrical signal, the brain cannot form as sharp an image as it can with signals sent from cones.

The second reason we don't use rods for daytime vision is that rods don't see colors as colors, only as shades of gray. You can demonstrate this by looking at a box of crayons with your rods—after sitting in the dark for 20 minutes or so to let your rods become activated. Now turn on a very dim light and you'll find it very difficult to distinguish the different crayons, particularly the red one, which looks black in dim light.

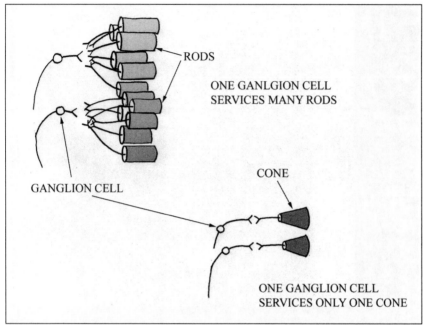

Figure 8

Can rods see color at all?

In a sense rods do see color. Rods are stimulated most intensely by blue-green light, but the brain interprets the messages from rods in shades of gray, not color. Rods are virtually blind to red light, and since the retinas of nocturnal animals are almost exclusively rods, nocturnal animals cannot tell when a red light is being shined at them. Zookeepers routinely fool nocturnal animals into foraging during the day by illuminating their cages with red lights. During World War II, fighter pilots had to be ready at a moment's notice to fly off into the night sky, so at evening time the pilots would put on red goggles. Being insensitive to red, their rods thought it was dark outside and pumped up the rhodopsin. That way, when the alarms rang and the pilots ran outside and removed their goggles, they had immediate night vision.

Nocturnal animals possess something behind their retinas that humans don't, namely, a layer of cells called the tapetum lucidum, which functions like a mirror. The tapetum lucidum reflects light passing through the retina back onto the retina for a second chance to be captured. Light shining off the tapetum lucidum gives nocturnal animals, including your pet dog, an eerie glow to their eyes.

How does the eye focus the center of our vision and blur everything else?

In the center of the retina is a small specialized patch of retina, called the macula, where images are superfocused. Remember that cones are much better at seeing fine detail because there is only one ganglion cell for every cone. Guess what: the macula is densely packed with only cones, no rods.

Why is the center of our vision the only area in sharp focus? Why can't the entire visual field be in focus?

In order to make the entire retina like the macula, the retina would have to be packed with cones, leaving no room for rods or night vision. Besides, if the entire visual field were in focus, you'd be distracted by everything you weren't looking directly at. Still, it would be cool to have your peripheral vision as sharp as central vision.

If you've ever walked your dog at night, you may have noticed that you see the dog better if you look slightly off to the side. Why is that?

Because the macula, where you see things most clearly, contains only cones and no rods, making the macula terrible for night vision. Right around the macula, though, the retina is packed with a doughnut of almost pure rods, so if you look slightly off to one side, the rods adjacent to the macula can see the target—but not as clearly as if you were using your macula in the daytime. In the more peripheral parts of the retina, beyond the doughnut of rods around the macula, the rods and cones are more mixed.

Does every color have its own cone?

No. There wouldn't be enough room in the retina if every color had its own cone. We have only three types of cones. One type of cone sees the color red best, another sees green best, and the third sees blue best. When the brain sees a light that stimulates the red and green cones, it interprets the light as yellow (see figure 9). If the red and green cones are both stimulated, but the reds cones are stimulated more, the light is interpreted as orange. A light that stimulates the green and blue cones is seen as cyan, and a light that stimulates the blue and red is seen as violet.

Artists utilize the same principles when mixing colors. Using a color wheel, the artist can predict the result of mixing two different colors. Blue and yellow make green, blue and red make purple, and red and yellow make orange. In a sense, we have the color wheel in our retinas. When a red light is shined into the eye for a long time, the cones that detect the

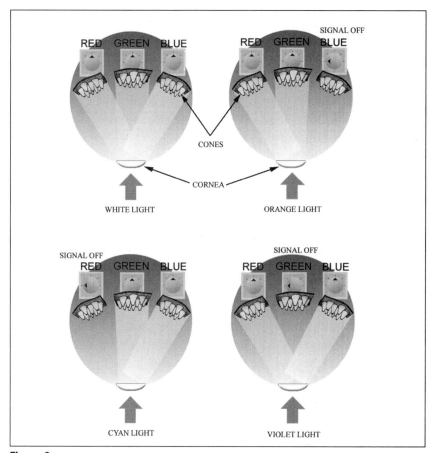

Figure 9

color red become exhausted from the intense stimulation. When the light is removed, the eye sees the color opposite red on the color wheel, namely, green. If a yellow light is shined in the eye, the afterimage is blue. Try it.

What is color blindness?

Some people are born with cones that can't see one of the primary colors. The most commonly defective cone is the one that normally detects green. People with defects in these cones have particular difficulty distinguishing reds from greens—hence the term "red-green" color blindness. The vast majority of color-blind people are men (8% of males versus only 0.5% of females are color-blind) for the following reason. Normally, a person suffers a genetic disease when that person has two defective genes, one defective gene from each parent. (A gene is a short segment of chromosome.) The gene for color blindness rests on the X chromosome. Women have two X chromosomes, so as long as they have one normal X chromosome, the normal gene will prevent color blindness (see figure 10). Very rarely, both X chromosomes in a woman will contain the gene for color blindness and that woman will be color-blind. Men, of course, carry an X chromosome and a Y chromosome. A Y chromosome is an X without its two legs. Those legs contain the gene for color vision, so a Y chromosome cannot counteract the color-blind gene on an X chromosome. Therefore, men need only one defective X chromosome to be color-blind while women need two—hence the discrepancy in color blindness between men and women.

Since the defective gene is on the X chromosome, and since men pass only their Y chromosome to their sons, sons born to color-blind fathers always have normal color vision. The daughters, however, are always carriers of the color-blind gene because one of their two X chromosomes is always defective (see figure 11).

Another example of an X-linked disease is hemophilia, a bleeding disorder in young boys resulting from a defect in the ability of blood to form blood clots.

What's a chromosome?

A chromosome is a long chain of DNA. Each link in the chain is a small bit of the DNA carrying the instructions for assembling one protein.

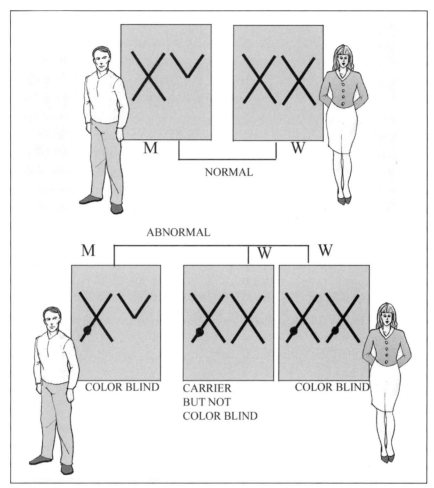

Figure 10

Humans have 46 chromosomes, 23 from each parent. Therefore, for every protein, there are actually two sets of instructions, one set on the chromosome derived from the mother and another on the chromosome derived from the father.

How does the cell know which parent's DNA to obey?

Both parents' DNA is used to make the protein at any one gene site, except for the two X chromosomes in a woman. In each cell of a woman's

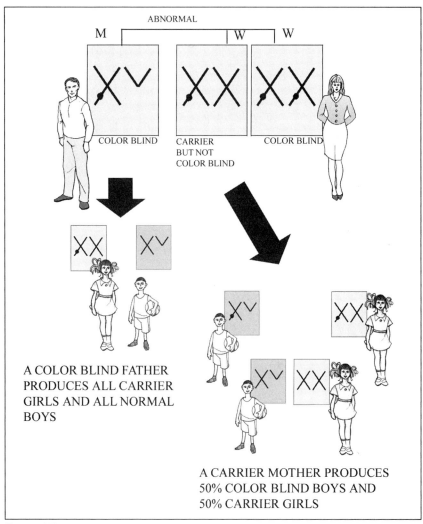

Figure 11

body, one of the two X chromosomes is randomly shut down so that, like a male cell, each female cell has only one functioning X chromosome.

What's the difference between recessive and dominant genes?

Each gene carries the instructions for making a single protein. Whenever the protein from a mother's gene is not identical to the protein made from the father's, one of the proteins may be more effective than its mate. Even if the less effective protein is completely inactive, the cell can function using its other effective protein. The gene that makes the less effective protein is called "recessive." If, however, the defective protein is detrimental to the cell, or if the cell somehow requires both genes to make their proteins, the cell will suffer, even die. Now the gene making the defective protein becomes "dominant." In other words, so long as the cell can survive with the defective gene product (a protein), that gene is recessive, but as soon as the gene product is detrimental to the cell—because the protein is toxic to the cell or the cell requires both genes to make its protein—the defective gene becomes a dominant gene.

Why is it dangerous to look at the sun?

Because the intense ultraviolet light rays of the sun can burn a hole in the macula and cause you to lose your sharp central vision. Sunlight is very high energy, and the only time we can safely look at sunlight is after it has been reflected off some object.

Why are carrots supposed to be good for your eyes?

Carrots contain lots of vitamin A, and rhodopsin is synthesized from vitamin A. As you'd expect, vitamin A *deficiency* causes night blindness.

How many of us have seen a retina?

You've all seen a retina because you've all seen a photograph of people with red eyes, which happens when light from the flash reflects off the red retina back to the camera. The way to avoid red eye is not to mount the flash above the camera lens but off to one side so that the retinal reflection doesn't return directly to the camera lens. Another way to prevent red eye is to make the pupil so small that only a little light gets into the eye to be reflected back from the retina. That's how most cameras work. A flash from the camera *before* the picture is taken causes the pupils to constrict, and then another flash actually illuminates the picture while the pupils are still constricted.

Why is the retina red?

The red is from blood circulating through the retina. Arteries carry blood away from the heart, branching to almost every spot in the body. Capillaries are the very terminal twigs of the arterial tree. After blood goes through the capillaries, it enters veins that carry it back to the heart. You can see the arteries and veins in your own retina by holding a pen light gently against the corner of your eye. The branching pattern you see is the blood vessels of the retina feeding the rods and cones.

Does the retina know what it's seeing?

No. The retina only sees the features of, say, a rabbit; it doesn't know that it's a rabbit. We interpret what we see in the brain only after the retina sends its signals to the brain for analysis. The brain recognizes the retinal image as a rabbit by comparing the new image with known past images. Because it is so important for us to distinguish what we've seen before from what we haven't, the brain is hardwired to be absolutely fascinated by new images. Watch a baby or early toddler stare with fascination at any new object. We never outgrow this fascination with things new.

So how does the retina tell the brain what it saw?

Remember the ganglion cells? The ganglion cells receive signals from the rods and cones. Axons of all the ganglion cells sweep along the surface of the retina to converge on a drain—the optic disc in the back of the retina. The axons pass through the optic disc into the optic nerve and, like a bundle of electrical wires, carry the electrical signals into the brain.

What is the blind spot?

The blind spot is a small area of vision where you cannot see anything. The blind spot is situated slightly to the outside of central vision and is best detected by closing one eye and holding your fully outstretched arm in front of you with the thumb up (see figure 12). Looking straight ahead, gradually drift the thumb to the side. The thumb will disappear at about 6 inches and then reappear as you move it beyond the 6 inches. The blind

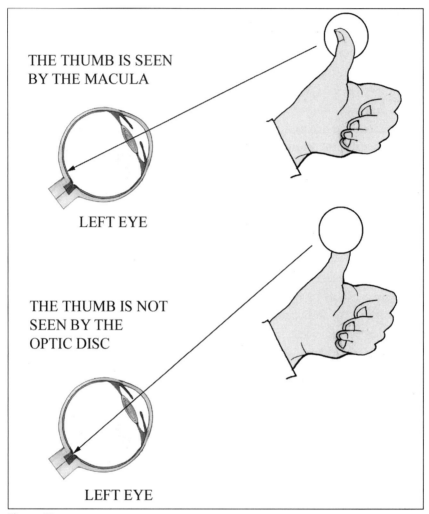

THE THUMB IS SEEN
BY THE MACULA

LEFT EYE

THE THUMB IS NOT
SEEN BY THE
OPTIC DISC

LEFT EYE

Figure 12

spot corresponds to the optic disc, the spot in the retina where the optic
nerve plugs into the back of the retina, a spot that has no rods or cones,
only ganglion nerve fibers connecting to the brain.

What is the instrument the doctor uses to look in the eye?

An ophthalmoscope. An ophthalmoscope contains a little flashlight that
shines a light through a small magnifying lens into the pupil. By looking

through the magnifying lens, a doctor can see the retina and the tip of the optic nerve plugging into the back of the retina.

Why do people have different-colored eyes?

The color of the eyes depends on the amount of pigment in the iris. The pigment is melanin, the same pigment that makes the skin brown. Brown irises have the most melanin and blue eyes have the least. Green, hazel, and gray eyes have amounts in between. Melanin is also situated in the retina and helps absorb light. The amount of melanin in the retina corresponds with the amount of melanin in the iris, so brown-eyed people with lots of melanin in the retina suffer less glare from bright sunlight than less-pigmented, blue-eyed people.

What's the difference between the pupil and the iris?

The iris (means rainbow in Greek) is the colored part of the eye surrounding the pupil. The pupil is not a physical structure, just a central space surrounded by the iris. The iris is a tiny loop of muscle that contracts in response to light, closing the pupil like a purse string. Other tiny muscles pull the iris open. The reason the iris contracts and dilates in response to the intensity of the light is to steady the amount of light striking the retina. (The pupil is called a pupil because a person can see himself reflected as a small person—a pupil—in the eye of another person.)

What does "20/20 vision" mean?

Having 20/20 vision means you can see at 20 feet what a normal person sees at 20 feet. If you have 20/50 vision, you see at 20 feet what a normal person can see at 50 feet, and if you have 20/10 vision you can see at 20 feet what a normal person has to get within 10 feet to see. Hawks have 20/5 vision because their retinas are packed more densely with rods.

Why do people have to wear glasses?

People need glasses to focus blurry images. The reason the images are blurry is that they are not being focused on the retina. Two structures focus images onto the retina: the cornea and a small lens inside the eye. If the eyeball front to back is either too short or too long, the cornea and the lens may not be able to focus the image on the retina at all.

When the image (without glasses) is focused in front of the retina, the person is called nearsighted, or myopic, unable to focus on images in the distance. When the image is focused behind the retina, the person is called farsighted, or hyperopic, unable to focus on images up close (see figure 13). Farsighted people need glasses that preconverge the image before it reaches the cornea, while nearsighted people need diverging lenses to prevent the image from focusing in front of the retina. Converging lenses, which are often rather thick, magnify the eyes, but divergent lenses barely affect the appearance of the size of the eyes.

Why does focusing an image on the retina make it look clear?

Every tiny detail of a viewed object reflects light in all directions. The light rays from every point on the object strike the viewer's eye more or less as a cone of light, passing through the entire length and width of the pupil. If there were no cornea or lens, the cone of rays would land on a wide swath of retina and the retina would be unable to pinpoint where the rays were coming from (see figure 14). In order for each detail of the object to be seen clearly, all the light rays emanating from each point must pass through the pupil and land on the exact same spot in the retina. The cornea and lens focus the cone of light rays onto one tiny spot in the retina. In this way, every detail of the viewed object is seen at only one spot in the retina and the retina can now transmit a clear image to the brain.

Because light rays have to pass through a sort of knot hole (the pupil), the image on the retina is upside down and reversed left to right. In other words, the brain sees things upside down and backward, but since it's been doing that since birth, it interprets the visual world correctly.

How does the cornea focus light?

Any time light traveling through air strikes a transparent structure, it slows down. If the light strikes the transparent structure, say glass, at an angle, the slowing down also causes the light to bend, or refract. The reason light coming from an angle bends as it slows is that light rays have

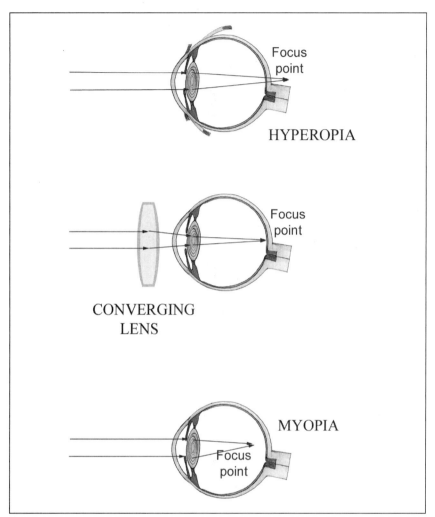

Focus point

HYPEROPIA

Focus point

CONVERGING LENS

MYOPIA

Focus point

Figure 13

some width to them, analogous to a rolling barbell (see figure 15). If the right side of the barbell strikes the glass first, the right side slows down before the left side and the track of the barbell, like the ray of light hitting the cornea, bends to the right. For this reason, the cornea's curved shape always causes light to converge toward the center.

The flip side of all this is that in order for the cornea to refract light, the light must slow down. In other words, the light must be traveling

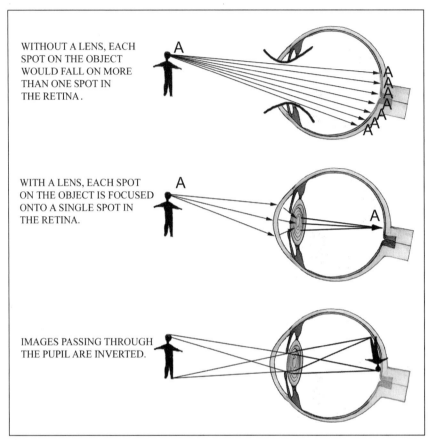

Figure 14

through something like air before it reaches the cornea. This principle is apparent to anyone who swims, because light travels through water at about the same speed as it does through the cornea. If you're not wearing goggles, light traveling through the water won't slow down when it strikes the cornea and therefore won't bend. No bending means no focusing, and no focusing means everything looks blurry until you reestablish an air–cornea interface by putting your goggles back on.

What's astigmatism?

Astigmatism is distortion of both close-up and faraway visual images because the cornea is elongated in one direction, like a football.

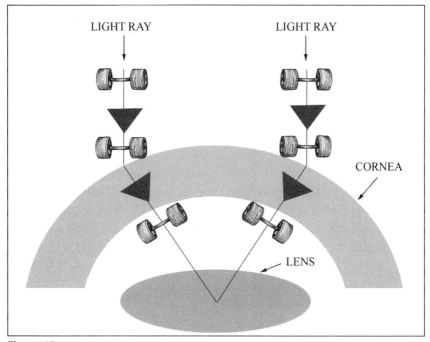

Figure 15

Why do you need a lens if you have a cornea to focus light onto the retina?

If you look at something far away and the image is sharp, then the image is focused on the retina. As you bring that image closer to the eye, however, the rays from the image reach the cornea from a greater angle and eventually the cornea alone will no longer be able to focus the rays onto the retina. The lens, which is situated right behind the iris, further focuses close-up images onto the retina. But depending on how close the image is to the eye, different-strength lenses will be needed to properly focus the image onto the retina. The lens solves this problem by changing its shape in order to adjust its focus for different close-up images. The rounder the lens, the more it refracts. The lens changes shape with the help of two little ciliary muscles attached to either side of the lens (see figure 16).

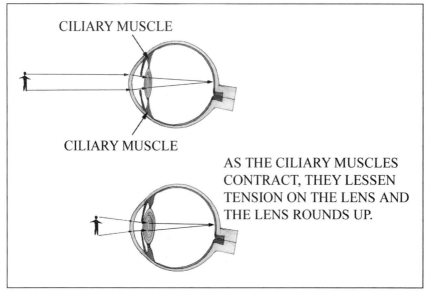

Figure 16

Why do people nearing the age of 40 have to start wearing reading glasses?

As we get older, the lens becomes less elastic and the ciliary muscles weaken. The ciliary muscles can no longer round up the lens when looking at something up close, so things up close go out of focus. This condition is called presbyopia. The solution: reading glasses for close-up vision.

How does lasik surgery work to help you get rid of glasses?

Lasik surgery changes the shape of the cornea so that images can now be focused on the retina. After the cornea is anesthestized with eyedrops, a sharp thin blade slices open a flap from the front of the cornea. A laser then molds the cornea into a new shape. The corneal flap is then pasted back up, leaving no scarring and a newly shaped cornea.

Instead of changing the shape of the cornea, can you change the shape of the lens or the shape of the eyeball?

So far, nothing can be done to change the shape of the lens or the eyeball.

When light travels through a cornea and gets refracted, why doesn't the light get spread out into the colors of a rainbow as it does when going through a prism?

White light from the sun is made up of all the colors in the rainbow. Each color has a different energy frequency. The faster the frequency, the more it slows when it hits a glass prism, and therefore the more it is bent. If the light strikes the glass at a high angle and leaves the other side of the glass at a high angle, too, the colors will be splayed out into the colors of the rainbow, with high-frequency blue on one side and low-frequency red on the other.

Unlike a glass prism, the angle of light entering the cornea is not particularly great, and since the front and back of the cornea are nearly parallel to each other, light exiting the cornea does not become spread out into the colors of the rainbow.

Why do things look clearer when seen through a pinhole?

Theoretically, you could focus without a cornea or lens by making the pupil so small that only one thin beam of rays from every detail of the viewed image enters the eye. The image would be dim, but clear, because each tiny spot on the image would fall on only one spot on the retina. And indeed if you look at something through a tiny pinhole punched in a piece of paper, the image does look clearer through the pinhole. In fact, a pinhole will suffice for a camera lens if you're willing to wait long enough for sufficient light to strike the film.

Taking this one step further, even things in front of and behind the image would be in focus with a pinhole pupil, because light rays from these images, too, would fall on only one spot in the retina. In other words, an ultratiny pinhole not only sharpens the image, but it also produces a very wide depth of field.

When looking at something up close, wouldn't it make sense for the pupil to become smaller in order for the eye to discern finer detail?

Yes. It makes so much sense that pupillary constriction when looking at something close up is hardwired into the brain as a reflex. Ask a friend to look at the tip of his nose and watch how the pupils constrict to allow the eye to discern fine detail up close. The combination of rounding up the lens and constricting the pupil for close-up vision is called the accommodation reflex. By maxing out the accommodation reflex, the Mokens, a population of sea gypsies living off the coast of Thailand, are able to sharpen their underwater vision well enough to locate sufficient food to sustain themselves.

Why do your eyes burn when you get soap in them or peel onions?

Unlike the conjunctiva (the white of the eye), the cornea has a rich supply of sensitive nerve endings. So while you can touch the conjunctiva pretty easily, you can't touch the cornea without quickly blinking. If you've ever gotten something in your eye like soap suds or onion fumes, the pain is coming from the cornea, not the conjunctiva (the fumes from onions form a mild solution of sulfuric acid in the tears). The best way to get burning chemicals out of your eyes is to wash them out with lots and lots of water.

Why do we have eyelashes?

To keep dust and other little particles from falling into the eye.

Why do we have eyebrows?

Probably to keep sweat from dripping into our eyes. They also help the face express our feelings.

What causes those red blotches that sometime develop in the white of the eye?

A red blotch in the conjunctiva is caused by a burst capillary, which spills less than a drop of blood. Not a big deal, because the blood gets absorbed, leaving no traces.

Why do we blink?

Two reasons. One is to wipe the eyeball clean. The other is to moisten the eyeball so it doesn't dry out. Blinking wipes a little teardrop across the eye.

Where do tears come from?

From a tear gland tucked up behind the upper eyelid. The tear gland squirts a tiny tear onto the surface of the eyeball and the eyelid spreads it over the eye.

If the tear gland is constantly dripping tears onto the surface of the eyeball, why don't the tears accumulate and make the eye watery?

Because the tears disappear down a drain at the inner corner of the eye. All night long, tears are slowly dripping over the eyeball and draining into the inner corner of the eye. When you wake up in the morning, there's a little spot of gunk in the corner of your eye that was too thick to get through the drain.

Where does the drain at the inner corner of the eye drain to?

Tears drain into a duct leading into the nose (a duct is any tube leading fluid from one place to another) (see figure 17), which is why you have to wipe your nose when you cry. Someday, if you're lucky, you'll meet a smoker who can blow smoke out his eyes by blowing against pursed lips and pinched nostrils, forcing smoke up the nose, into the tear ducts, and out through the eyes. Cool.

Why do we cry when we're sad?

No one really knows why we bawl when we're sad. Perhaps we cry because tears are an effective attention grabber at a time when attentive concern is most needed.

How do you move your eyeballs?

The same way you move anything in the body—with muscles, in this case

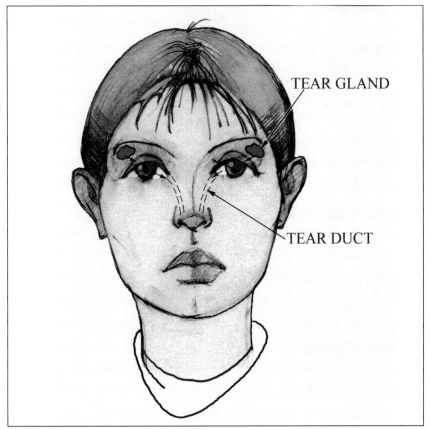

TEAR GLAND

TEAR DUCT

Figure 17

muscles attached to the eyeball (see figure 18). The nerves controlling eye movements are located in the oldest part of the brain—the brainstem. The brain is like an ice cream cone. The ice cream part is the cerebral hemispheres, where we interpret what's going on around us, think about things, and plan our actions. The cone part, or brainstem, is the oldest part of the brain, which controls ancient functions shared by all animals: consciousness, sleep, eye movements, pupillary reaction, eye closure, facial sensation, facial movement, hearing, swallowing, articulation of sounds, rotating the head, tongue movements, blood pressure, pulse rate, and respiration. See chapter 15.

What happens if one of the eyeball muscles is weak?

The eyeballs won't move together. The eyeball that doesn't move so well is called a "lazy" eye. The scientific term is strabismus.

How do you strengthen a weak eye muscle?

How do you make any muscle stronger? By exercise. To encourage the weak eye to exercise, the good eye is covered with a patch so the kid has to use his lazy eye.

Why do we have two eyes? A lot of people lose one eye and can still see. What do two eyes do better than one eye?

First of all, two eyes give us a wider visual field. Hold up your left hand next to your left shoulder and wiggle your fingers. Now close your left eye and suddenly your wiggling fingers are gone.

The other reason we have two eyes is that each eye has a slightly different view of the world. This is why you close one eye when aiming a gun—it's too distracting to see another image when trying to concentrate

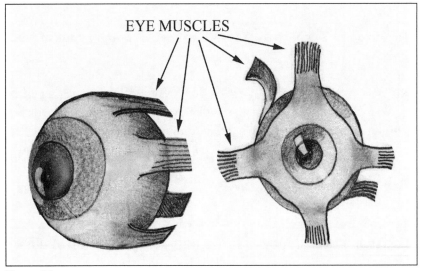

EYE MUSCLES

Figure 18

on the target. With both eyes open, however, the brain can overlap the two images and see a much richer three-dimensional image (see figure 19). Close one eye and look at something far way. Monocular vision is okay, but now try it with both eyes—binocular vision—and see how much easier it is to judge distance. This works better for looking at objects close-up, when the retinal images are very different.

Without three-dimensional vision, it is more difficult to judge how far objects are from us. A person with only one eye has to rely more on the size of an object, its brightness, the eye's internal focusing system, or how fast the image moves across the retina (close-up images move faster across the retina than faraway images) to judge how far away the object is.

Suppose one eye is really lazy, so lazy that it can't be yoked to the other eye and the two eyes produce different images. How does the brain form a single image if it's receiving two nonoverlapping images?

It doesn't. If one eye is so lazy that the images from each eye cannot be fused into a single three-dimensional picture, the brain will ignore the information coming from the lazy eye. If the problem is present in a toddler and the eye doctor doesn't correct it within a couple of years, the brain will eventually ignore that eye forever and the person will become blind in that eye.

Why do some people's eyes look like they're popping out of their heads?

The most common reason for eyes to bulge is that they are being pushed out of their sockets by inflamed, swollen eye muscles. The most common cause for this is Graves' disease, an autoimmune disease that attacks the thyroid and the eye muscles.

What are "floaters" in the eye?

The eye is like a basketball in that it needs something inside it to keep it pumped up nice and round. That something inside the eye is vitreous humor, a clear, colorless jelly. It's clear and colorless because light has to travel through it on its way to the retina. Sometimes, cellular debris floats

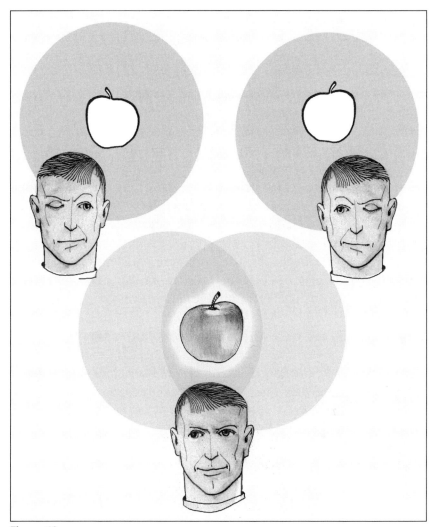

Figure 19

around in the vitreous humor, which you see as tiny floaters in your visual field. Eventually, they go away.

What is glaucoma?

In glaucoma, pressure inside the eye starts to rise. Rising pressure inside the eye presses hard against the tip of the optic nerve at the optic disc.

Eventually, as the high pressure kills the ganglion nerve fibers entering the optic nerve, the person slowly becomes blind in that eye. The gradual rise in intraocular pressure is a painless process ("intra" mean inside and "ocular" means eye). That's why the eye doctor checks the pressure in your eyes even if you're not complaining of anything.

The treatment for glaucoma is to lower intraocular pressure. The reason for the rise in intraocular pressure is blockage of fluid circulating in front of the lens and iris. Normally, watery fluid (called aqueous fluid) is made by a tiny gland situated behind the iris where the iris meets the ciliary muscle. Aqueous fluid flows from behind the iris through the pupil to the front of the iris, where it is absorbed between the iris and the cornea (see figure 20). In glaucoma, the absorption site is blocked, damming up fluid in the front, or anterior, chamber and raising intraocular pressure. Treatments include medications to slow the production of aqueous fluid, surgery to open up the drain site, or surgery to make a new drain through a different part of the conjunctiva.

Why do people see stars when they are hit in the head?

When a person is struck in the head, he suddenly closes his eyes very tightly, causing a sudden sharp rise in intraocular pressure. The sudden rise in intraocular pressure taps against the rods and cones, causing them to send isolated signals to the brain as "stars."

What's a cataract?

It's pretty amazing for a biological substance to be completely transparent. The lens is transparent because of the help of a special protein matrix. When the protein is damaged or is genetically defective, it begins to unravel and clump together, causing the lens to become a cloudy cataract ("cataract" means waterfall in Latin). Cataracts are common in old people. Ultraviolet light is particularly damaging to the delicate protein matrix in the lens. For this reason, it is best to wear glasses and sunglasses that are coated with an ultraviolet filter. Wearing sunglasses without an ultraviolet filter coating may be worse than no sunglasses at all. By blocking out light, sunglasses encourage the pupil to open up and allow more light, including ultraviolet light, into the eye.

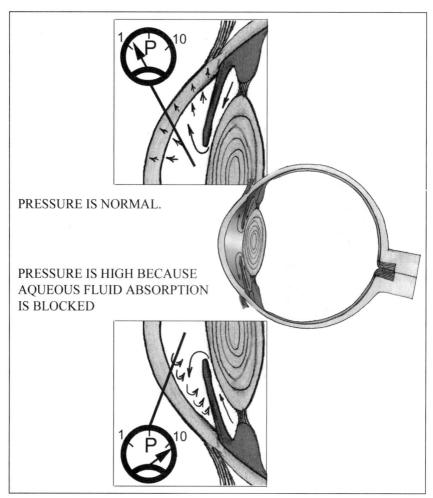

PRESSURE IS NORMAL.

PRESSURE IS HIGH BECAUSE
AQUEOUS FLUID ABSORPTION
IS BLOCKED

Figure 20

How do you treat cataracts?

The solution for cataracts is to take out the lens, which of course prevents images from being focused on the retina. The solution to that problem is to get thick glasses that can really refract light, but they make the eyes look super big. A better solution is to take out the cloudy lens and replace it with an artificial one.

When do they transplant corneas?

If trauma or disease causes the cornea to becomes cloudy, scarred, or mis-
shapen, it's a relatively straightforward operation to cut out the old
cornea and replace it with a donor cornea from a cadaver. In fact, the first
corneal transplant was performed almost 100 years ago, in 1906. The risk
of corneal rejection is not very high, because the cornea does not have a
blood supply (otherwise it wouldn't be crystal clear). Instead, the cornea
receives its nutrients by diffusion from the ocular fluids.

5

EARS

The ears, or otolaryngologic system, were developed to detect sounds and to help with balance. The inside apparatus of the ear is protected deep in the temporal bone of the skull.

Why are our ears shaped so funny?

The outside of the ear, called the pinna, collects sounds from the air and funnels them into the ear canal. The small triangular flap in front of the external ear canal is called the tragus. All the funny little curves in the ear help collect sounds of different frequencies.

Why do we have earwax?

Earwax, or cerumen, is made by glands lining the wall of the ear canal. The sticky earwax collects dust to keep the eardrum clean. Cleaning out the earwax with a cotton tipped stick is not a good idea because you may end up packing the earwax, which only obstructs the external ear canal and impairs hearing. Special solutions available at drugstores soften the earwax and allow it to be washed out with a bulb syringe.

What happens to sounds as they enter the ear canal?

First the big picture. Sounds beat against the eardrum, and the vibrations of the eardrum stimulate nerves deep inside the ear. These nerves transmit signals to the brain, which interprets the signals as sound, determines the nature of the sound and its direction, and then decides what to do about it.

Now let's take a closer look using an otoscope—a magnifying lens with an attached flashlight. Sliding the otoscope into the external auditory canal, the doctor can see the eardrum, or tympanic membrane. The tympanic membrane does look like a drum, but it's not perfectly flat, because there's a tiny bone sticking into the eardrum from the other side. Viewed from the other side of the eardrum, that bone looks like its name, malleus ("hammer" in Latin) (see figure 21). When the eardrum vibrates, the malleus picks up the vibrations and hammers them against another bone, the incus, or "anvil" in Latin, which transmits the vibrations to a third bone, shaped like a stirrup and called the stapes (stirrup in Latin). The area containing the malleus, incus, and stapes is known as the middle ear.

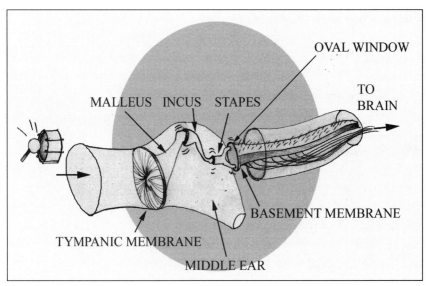

Figure 21

What makes the tympanic membrane vibrate?

Sounds in the air. Air is made up of molecules of nitrogen, oxygen, and carbon dioxide. These molecules are constantly in motion, jiggling back and forth. A sound occurs when something sets the air in motion in such a way that a wave of air molecules vibrates in synchrony. It's like a crowd at a football game. Everyone is jiggling about in their seats, but when they decide to do a wave, everyone in a column of the stadium stands up and then sits down together. The wave you see moving through the crowd could just as well be air molecules. The tympanic membrane is so sensitive to vibration that it can feel tiny waves of moving air molecules.

Sound waves travel through air considerably slower than light waves. The most obvious example of this is sitting in the bleachers and watching a pitcher warm up. You see the ball hit the catcher's mitt well before you hear it. Which raises one of the famous problems haunting baseball: first-base umpires call runners out by comparing what they see (the runner's foot striking the bag) with what they hear (the ball striking the first baseman's glove). Since sound travels slower than light, what the umpire hears actually took place a split second ago. So what he thinks is a tie is really an out.

Why are some sounds high pitched and some low pitched?

The pitch of a sound is determined by how fast air waves are generated. Let's go back to the stadium. Pretend each time a column of spectators stands up and then sits down, they generate a wave of air molecules. If everyone stands up and sits down once a second, the sound wave frequency would be one cycle per second. If everyone stands up and sits down ten times a second, the sound wave frequency would be ten cycles per second. The human ear hears sounds best when the sound pitch is between 1,000 and 3,000 cycles per second, which is about the range of normal speech. The highest pitch a human can hear is about 23,000 cycles per second. A dog can hear sounds up to 45,000 cycles per second—in the range of dog whistles. Whales are capable of hearing sounds as high as 100,000 cycles per second.

How is the loudness of sound measured?

The unit of sound is called a bel, after Alexander Graham Bell, the inventor of the telephone. One-tenth of a bel is a decibel. The human ear is capable of detecting changes of one decibel. Normal speech ranges from about 42 decibels to 70 decibels.

What happens after sounds vibrate the tympanic membrane and the vibrations are picked up by the malleus, incus, and stapes?

The third bone, the stapes, rests against another drum called the oval window, which is very similar to the tympanic membrane. In this way, vibrations from the tympanic membrane cause the oval window to vibrate. On the other side of the oval window, and attached to it, is a long diving-board-shaped membrane called the basement membrane (see figure 22). Sitting along the length of the basement membrane in a bath of fluid is a row of about 20,000 little hairs. The vibrating oval window causes the basement membrane to vibrate. High-frequency sounds make the first part of the basement membrane vibrate most, and low-frequency sounds make the more distant parts of the basement membrane vibrate most. At the bottom of each hair is a nerve connected to the brain, so that each time the hair vibrates, a signal is transmitted to the brain. By knowing which hair along the basement membrane is vibrating, the brain is able to figure out whether a high-pitched or a low-pitched sound is being heard. To save space, the basement membrane is rolled up like a conch shell into a structure called the cochlea. The space deep inside the ear containing the cochlea is called the inner ear.

If you already have a tympanic membrane, why go through all the trouble of vibrating three tiny bones to make another eardrum vibrate? Why not have sound vibrate the oval window directly?

Here's the problem. The cochlea is filled with a clear fluid, so the basement membrane and hair cells are essentially underwater. Any time sounds traveling through air pass into water, they lose strength, which you can attest to if you've listened to someone talking to you while your head was submerged in a bathtub. To make up for the loss of strength as

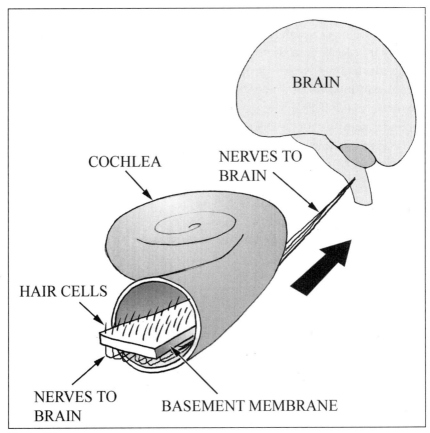

Figure 22

sounds enter the fluid-filled inner ear, bones in the middle ear mechanically preamplify the sounds by taking the energy being exerted against the tympanic membrane and concentrating it onto the much smaller oval window.

Another important function of the malleus, incus, and stapes is to dampen loud, low-pitched sounds and thereby protect the delicate hairs in the inner ear. Tiny muscles attached to the malleus and stapes contract in response to loud, low-pitched noises, causing the stapes to lift slightly away from the oval window. This protective mechanism is also important when you're trying to listen to your date at a noisy party and need to filter out low-frequency background noise. As we age, the dampening apparatus becomes less flexible, which may explain why old people are so intolerant of loud, raucous noise.

The dampening system in the middle ear is only so good. Prolonged exposure to loud noise—including loud music—will eventually damage the delicate hair cells in the inner ear. Partial hearing loss is a real occupational hazard for rock musicians. The dampening system in the middle ear is also a bit slow, so it doesn't protect against sudden loud noises such as a shotgun blast or a firecracker. The only real protection in that situation is earplugs or earmuffs such as the ones worn by airport personnel working around loud jet engines.

Why do your ears pop when you ascend in an airplane or climb a mountain?

The popping sound is air rushing out of the middle ear. Air rushes out of the middle ear through a tiny tube called the eustachian tube, which connects the middle ear to the back of the throat (see figure 23). The purpose of the eustachian tube is to maintain equal air pressure on either side of the tympanic membrane. The tympanic membrane completely covers the ear canal, so air cannot pass from the external auditory canal directly into the middle ear. This does not present a problem so long as air pressure in the external auditory canal and the middle ear are equal— the tympanic membrane in that case won't be pushed in either direction.

The problem is that we live at the bottom of a sea of air. Air seems light, but on the surface of the Earth the ocean of air weighs down on us with a pressure of almost 15 pounds per square inch. As we ascend into thinner air, there's less air weighing down on us and therefore less air pressure. Even inside airplanes flying at high altitude, air pressure is less than at ground level because the cabins are not pressurized to ground level, only to about 5,000 feet. (You can prove this by bringing a sealed bag of potato chips on board. As the plane ascends, the air inside the bag will expand and make the bag taut as a drum. For this reason, you have to be careful flying in airplanes with an air cast around the ankle. The air inside the cast can expand and cut off circulation to the foot.) So, at sea level, equally high pressure on either side of the tympanic membrane pushes equally hard against the tympanic membrane. As you ascend, and

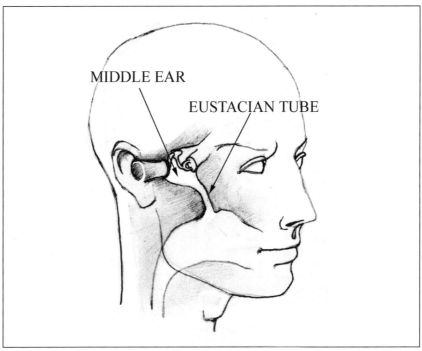

MIDDLE EAR

EUSTACIAN TUBE

Figure 23

air in the external ear canal exerts less and less pressure against the tympanic membrane, high-pressure air in the middle ear will press against the tympanic membrane until it is allowed to escape through the eustachian tube and connect with the outside air. Until that happens, your ears feel stuffed and your immediate reaction is to open your jaw wide. This opens the eustachian tube and vents the high-pressure air in the middle ear into the back of the throat. The air rushing out of the middle ear is audible as a pop. Another way to open the eustachian tube is to gently blow against closed lips while pinching your nose shut. You must do this gently to prevent rupturing the delicate membranes in the inner ear.

The opposite situation occurs when you descend in an airplane. The outside air pressure begins to increase, pushing the eardrum inward. Inward movement of the eardrum is more painful than outward movement, so descending is more painful than ascending. The solution is the same: open your mouth or blow gently against closed lips to open the eustachian tubes. Now the popping sound you hear is air rushing into the middle ear.

Have you ever had a middle-ear infection? How does a doctor detect an infection building in the middle ear?

The doctor looks into your ear with an otoscope and sees changes in the tympanic membrane. The most obvious change is reddening of the tympanic membrane, representing tiny blood vessels dilating to carry blood to fight the infection. As the infection develops, fluid and then pus accumulate in the middle ear and begin to push outward against the tympanic membrane, which the doctors sees as bulging. If antibiotics can't stop the middle-ear infection, the doctor may try to drain the pus by puncturing the tympanic membrane (it's not that painful) to allow the pus to ooze out from the middle ear into the ear canal, where it can be washed away. After the infection has cleared, the tympanic membrane usually seals shut, sometimes leaving scars at the puncture site. If enough scars accumulate, the tympanic membrane may become a bit stiff and the ear won't hear as well. If the hole does not seal shut, the eardrum may be left with a perforation. Perforated eardrums pose some risk to further middle-ear infections, so it's best not to pour things into your ear if you have a perforated eardrum, since this could cause infection.

How does one get a middle-ear infection?

The middle ear is lined with moist mucosa. Excess moisture drains out of the middle ear through the eustachian tube. When you get a cold, the mucosa in the back of your throat swells and partially obstructs the opening of the eustachian tube. Fluid now begins to back up into the middle ear. Bacteria in the back of the mouth—the mouth always has lots of bacteria—simply travel up the eustachian tube to bathe in the fluid collecting in the middle ear. White blood cells cannot reach the bacteria because blood vessels only travel along the mucosal walls, not in the fluid collecting in the middle ear, leaving the bacteria free to multiply. Infants get more middle-ear infections than adults because their eustachian tubes are much shorter, making it easier for bacteria to reach the middle ear.

Also, infants often drink milk while lying on their back, which allows the milk to drain partway into the eustachian tubes and deliver bacteria there.

What is so dangerous about a middle-ear infection?

Inflammatory cells fighting an infection leave scar tissue in their wake. In middle-ear infections, the scar tissue restricts mobility of the malleus, incus, and stapes, causing hearing loss. Also, before the days of antibiotics, kids used to get lots of serious ear infections that would often spread into the adjacent mastoid bone, causing mastoiditis, and from there into the brain, where inflammatory cells would wall off the infection as a brain abscess. In the 1880s and 1890s, Dr. William Macewen, a pioneering Scottish neurosurgeon, would operate on brain abscesses by sawing out a section of skull bone and cutting open the wall of the brain abscess (which was usually near the surface of the brain). To prevent pus from reaccumulating in the abscess cavity, he needed to devise a way to keep the pus draining. His solution was to stick a sterilized, decalcified (that is, with the calcium removed) chicken bone into the abscess cavity for a few weeks to allow the pus to work its way up the spongy bone marrow cavity. Once the drainage stopped, the bone was removed. This was long before antibiotics, but to this day Macewen still has one of the best, if not the best, record for curing brain abscesses of any neurosurgeon in the world.

Why do you get dizzy after being spun around?

Because you are disturbing the balance system in the inner ear. This balance system is called the labyrinth. The labyrinth consists of three tubes, or canals, each in the shape of roughly half a circle, so the other name for the labyrinth is semicircular canals. The three canals are at right angles to each other, one for each plane of space (see figure 24). All the twists and turns in the semicircular canals resemble a labyrinth (a maze), hence the name.

With these three semicircular canals, the brain can tell whether our head is rocking forward, rocking backward, being tilted to the left or right, or being twisted around. Here's how it's done. Lining the inside of

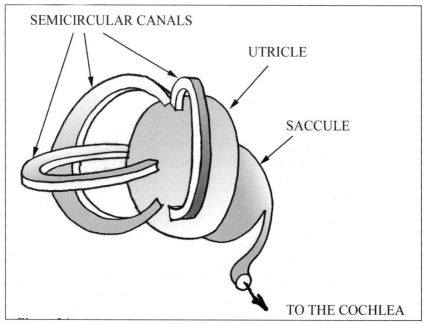

SEMICIRCULAR CANALS

UTRICLE

SACCULE

TO THE COCHLEA

Figure 24

each semicircular canal are cells with tiny hairs. Each semicircular canal is filled with fluid. When we turn our head, the fluid inside the semi-circular canals moves, moving most vigorously in the semicircular canal lying in the plane of movement. So, if you rock your head back and forth like you are nodding yes, the fluid in the sagittal semicircular canal will move most. If you tilt your head from side to side, fluid in the coronal canal will move most. And if you twist your head to look over your shoulder, fluid in the horizontal canal will move most. At the bottom of each hair is a nerve that tells the brain each time the hair is moved. By calculating which hairs are moving and the direction they're moving, the brain can then tell what direction and how fast the head is moving.

When you first spin around, the fluid inside the spinning semicircular canal lags behind, causing the hair cells to bend. After 30 seconds of spinning, though, the semicircular fluid catches up. Then, when you stop, the fluid keeps on spinning, bending the hairs in the opposite direction and causing that dizzy sensation known as vertigo.

Once in a while, debris collects in one of the semicircular canals, preventing the free flow of semicircular fluid. Patients suffer vertigo when moving their head in the plane of the clogged semicircular canal. Head positioning exercises can usually dislodge the debris.

As important as it is to know where our head is in space, this was probably not the reason the semicircular canals evolved. As soon as nerves from the semicircular canals enter the brainstem, they go directly to the nearby eyeball control centers. The reason for the intimate connection between head motion and eye movement is that when our head turns in any direction, the semicircular canals instruct the eyeballs to turn in the opposite direction to keep the eyes locked on target. Of course, if the target is moving while our head is moving, we don't want our eyes moving in exactly the opposite direction of head motion. When the target is moving, special brain cells inhibit the semicircular control of eye movements. God thought of everything.

What if the head isn't moving? How does the brain tell in what position the head is being held?

At the bottom of the three semicircular canals are two large, hollow chambers called the saccule and utricle. Inside them are thousands of little hairs, again, each one connected to the brain by a nerve at the base of the hair. Rattling around inside the saccule and utricle, and stimulating the hairs, is a tiny chip of calcium. Depending on where the calcium lies, the brain figures out whether our head is vertical or not. For example, if the chip is lying at the very bottom of the sacs, our head is vertical, but if the chip is lying off to the side, the brain understands that our head is being held in a titled position. Sometimes a tiny piece of the calcium chip breaks off, so there are now two chips of calcium rattling around inside the utricle or saccule. This confuses the brain about where our head is situated and we feel dizzy.

Why do you need two chambers—a saccule and a utricle—to determine if your head is upright?

You don't. We need two sacs to do something else: the saccule and utricle detect head movement when the neck is held rigid. The resting chip of

calcium in the saccule bends its hair cells when the head moves up and
down or when it moves—not tilts—forward and backward. Similarly, the
utricle detects a rigid head moving from side to side.

Why do scuba divers sometimes get disoriented and swim downward when they really want to swim to the surface?

This happens when the utricle and saccule have been damaged. Without
these two structures to tell them which way is up, scuba divers must either
maintain visual contact with the surface of the water or watch which way
their expired bubbles float. Diving in deep murky water prevents divers
from seeing the surface or the direction their expired bubbles travel. Even
with a normal vestibular system, in deep water buoyancy lightens the
weight of the calcium chips in the saccule and utricle (just as it lightens
the weight of the diver) and weakens the sensation of moving up or down.

What is Meniere's disease?

Meniere's disease is an illness characterized by sudden bouts of severe
vertigo (often throwing patients to the floor), tinnitus (ringing in the
ears), and slowly worsening hearing loss, usually in one ear. The fluid that
bathes cochlear hair cells is connected through a tiny tube to the fluid
bathing the semicircular canals, saccule, and utricle. The volume of fluid
is regulated by a tiny peninsula containing the fluid called the endolymphatic sac. In Meniere's disease, the endolymphatic sac somehow malfunctions and fluid backs up into the cochlea, semicircular canals, and
saccule and utricle, eventually damaging these chambers with high
pressure. Damage to the cochlea causes hearing loss, tinnitus, and high
pressure in the semicircular canals causes bouts of vertigo.

Why should the balance system—the semicircular canals—be con-nected to the hearing apparatus?

When animals were first being created in the sea and developing the
ability to move their heads, they needed a sensing apparatus to detect
how far, how fast, and in what direction they were turning their heads.
The semicircular canals were perfect for telling the animal what its own

head was doing, but these animals also demanded a means of detecting what the water *around them* was doing. A reasonable request, and so developed a set of hairs that could detect movement of the water. When sea animals came onto land, this apparatus was modified a bit to detect movement of the air, which is what sound is. The cochlea, semicircular canals, utricle, and saccule still pay tribute to their sea origins by being immersed in fluid.

What would happen to your balance if a virus destroyed the semi-circular canals?

Probably not much, so long as the brain's two other balance mechanisms were still intact. The two other balance mechanisms are vision and joint position sense. However, since the semicircular canals were designed to keep our eyes on target when our head is moving, damage to the semicircular canals prevents us from doing so. Patients with this condition, called oscillopsia, complain of a jiggling world when, for example, riding in a bumpy car.

Visual input is very important for balance. Admittedly, blind people with intact joint position sense and intact semicircular canals walk fine, but for those of you not used to being blind, try getting up from the floor in total darkness. Not so easy. Better yet, try flying a small airplane into clouds. Within one minute of flying without visual input, simply flying by the seat of his pants, any pilot, no matter how experienced, will be flying upside down or steering his plane into a death spiral.

Joint position sense is monitored by tiny nerves in and around every joint. By getting continuous feedback from joints, the brain is able to monitor our movements. Without joint position sense—hard to imagine, isn't it?—the brain miscalculates how far and how fast to move the limbs. The feet slap against the floor thinking they still have another 2 or 3 inches to go, and the legs are lifted too high when taking a step, like those prancing Austrian horses. But though the gait is odd, the balance is pretty good, because the semicircular canals and vision are still intact.

Balance becomes a serious problem when two out of the three balance systems fail to work properly. For example, if the semicircular canals are damaged and you close your eyes (or get up in the middle of the night to go to the bathroom), balance will be markedly impaired.

6

RESPIRATORY SYSTEM

The respiratory system, extending from the nose to the lungs, is responsible for moving air in and out of the lungs and smelling it along the way.

Where does the actual smelling take place?

The technical term for smell is olfaction. Molecules of, say, french fries float into the air and enter and float all the way to the top of the nose, where the actual smelling takes place. The smell apparatus consists of tiny hairs hanging down from the very top of the nasal chamber. The hairs that hang out of old people's noses are not the ones that do the smelling. The smelling hairs are way high up in the nose. Don't bother to look up your friend's nose, because you won't be able to see them. Olfactory hairs are actually nerve cells extending down from the brain itself. The olfactory hairs poke into the nasal cavity through tiny holes in the bony roof of the nose called the cribriform plate ("cribriform" means sieve in Latin) (see figure 25).

It makes sense that the olfactory fibers should be high up in the nose, because that's where the brain is, but why should the entrance to the nose be so far away from the site where smell actually occurs? Why not put the nostrils higher, closer to the eyes?

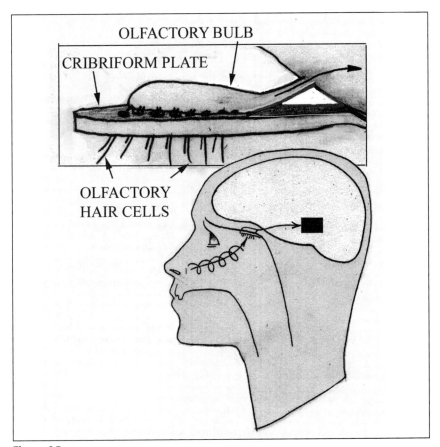

Figure 25

One of the most important purposes of smell is to detect spoiled food, and what better place to put the nose but over the mouth to sniff what you're about to eat.

How are molecules smelled by the nose?

All along the olfactory hairs are millions of tiny receptors just waiting to be stimulated by molecules floating in the air. Humans can detect maybe 10,000 different odors, with women having a keener sense of smell than men. Instead of having 10,000 different receptors for every smell, there are only about 1,000 receptors, and each nerve cell carries only one type of receptor. One theory of olfaction is that odors attach to more than one receptor. If an odor molecule attaches to receptors 1 and 500, the brain interprets that as one odor, while another odor molecule attaching to receptors 1 and 450 is interpreted as something else. So from 1,000 receptors the brain can receive enough information to distinguish among many thousands of different odors.

What happens if we damage the olfactory hair cells?

If we lose the olfactory hair cells, we can't smell anything. We can't taste either, because most of taste is smell. The only things our tongues taste is salt, sweet, bitter, and sour. Everything else we "taste" is via the nose. That's why you pinch a child's nose when spoon feeding him a bad-tasting medicine. People who lose their sense of smell are miserable. It's surprising how much enjoyment of life comes through savoring the fragrance and taste of food.

What's the most common way to lose your sense of smell?

Smoking dulls the sensitivity of the olfactory hair cells, but the quickest way to lose the sense of smell is to forget to wear a seatbelt. As you smack your head against the windshield, the brain is thrust forward, shearing off the olfactory hair cells poking through the cribriform plate in the roof of the nose.

Does everything have a smell?

No. In order to be smelled, molecules have to float into the air and travel up the nose. Anything shedding molecules of itself into the air is called volatile, and most things are not volatile. Heat makes things more volatile, which is why hot food smells so much better than cold food.

What happens after a molecule of some fragrance stimulates a smell receptor? Do the olfactory nerves recognize the smell of french fries?

No, like with the retina, signals from the olfactory hair cells first have to go into the brain and the brain recognizes the smell. Smell signals from the olfactory bulb go directly into the temporal lobe, where they hook up with the brain's new memory centers—the hippocampus and adjacent structures. Of all the five senses—vision, hearing, taste, smell, and touch—only smell has a straight shot into the hippocampus and neighboring memory structures. All the other senses have to stop at other places in the brain for analysis before reaching the temporal lobe's new memory structures.

Why should smell have such a ready access to memory centers in the brain?

Because most animals sniff their way through the world. They need to remember what's good to eat, what they need to run away from, where their home is, who their mother is, and where's a good place to find food. If you have ever encountered a fragrance in the air that evoked an immediate memory of some past experience, that's a remnant of the ancient connection between smell and memory.

Why do we need a nose to breathe in air if we already have a mouth? Why can't the mouth do the breathing?

First of all, if you don't have a nose, you can't breathe while your mouth is full of food. Second, the nose does things to the air as you breathe: it heats up and moisturizes the air. Inside the nose are little fins called turbinates that have a rich blood supply. Since blood is warm, as the air flows over and under and around the turbinates, it is warmed by the blood flowing in the turbinates. Meanwhile, moisture along the nasal mucosa—the soft pink lining of the nose—evaporates into the air passing by.

A third thing the nose does is clean the air so you don't breathe dirty air into the lungs. Small hairs sticking out from the mucosa collect dust particles. The nasal mucosa also cleans the air by secreting a thick, sticky fluid called mucus, which traps air particles. When enough of the junk accumulates in the mucus, you pick it out of your nose as a booger. If something is particularly irritating to the nose, we sneeze it out.

Why do we snore?

Snoring is the sound made by the soft palate (the flip-flop part of the roof of the mouth) flapping against the tongue or against the walls of the pharynx (see figure 26). It happens more commonly in fat people because the fat in their necks encroaches on the airway. This encroachment is especially severe during sleep, as the muscles in the back of the throat relax. Air passing through the narrowed pharynx travels faster, causing the soft palate to flap back and forth.

Can a collapsing pharynx completely obstruct the airway during sleep?

Yes, and it's not healthy. In response to the sudden cutoff of air, sometimes for 30 seconds or more, patients who suffer from this problem thrash about and usually awaken. The name of this condition is sleep apnea ("apnea" means no breathing). Repeated bouts of awakening like this through the night leave the patient exhausted the next day. Eventually, for reasons probably related to the lowered blood oxygen level during the apneic spells, these patients also develop high blood pressure.

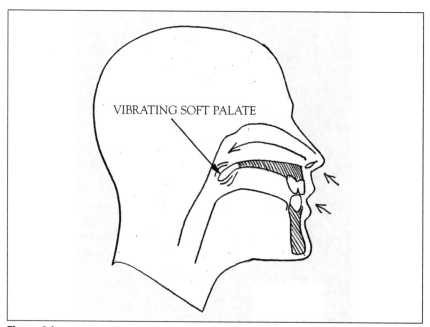

Figure 26

The treatment for sleep apnea is to relieve the obstruction. If the soft tissues in the nose and pharynx are swollen because of hay fever, the hay fever has to be treated. If the person is fat, he or she should lose weight. When all else fails, ear, nose, and throat surgeons can remove the extra flabby tissue in the back of the throat, including the uvula. An even more drastic approach is to surgically place a hole in the trachea through the front of the neck so that air avoids the pharynx altogether. This procedure is called a tracheostomy. ("Otomy" means to make a hole; "ostomy" means to make a hole in an internal organ and bring that hole to the skin surface; "ectomy" means to remove from the body.)

Why when we drink something do we sometimes suddenly start coughing and choking?

Both air and food have to get into our bodies by passing through the back of the throat—the pharynx. Air must get to the lungs and food must get to the stomach. There's a tube for each one—a trachea to carry air to the lungs and an esophagus to carry food to the stomach. The trachea is the bumpy tube in the front of your throat. The esophagus sits behind the trachea and can't be felt. Only air, and no food or drink, is supposed to go into the trachea. At the top of the trachea is a little toilet-seat-shaped flap made of cartilage, called the epiglottis, that moves up and down to cover the opening of the trachea. The epiglottis is attached to the back of the tongue. Each time we swallow food, the back of the tongues pushes food to the back of the throat and at the same time pushes downward on the epiglottis to close the trachea (see figure 27). The closure of the epiglottis is why you have to stop talking when you take a swallow of food.

If food or drink does accidentally get into the trachea, called aspiration, we immediately try to cough it out of the trachea (see figure 28). This coughing is an involuntary reflex—we have no control over it because a wide open trachea is too important to leave to voluntary protection. If we can't cough up the aspirated food, Dr. Heimlich described a procedure to make you cough (see figure 29). Standing behind the choking victim, wrap your arms tightly around his abdomen and lock your fists under the sternum (breastbone). Then yank as hard as you can to force the diaphragm upward and squeeze the lungs, sending a jet of air up the trachea to dislodge the aspirated food. Forceful pounding on the back may also send a jet of air up the trachea to dislodge the food.

How do lions kill their prey?

Lions cleverly kill their prey by simply grabbing the trachea and squeezing it shut, suffocating the animal to death.

Is that how hanging kills—by squeezing the trachea?

No. When a person is hung, the knot of the noose is carefully positioned underneath the chin. When the person falls through the trap door, the sudden jolt at the end of the rope yanks the knot upward, snapping the head back so hard that it breaks the neck and severs (or severely damages) the spinal cord.

The spinal column has two jobs: to provide us with a backbone so we can stand up, and to protect the spinal cord. The backbone part is provided by

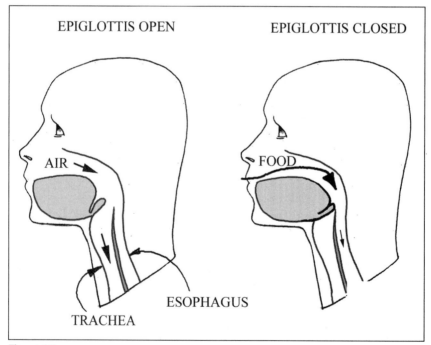

Figure 27

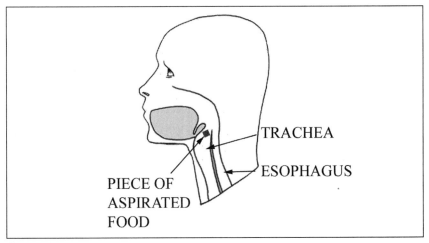

Figure 28

vertebral bodies—cubes of bone stacked one on top of the other with inter-vertebral discs made of cartilage in between. Protecting the spinal cord is a ring of bone connected to the back of each vertebral body. The entire column of rings acts like an elevator shaft down which the spinal cord

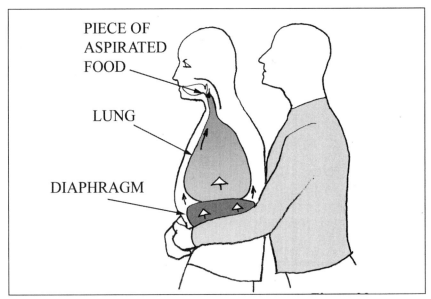

Figure 29

descends behind the vertebral bodies. The vertebral bodies, like all bones, are connected to each other by tough fibrous bands called ligaments. Hanging snaps the ligaments connecting the first and second vertebral bodies, allowing the first vertebral body to slip forward, effectively severing the spinal cord at C1–2 ("C" stands for cervical, which means neck in Latin) (see figure 30). Hanging victims become instantaneously paralyzed from the jaw down, unable to move their arms, legs, or chest muscles, and unable to move their diaphragm, so they suffocate to death.

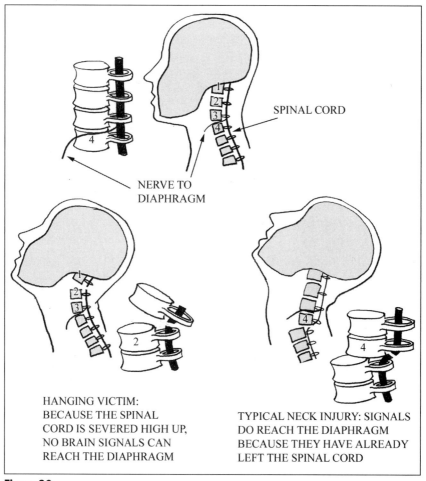

SPINAL CORD

NERVE TO DIAPHRAGM

HANGING VICTIM: BECAUSE THE SPINAL CORD IS SEVERED HIGH UP, NO BRAIN SIGNALS CAN REACH THE DIAPHRAGM

TYPICAL NECK INJURY: SIGNALS DO REACH THE DIAPHRAGM BECAUSE THEY HAVE ALREADY LEFT THE SPINAL CORD

Figure 30

How can any person breathe if he's quadriplegic (paralyzed from the neck down)?

The nerves to the diaphragm leave the spinal cord primarily between the third and fourth cervical vertebrae, while nerves to the arms and legs leave below C4. If a spinal cord injury occurs anywhere below C4, the diaphragm still works. A spinal cord injury above this level, as happened to Christopher Reeves when he fell off his horse, requires a person to be on a ventilator to push air into the lungs.

How do we breathe?

We inhale air through the nose and mouth past the open epiglottis, past the vocal cords, and into the trachea. Behind the sternum, the trachea divides into two large bronchial tubes, one for each lung. The bronchial tubes branch many more times into tiny bronchioles, until finally air reaches actual lung tissue.

Air is actually sucked into the lungs by the downward movement of the diaphragm (see figure 31). Imagine a large barrel with the bottom cut out and replaced with a broad thin sheet of rubber. Drill a hole in the top of the barrel and then pull down on the rubber sheet. Air will be sucked through the hole into the barrel.

Why does pulling down on the rubber bottom suck air into the barrel?

The easiest way to understand this is to plug up the hole in the top of the barrel and then pull down on the rubber bottom. By making the volume of the barrel bigger, the same number of air molecules are now distributed over a larger volume, meaning the air is now less dense and therefore under less pressure. When the plug is removed, the dense, high-pressure air outside the barrel forces its way into the low-pressure barrel. Air is not actually sucked into the barrel; it pushes its way into the barrel.

What does this have to do with the lungs?

Lift up the top of the barrel and, from inside the barrel, attach a trachea and set of lungs to the hole. Close the cover back up and again pull down

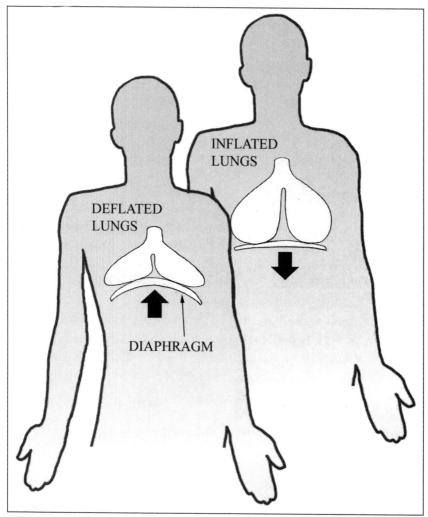

INFLATED
LUNGS

DEFLATED
LUNGS

DIAPHRAGM

Figure 31

on the rubber sheet. The air will still enter the hole but it will now be directed down the trachea and into the lungs. The barrel, of course, is your chest and the rubber bottom is your diaphragm—a large, broad, thin muscle separating the entire chest from the abdomen. The diaphragm is bowed upward toward the chest, and when it contracts—it's a muscle, remember—the diaphragm moves downward, sucking air through the trachea and into the lungs.

When quietly breathing, feel your lower ribs and abdomen expand outward each time you breath in. Why does this happen?

The easy part is the abdomen bulging outward: with each inspiration, the diaphragm contracts and exerts downward pressure on the abdomen, pushing the abdomen forward. The lower ribs expand for the same reason. Here's why. At rest, the diaphragm is bowed upward into the chest cavity. In other words, the sides of the diaphragm course upward along the chest wall for a few inches before spreading out to form a broad dome across the upper abdomen. This means that the lower ribs surround the upper reaches of the abdomen—the abdominal contents up under the diaphragm. So when the diaphragm contracts and pushes downward on the abdomen, not only does the abdomen bulge forward but also the lower ribs bulge out to the sides.

Why can't you stick your fingers between your ribs and touch your lungs?

Take a big breath and feel how your ribs expand outward. When you need to take a deep breath, intercostal muscles between the ribs contract and lift the ribs upward and outward, expanding the volume of the chest. Those intercostal muscles prevent you from slipping your fingers between the ribs. The topmost ribs are lifted up by our neck muscles. Next time someone is breathing heavily, watch carefully for those contracting neck muscles, called the accessory muscles of respiration. Snakes make great use of their intercostal muscles to propel themselves along the ground by rapidly moving their ribs up and back. That fearsome hood that the cobra spreads is spread by specialized ribs.

What muscles do you use when you cough?

To expel air rapidly from the lungs, you need to contract the chest suddenly. This is done without the help of the diaphragm, because the diaphragm is only capable of pulling downward and expanding the volume of the chest cavity. Two sets of muscles coordinate a cough. One set is the abdominal muscles, which by rapidly contracting rapidly shove the diaphragm up into the chest. While this is being done, parallel rows of intercostal muscles—angulated in the opposite direction to the chest-expanding intercostal muscles—contract to pull the ribs together. Try coughing—you will feel your abdomen tighten and your ribs pull together.

What are hiccups?

Hiccups are a sudden involuntary contraction of the diaphragm that causes a sudden rush of air into the trachea that is abruptly terminated by the sudden closure of the epiglottis.

What is epiglottitis?

If the epiglottis becomes infected, from say a strep throat, it can swell enough to obstruct the top of the trachea and suffocate the patient. ("Strep" is short for the bacterium streptococcus.) As the epiglottis swells and the opening to the trachea narrows, you can hear the air whistling through the narrowed opening. Impending obstruction from epiglottitis is a medical emergency requiring a tracheostomy.

Can someone be kept alive if he can't breathe on his own?

Yes, if he is placed on a breathing machine, or ventilator.

How does a ventilator work?

A ventilator is a pump, and like any pump it takes in whatever it's pumping—in this case, air—into a chamber, or bellows, and then rapidly squeezes the bellows to force the air out through a tube. Lots of people still use a bellows to blow air into a fire and provide the fire with more oxygen so it will burn brighter and hotter.

How does the air coming out of the ventilator get into the lungs?

Doctors can't allow the ventilator to simply pump air into the mouth, because much of the air would go down the esophagus into the stomach and blow up the stomach. To get air from the ventilator to go into the trachea, the doctor inserts a tube into the trachea and then connects the ventilator to the tube. This is called an endotracheal tube ("endo" means inside).

How do you get the endotracheal tube into the trachea?

By intubating the trachea—inserting the endotracheal tube through the back of the throat into the trachea. Because most people will gag when something is thrust into the back of their throat, the back of the throat is first sprayed with an anesthetic, or the patient is put to sleep with a mild anesthetic. The endotracheal tube is then slid through the pharynx to the top of the trachea.

Normally, the top of the trachea is covered by the epiglottis, which is there to protect the trachea from anything accidentally falling into the trachea. To get the epiglottis to open, the anesthesiologist tilts the head back and pulls the jaw forward. This maneuver, which lifts open the epiglottis, is why you tilt the head back and pull the jaw forward when giving mouth-to-mouth resuscitation—to ensure that air is getting into the trachea. Conversely, when you get a bloody nose, don't tilt your head back, because blood may run down the back of the throat into the now open trachea. Tilt your head forward so the blood will drain out the nostril and the epiglottis can close off the top of the trachea. This same principle applies to swallowing pills. While you may want to tilt your head back to jostle the pills to the back of your throat, you should then tilt your head forward to close the epiglottis when you actually swallow the pill. (People with impending tracheal obstruction from epiglottitis often tilt their heads back in a desperate attempt to keep the trachea open.)

How does the anesthesiologist direct the endotracheal tube past the epiglottis into the trachea without inadvertently intubating the esophagus?

This problem is magnified by the tongue, which in a supine patient (a patient lying on his back) flops down and obstructs the view of the tracheal opening. To lift the tongue out of the way and provide some light to see the tracheal opening, the anesthesiologist first inserts a long flashlight attached to a speculum (a long, flat blade)—the instrument is called a laryngoscope—into the mouth and advances it to the back of the throat. By lifting the speculum to get the tongue out of the way (the patient is on his back), the anesthesiologist is able to see the opening to the trachea.

What do you suppose those two white bands are at the top of the trachea?

The vocal cords (see figure 32). The anesthesiologist slips the endotracheal tube between the two vocal cords and down a few inches into the trachea.

How do you make the endotracheal tube fit snugly inside the trachea so that when air is pumped through the endotracheal tube into the trachea, the air doesn't escape back out of the trachea around the sides of the endotracheal tube?

Wrapped around the outside of the endotracheal tube is a tiny balloon cuff. After the endotracheal tube is inserted into the trachea, the anesthesiologist blows up the balloon cuff. As the cuff inflates, it seals off the space around the endotracheal tube so that no food or saliva can slip down past the sides of the endotracheal tube into the lungs, and no air being pumped into the trachea can do a U-turn and escape out the top of the trachea. The inflated cuff also secures the endotracheal tube so it won't slip up or down. Remember Dr. Macewen who was curing brain abscesses before the advent of antibiotics? He was also the first doctor to push for intubation of the trachea to deliver continuous anesthesia during surgery.

What are the vocal cords for?

The vocal cords generate the sounds of our voice. The voice box, or larynx, is located at the top of the trachea, inside our Adam's apple.

How do the vocal cords inside the larynx make sounds?

The vocal cords vibrate back and forth as we exhale air up the trachea. The faster the vocal cords vibrate, the higher the pitch. Try this with a rubber band. The more you stretch the rubber band, the higher the pitch when it's

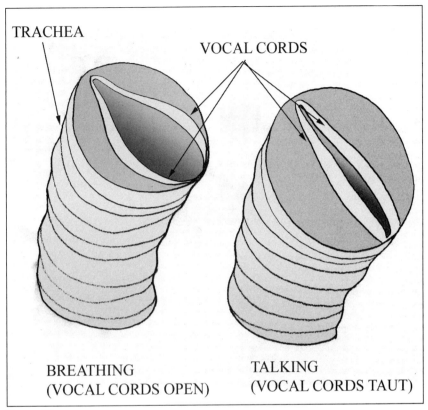

TRACHEA

VOCAL CORDS

BREATHING
(VOCAL CORDS OPEN)

TALKING
(VOCAL CORDS TAUT)

Figure 32

plucked. The vocal cords are longer and thicker in men than in women, which is why men have lower voices and bigger Adam's apples than women. Many musical instruments also generate sounds with a vibrating string—guitar, banjo, and bass fiddle by plucking a string; a piano by tapping a string; and a violin, viola, cello, and base fiddle by stroking a string.

How do the vocal cords change the frequency of vibration—faster for high-pitched sounds and slower for low-pitched sounds?

There are two muscles inside the larynx, one for each vocal cord. When the muscles contract, they pull the vocal cords tauter to make them vibrate faster as air rushes by.

Why do we sound hoarse when we have a cold?

When we get a cold, snot drips down from our sinuses and throat onto the vocal cords. The wet, swollen vocal cords can't vibrate very well, so we sound hoarse.

Why does the pitch of our voice rise when we breathe helium?

Molecules of helium are lighter than molecules of nitrogen, oxygen, and carbon dioxide, which make up the air. Being lighter, helium molecules move faster when set in motion by vibrating vocal cords. Faster-moving molecules produce a higher pitch. The opposite effect occurs when a person breathes gases heavier than air—the pitch drops and it sounds like the devil himself is talking.

Breathing gases heavier than air can get a little tricky, because a heavy gas, being heavy, settles in the lungs and is difficult to breathe out unless you literally stand on your head. Breathing helium can also be a problem if you don't take time between breaths to breathe oxygen, too. Breathing helium from a *pressurized* tank is a definite no-no because enough helium can be forced into the bloodstream to form helium bubbles. Bubbles of any gas in the blood can act like a blood clot, cutting off the blood supply to a section of the heart, brain, or other vital organ.

What is decompression illness?

As deep-sea divers descend into deepwater, the high water pressure forces the nitrogen in the air (air is 80% nitrogen) into the body's tissues. The deeper and longer the dive, the more nitrogen is driven into the body's tissues. If the diver ascends to the surface too rapidly, tissue nitrogen emerges from the tissues as bubbles, akin to a bottle of soda when its cap is popped off. Having bubbles of nitrogen collecting in joints is quite painful and forces divers to bend over in pain, hence the term "bends" for this condition. Nitrogen bubbles in the bloodstream are usually trapped by the small capillaries in the lungs and exhaled into the air. If the bubbles slip through the lungs into the arterial bloodstream, they can obstruct arteries in the brain, spinal cord, heart, and other vital organs. The treatment for such blocked arteries (and for the bends) is to drive the nitrogen back into the tissues by placing the diver into a diving chamber and jacking up the atmospheric pressure. The atmospheric pressure can then be lowered gradually, allowing the nitrogen to escape without forming dangerous bubbles.

What are the sinuses?

The sinuses are hollow chambers in the skull (see figure 33). Instead of solid bone, the skull has a number of large air pockets, or sinuses, to lighten its weight. Sinuses are lined with the same mucosa that lines the inside of your mouth. It's always a little wet inside the sinuses, so there's a hole at the bottom of each sinus for the moisture to escape. When you get a cold, the swollen mucosa may obstruct the hole, causing fluid to back up into the sinus and become infected, a condition called sinusitis. Pus collecting in a sinus can linger on because there are no arteries in the cavity of the sinus to deliver white cells or antibiotics into the pus. Decongestants are used in sinusitis to shrink the mucosa and open up the drain hole for the pus to drain out. If antibiotics and decongestants fail, an otolaryngologist may have to drill out another drain hole in the sinus wall.

Why do we gag when the doctor sticks a tongue depressor in the back of our throats?

The gag reflex kicks things out of the pharynx before they can be aspirated.

What would happen if we didn't cough when food was aspirated?

Aspirated food would tumble down the trachea until it lodged in one of the bronchial tubes. Bacteria in the mouth picked up by the food would start growing on the particles of food, and if the bacteria were able to spread into the lungs, pneumonia would develop.

The possibility of aspiration is why you are not allowed to eat or drink before surgery. Your stomach needs to be empty of all food and drink, because the anesthetic relaxes all muscles in the body, including those that close the epiglottis. It's not uncommon for patients to feel nauseated coming out of anesthesia, and vomiting is the last thing you need to do when the epiglottis is too drugged to protect the trachea from aspiration.

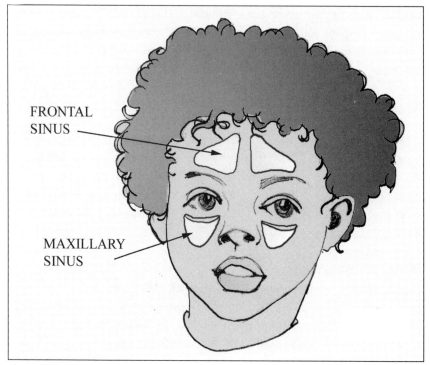

FRONTAL
SINUS

MAXILLARY
SINUS

Figure 33

Why do we breathe?

To get oxygen inside our bodies and to get rid of carbon dioxide. How much carbon dioxide we breathe off affects the acidity of the blood.

How do the lungs know *when* to breathe?

Breathing is controlled by the brain. Because breathing is such an important function for all animals, the respiratory center is in the oldest part of the brain, the brainstem, which all animals possess. The respiratory center rhythmically stimulates the diaphragm to contract. The respiratory center can itself be stimulated by a rise in carbon dioxide in the blood. Conversely, it can be depressed by drugs such as morphine, heroin, and barbiturates, which is why patients die from overdoses of these drugs—the victims stop breathing. The treatment for an overdose victim is relatively simple: mouth-to-mouth resuscitation until you can get them on a ventilator. Eventually, the drugs will be metabolized (broken down) by the liver and breathing will spontaneously recover.

While the brainstem respiratory center controls automatic breathing, we can voluntarily bypass the respiratory center, for example, by simply taking a deep breath. Damage to the brainstem respiratory center results in Ondine's curse. Ondine, legend has it, cast a spell on her unfaithful husband, destroying, among other things, his ability to breathe unless he thought about it. He died in his sleep, as would patients today with Ondine's curse if they were not hooked up to a ventilator at night.

As you might expect, the brainstem is also responsible for other basic functions shared by all animals such as consciousness, blood pressure, temperature control, eye movements, facial sensation, facial movement, balance, and swallowing.

What is the hyperventilation syndrome?

The hyperventilation syndrome is a state of high anxiety leading to over-breathing and blowing off too much carbon dioxide. The resulting chemical changes in the blood lead to a slew of symptoms, such as dizziness, lightheadedness, chest pain, tingling in the hands and feet, wheezing, and if it's severe, involuntary contractions of the hands. To raise the carbon dioxide level back to normal, patients are asked to breathe into a paper bag, which forces them to rebreathe their own carbon dioxide. Once things have calmed down, the cause of the anxiety state has to be sorted out.

What is oxygen?

Oxygen is a molecule made up of two oxygen atoms hooked together, symbolized as O_2. It makes up 21% of the air we breathe. Oxygen molecules breathed into our lungs are picked up by capillaries in the lungs and carried throughout the body.

Why do we need oxygen?

In the process of breaking down food to make energy molecules, two byproducts are released: CO_2 (carbon dioxide) and hydrogen. Carbon dioxide is discarded by breathing it away. The hydrogen is disposed of by combining it with the oxygen we breathe to form water—H_2O—which is urinated away.

Animals breathe in oxygen and breathe out carbon dioxide. What do plants do?

Exactly the opposite. Green leaves take in carbon dioxide from the air and exhale oxygen. How convenient; plants and animals use each other's garbage. Obviously, then, we need green plants and trees to generate a large supply of oxygen for the planet.

What do the lungs do with the air breathed in?

At the end of each tiny bronchiole is a cluster of bubbles, such as the ones that form at the end of a toy bubble pipe. Each individual bubble is called an alveolus. The walls of an alveolus are very thin—thin enough for tiny capillaries to travel in. Oxygen from the air moves across the alveolar wall, across the capillary wall, and into red blood cells, where hemoglobin molecules pick up the oxygen and carry it to distant parts of the body (see figure 34). While this is happening, carbon dioxide circulating in the blood moves from alveolar capillaries into the alveolus, where it is blown out of the lungs with each breath.

What does smoking do to our lungs?

The more alveoli we have, the easier it is to take in oxygen and get rid of carbon dioxide. The fewer alveoli we have, the harder it is. Smoking reduces the number of alveoli by destroying the delicate walls separating alveoli, so you end up with a few large alveoli instead of a lot of small ones (see figure 35). Marijuana smoke is considerably more damaging than cigarette smoke. Three or four joints does the same amount of damage to the alveoli as an entire pack of cigarettes. Without alveolar walls, there's no place for capillaries to take up oxygen into the blood. When enough alveolar walls are destroyed, you feel short of breath, and when still more alveolar walls are destroyed you end up dragging a tank of oxygen. The disease that destroys alveolar walls is emphysema.

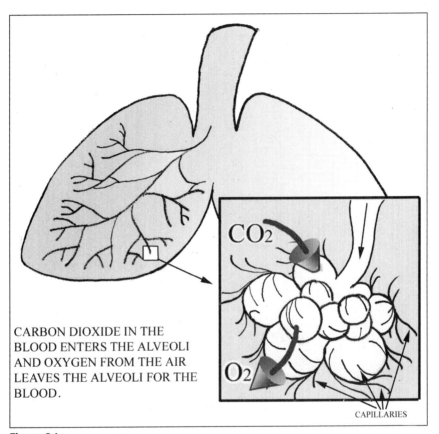

CARBON DIOXIDE IN THE
BLOOD ENTERS THE ALVEOLI
AND OXYGEN FROM THE AIR
LEAVES THE ALVEOLI FOR THE
BLOOD.

CO_2

O_2

CAPILLARIES

Figure 34

If the alveoli are so delicate and billowy, in the same way that a large bubble of bubble gum is delicate and billowy, how come the alveoli don't collapse each time you exhale?

Yeah, that would be a problem if the alveoli collapsed each time you exhaled, because the walls of the collapsed alveoli would stick together and wouldn't easily reinflate with the next breath. We have two tricks to avoid this problem. The first involves a simple principle called surface tension. If you take two flat pieces of glass, drip some water between them, and then lay one on top of the other, they can't be pried apart. The only way to separate them is to slide one past the other. Surface tension keeps the lungs inflated by a layer of sticky mucus between the outside

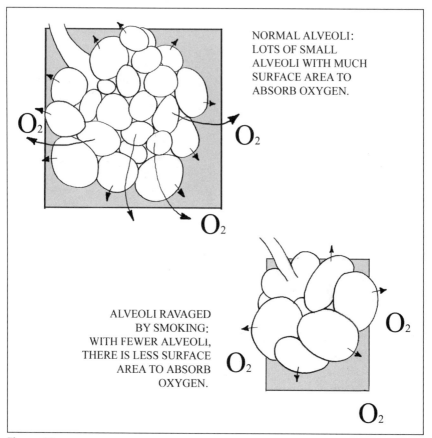

NORMAL ALVEOLI:
LOTS OF SMALL
ALVEOLI WITH MUCH
SURFACE AREA TO
ABSORB OXYGEN.

O_2

O_2

O_2

ALVEOLI RAVAGED
BY SMOKING:
WITH FEWER ALVEOLI,
THERE IS LESS SURFACE
AREA TO ABSORB
OXYGEN.

O_2

O_2

O_2

Figure 35

surface of the lung, called the pleura, and inside surface of the chest wall. So now, each time we exhale, the lungs don't collapse, because surface tension is keeping them stuck against the chest wall. On deep inhalation, the expanding chest wall drags the lungs with it, helping the diaphragm to suck in even more air.

The second trick to keep our lungs inflated after exhaling is not to empty all the air out of our lungs each time we exhale. Even if we inhaled fully and then exhaled as hard as possible, 20% of the air would still be left in the lungs to keep them inflated. After heavy exercise, we keep our alveoli open by pursing our lips with each expiration to put a little back pressure on the alveoli. People with emphysema have to purse their lips with every breath to keep their flimsy alveoli open.

What happens when you get the wind knocked out of you?

A sudden blow to the stomach or chest forces all of the air out of your chest, including some of that 20% reserve. According to one explanation, until the 20% reserve is refilled, which takes a few seconds, the brain cannot—for unclear reasons—initiate a new breath. The other explanation is that a sudden blow to the abdomen or chest temporarily paralyzes the diaphragm, preventing it from sucking any air into your lungs—until the diaphragm recovers and starts contracting again.

Why do premature babies have such a hard time breathing?

Premature lungs have tiny alveoli. Tiny alveoli tend to collapse on expiration, because water molecules lining the alveolar walls attract each other and pull the alveolar walls together. This is the same reason water droplets spilled onto a countertop remain as droplets instead of spreading out as a thin sheet of water. The hydrogen side of the water molecule is more positive than the oxygen side, so one molecule's hydrogen side is attracting another molecule's oxygen side. At the edge of a water droplet, water molecules are being attracted toward all the other water molecules in the interior, creating surface tension, which prevents the droplet from spreading out on the countertop. Agents that break up this surface tension are called surface active agents, or surfactants for short. Soap is a good surfactant, which you can demonstrate by dropping a bit of liquid soap on a water droplet.

Soaps, detergents, and surfactants break apart water molecules and keep them separated from each other by using a long molecule, with one end water soluble and the other end fat soluble, or water insoluble. The water molecules mix with the water-soluble end of a surfactant but are kept apart from each other by the water-insoluble end, which acts as a coat of water-insoluble fat, or lipid. Soap traps greasy dirt the opposite way: by trapping grease molecules in its fat-soluble end and dragging grease down the drain with its water-soluble end.

In the lungs, the attraction force of alveolar surface tension, which wants to collapse alveoli, is broken up by a surfactant coating the interior of the alveoli. By breaking up alveolar surface tension, surfactant prevents alveoli from collapsing on expiration. Premature babies don't make enough surfactant. Nowadays, doctors spritz a man-made surfactant down the trachea into the lungs to substitute for natural surfactant until the lungs mature enough to make their own surfactant.

What is a collapsed lung?

A collapsed lung, or pneumothorax ("pneumo" means air and "thorax" means chest, hence air in the chest outside the lung), is a lung that's lost the surface tension between the surface of the lung and the chest wall, allowing the lung to collapse away from the chest wall. Anything that permits air to enter the pleural space, the space between the pleura covering the lung and the pleura lining the chest wall, can do this. Sometimes, for example, a lung will suddenly pop a congenital (meaning from birth) bleb (a very delicate bubble) on the surface of the lung. When the bleb bursts, air escapes from the lung into the pleural space, breaking the surface tension keeping the pleura and chest wall stuck together. Without that surface tension, the lung collapses, sometimes only a little, sometimes a lot.

The risk of a pneumothorax requires scuba divers to exhale as they ascend from a deep dive. The air inhaled in deep water is compressed by the high underwater pressure, but as a diver ascends to the low-pressure surface, the air in his lungs expands. If the diver fails to exhale during the ascent, the dense air can expand enough to burst a lung.

How do you reexpand a collapsed lung?

You can't just take a big breath, because there's a hole in the lung and the inhaled air will just pass into the pleural space between the lung and chest wall. Even if the hole seals up, inhaling deeply won't help, because the collapsed lung needs surface tension to keep itself plastered against the chest wall. To reexpand a collapsed lung and keep it reexpanded, we need to get the air out of the pleural space so that the lung can reattach itself to the inside of the chest wall.

To get the air out of the pleural space, simply stick a sterile tube into the chest and suck out the air. First, you feel for a spot between two ribs and clean it of all bacteria. The best killer of bacteria is iodine, so the skin is painted with an iodine solution. Then you make a cut in the skin and push a thin sterile rod through the chest wall between two ribs. The last step is to remove the rod and insert a sterile plastic tube through the hole into the pleural space. Don't worry too much about puncturing a lung, as it has already collapsed and is situated far away from the chest wall. The other end of the chest tube is attached to a suction machine to suck the air out of the pleural space. If you don't have a suction machine, not to worry. Simply place the other end of the tube in a jar of water. As the lung slowly reexpands, it pushes air out the chest tube into the water in the form of little bubbles, which escape to the surface of the water. Eventually, all the air in the chest cavity is trapped by the water, the pleura reestablishes surface tension with the chest wall, and the lung remains inflated.

Is a pneumothorax dangerous?

Most of the time, a sudden pneumothorax is not too dangerous even if left untreated. Over a few months, the lung will reexpand as the hole in the lung is sealed off naturally and the air inside the chest cavity is reabsorbed by the body. And don't forget that the other lung is still breathing. Once in a while, though, a pneumothorax can be very dangerous, for example, when the person has been a smoker for a long time and needs both lungs to oxygenate his blood.

A pneumothorax becomes life threatening when the hole in the lung is covered over by a little flap of tissue, like one of those flap valves at the top of a chimney exhaust pipe on a tractor-trailer. The flap of tissue allows air to escape from the lung into the pleural space, but prevents air in the pleural space from reentering the lung. With each breath, more and more air enters the pleural space. Eventually, all that air entering the pleural space begins to shove against the heart. This dangerous situation is called a tension pneumothorax. As the heart is shoved to the side, it becomes less effective at pumping blood and the blood pressure begins to fall. Without adequate blood pressure, all the internal organs begin to suffer from lack of oxygen and glucose, and the whole body begins a downward death spiral. The same thing can happen if the pneumothorax is caused by a hole in the chest wall and a flap of tissue along the inside of the chest wall allows air to enter the pleural space but not escape.

A tension pneumothorax is a medical emergency. The air has to be gotten out immediately. Fortunately, it's easy to do. Just insert a large bore needle between two ribs into the pleural space and the air will whoosh out under high pressure. You don't have to worry about the needle hitting the lung because the whole side of the chest is filled with air.

Not long ago, a woman on an airplane suffered sudden chest pain and shortness of breath. God was watching over this woman, because there was a surgeon on board the plane who, without a stethoscope or a chest X-ray, quickly recognized her problem as a pneumothorax (or perhaps a tension pneumothorax). It was clear that a chest tube had to be inserted before the plane landed. The surgeon concocted a chest tube using the tubing from one of the plane's oxygen masks. He cleaned the skin, cut a hole, inserted the tube into the chest, and then stuck the other end of the tubing into a glass of water. The doctor's quick thinking, willingness to improvise, and courage to insert a tube into a woman's chest at 30,000 feet saved her life.

What's the name of the instrument a doctor uses to listen to your chest?

A stethoscope, the same instrument safecrackers use to listen to tumblers falling into their chambers as the dial is turned.

Why does a doctor listen to the lungs with a stethoscope?

In a normal person, the doctor hears air entering the alveoli with each inspiration. When there's an infection in the lung—pneumonia—the alveoli become filled with white blood cells and mucus, that is, pus. The sticky infected fluid makes the walls of the alveoli stick together. With each breath, the alveoli snap open, which the doctor hears as a crackling sound with each inspiration.

As the pneumonia worsens, instead of being light and airy, the lung becomes waterlogged and heavy. Now when the patient inhales, there's no air entering the alveoli at all. Instead of hearing the alveoli filling with air, the doctor hears air traveling through the bronchial tubes. In a normal lung, he wouldn't hear air traveling through the bronchial tubes, because those sounds are muffled by the air-filled alveoli. In an infected lung, which is now waterlogged and solid, the low-pitched sounds from air rumbling down the large bronchial tubes pass right through the lung to the doctor's stethoscope.

In a pneumothorax, the breath sounds are diminished or absent on one side of the chest because less air is getting into the partially collapsed lung and the lung is no longer up against the chest wall.

What would the doctor hear if the bronchial tubes were suddenly constricted so that only a tiny stream of air was able to get through at a very high speed?

Try blowing air out of your mouth with your lips wide open. Now try it with your lips pursed. That whistling sound you make is the same sound the bronchial tubes make when they're constricted—wheezing.

What disease constricts the bronchial tubes?

Asthma. Sometimes the constriction is so severe that you can hear the wheezing even without a stethoscope.

How are the bronchial tubes—the bronchioles—able to constrict?

In the walls of every bronchiole is a layer of muscle. When these muscles contract, the bronchioles constrict (see figure 36). We normally use these muscles when we want to generate a fast blast of air, like a cough.

What causes an asthma attack?

Asthma is more than bronchiole constriction—there's inflammation in the bronchial walls, too. In an asthma attack, capillaries leak fluid into the walls of the bronchial tubes, thickening the walls and narrowing the lumen (the hollow center) of the bronchioles. To make matters worse, the lumen of the bronchioles become plugged with mucus, white blood cells, and fluid leaking from small blood vessels. The net result is air can't get in and out of the lungs.

The initiator of an asthma attack is an antigen coming in contact with the bronchioles. The antigen can reach the bronchioles through the air,

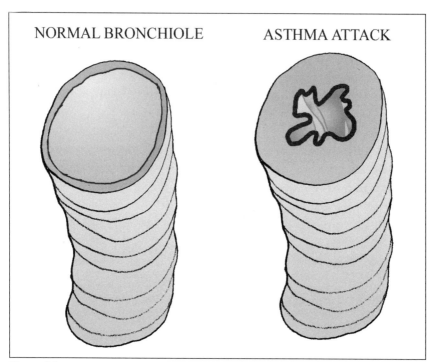

NORMAL BRONCHIOLE   ASTHMA ATTACK

Figure 36

such as pollen, or through the bloodstream as a food antigen, such as peanuts. Lining the walls of bronchioles are very sensitive white blood cells called mast cells (the same cells that in the skin trigger poison ivy). When the antigen is inhaled, antibodies attached to the surface of mast cells latch onto the antigen and trigger the mast cells to release histamine and leukotrienes, which stimulate the bronchiole muscles to contract, blood vessels in the bronchioles to leak fluid, mucus-making cells to work overtime, and inflammatory white blood cells to flood the area. As their bronchial tubes constrict, asthmatics cough and cough to clear their bronchioles of all the extra fluid and mucus. If the antigen is eaten, like peanuts, the release of histamine and leukotrienes by mast cells lining the gut wall can also cause abdominal cramping, pain, vomiting, and diarrhea.

What's anaphylaxis?

Anaphylaxis is a life-threatening allergic reaction that starts out as a typical allergic reaction, with bronchiole constriction and congestion resulting from capillary fluid leaking into bronchiole walls. As more and more blood vessels throughout the body begin to dilate and leak, the blood pressure drops. Fluids leaking from blood vessels in the throat cause the tongue and epiglottis to swell and close off the entrance to the trachea. Between the falling blood pressure, the blocked trachea, and the narrowed bronchial tubes, a person can die in less than 10 minutes from an anaphylactic reaction.

The best way to counteract the effects of histamine and leukotrienes is to give a shot of epinephrine, which opens up the bronchial tubes and squeezes the dilated arteries back down to normal. It's recommended that people highly allergic to bee stings and peanuts carry with them an epinephrine injection kit to hold them over until they can get to an emergency room. Even if the symptoms begin to wear off, it's vital that the victim get to an emergency room because, for unclear reasons, the deadly symptoms often recur within a few hours.

What is mountain sickness?

Mountain climbers obviously get short of breath as they ascend into air with less oxygen in it, but in some climbers the low oxygen and low atmospheric pressure allow capillaries to leak fluid into the alveoli, resulting in pulmonary edema and severe shortness of breath. Likewise, capillaries in the brain can leak fluid, resulting in a waterlogging of the brain called cerebral edema. The rising intracranial pressure causes headaches, dizziness, nausea and vomiting, and ataxia (staggering gait), culminating in confusion, stupor, coma, and finally death.

What is cystic fibrosis?

Cystic fibrosis is a genetic disease in which thick mucus is continually secreted by the walls of the bronchial tubes. The collecting mucus plugs up the bronchial tubes and becomes repeatedly infected. Eventually, the recurrent bronchial infections thicken the bronchial walls and injure adjacent lung tissue. Nowadays, with medications to thin out the mucus, vigorous chest physical therapy to clear the clogged mucus, and prompt antibiotic treatment, kids with cystic fibrosis do pretty well.

Why does smoking cause lung cancer?

Cigarette smoke has a lot of black tar in it. You can't see the tar unless you smoke through a kleenex and allow the tar to collect as a black stain on the kleenex. This tar contains cancer-causing agents, or carcinogens.

What is the difference between "cancerous" and "malignant"?

Malignant is synonymous with cancerous. If you cut your skin, the skin on either side grows together and the cut heals. How does the skin know when to stop growing? Whatever that feedback signal is, it isn't working in cancer.

What is the difference between a benign and a malignant tumor?

A tumor is a lump of tissue that grows larger and larger. A benign tumor is one that stays localized to one site in the body and can be removed in its entirety. "Benign" does not mean the tumor won't kill—it will if it's in the right location and isn't removed. Malignant tumors are different. Instead of staying localized, they can spread—metastasize—through the bloodstream to distant parts of the body. Even when they don't metastasize, they often cannot be fully removed, because malignant tumors grow as long tentacles reaching off in all directions, kind of like a crab, with a central mass of malignant cells and little arms extending out into the surrounding tissue. In astrology, the crab is cancer, hence the name for this disease. Among doctors, the slang term for cancer is "crab."

Why are people with cancer given radiation?

Rapidly growing cancer cells are busy using their DNA to make proteins for cell growth. Radiation interferes with DNA's synthesis of proteins in all cells, but because cancer cells grow the fastest, they are the ones most hurt by the radiation.

7

CARDIAC SYSTEM

To make energy and run the machinery of the body, the peripheral tissues and internal organs must extract oxygen from the blood, leaving the blood deoxygenated. Before returning to the peripheral tissues and internal organs, the blood must be reoxygenated by the lungs. The heart serves to pump blood through the lungs and then back out to the periphery.

The heart has an important physiological problem to work out. High pressure is needed to pump blood from the heart to all the distant parts of the body, but delicate capillaries can't handle high pressure. The problem is easily solved for capillaries in peripheral tissues, because by the time arterial blood reaches delicate capillaries out in the periphery the blood pressure has fallen off tremendously. However, capillaries in the lungs aren't out in the periphery. How can blood be pumped under high pressure to reach the periphery without damaging delicate capillaries in the closely situated lungs?

The solution was to divide the heart into two separate pumping chambers, or ventricles, one to pump blood out to the periphery under high pressure and another to pump blood to the lungs under low pressure. As a result, the heart consists of two hollow muscles separated from each other by a baffle, or septum. Deoxygenated blood from the peripheral organs returns to the right ventricle, is pumped to the lungs, and returns to the left ventricle freshly oxygenated (see figure 37). With each contraction, the left ventricle pumps about a third of a cup of oxygenated blood into a very large artery, called the aorta, and down the aorta into smaller and smaller arteries, the blood losing pressure along the way, until finally reaching tiny capillaries in the body's tissues under low pressure. Once through the capillaries, blood returns to the heart through larger and larger veins, eventually reaching the large inferior vena cava from the lower body and the superior vena cava from the upper body, before reentering the right side of the heart. The typical heart beats 70 times a minute, pumping a little more than 20 cups of blood, or about 5 quarts. Since our total blood volume is about 5 quarts, every minute all the blood is circulated once around the vascular tree. ("Artery" means windpipe in Greek. The ancient Greeks thought that arteries carried a creative, airborne spirit inhaled by the lungs. Back then, what explanation would you have given for breathing?)

If the heart is simply a hollow muscle, how is it able to pump blood forward into the aorta without also squirting it backward into the inferior vena cava?

Obviously, the heart needs some valves, which are best seen by opening the two sides of the heart. The heart has two main pumping chambers—a left and a right ventricle ("ventricle" means belly in Latin). Both ventricles have an inlet valve where blood enters and an outlet valve where blood leaves the ventricle. In the left ventricle, the intake valve is called the mitral valve because it looks just like a miter—a tall pointed hat worn by bishops. The left ventricular outlet valve is called the aortic valve. In the right ventricle, the intake valve is the tricuspid valve, so-called because it has three (tri) flaps (cusps). The right ventricular outlet valve is known as the pulmonic valve because right ventricular blood is being pumped to the lungs.

Each time the heart squeezes, rising pressure inside the right and left ventricles shuts the intake valves (see figure 38B). As the pressure continues to rise, both outlet valves are simultaneously forced open, permitting blood to flow outward—to the lungs from the right ventricle and to the peripheral organs from the left ventricle.

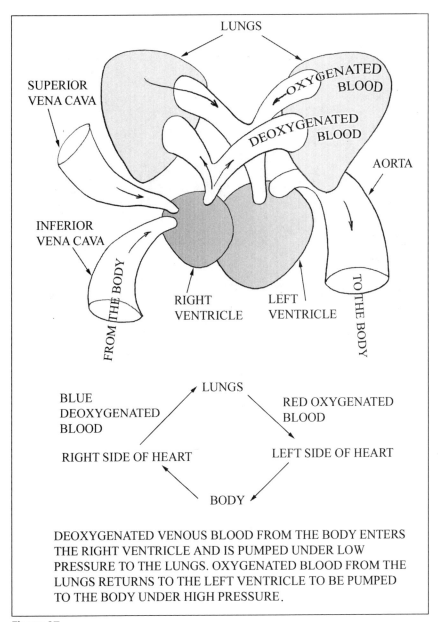

DEOXYGENATED VENOUS BLOOD FROM THE BODY ENTERS
THE RIGHT VENTRICLE AND IS PUMPED UNDER LOW
PRESSURE TO THE LUNGS. OXYGENATED BLOOD FROM THE
LUNGS RETURNS TO THE LEFT VENTRICLE TO BE PUMPED
TO THE BODY UNDER HIGH PRESSURE.

Figure 37

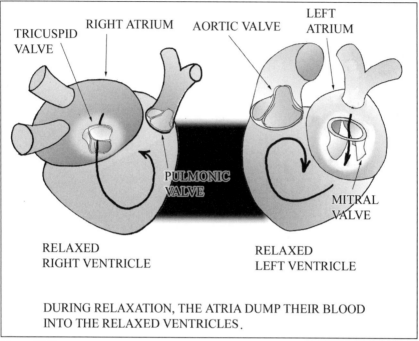

Figure 38A

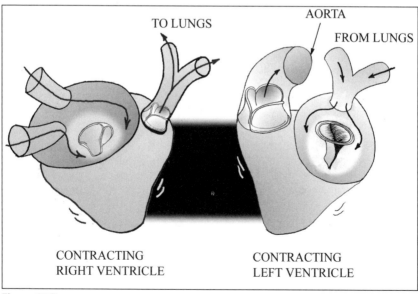

Figure 38B

After a third of a cup of blood is pumped from both the right and left ventricles, the pulmonary and aortic valves simultaneously close so that none of the blood in the pulmonary artery or aorta gushes back into the ventricles. Meanwhile, the tricuspid and mitral valves have already opened to allow the ventricles to fill up with blood again (see figure 38A).

What do you see in figure 39 as the major difference between the walls of the right and left ventricles?

The thickness of the walls. The left ventricle needs a thick, muscular wall because it's pumping under high pressure to get blood to all the distant sites in the body.

The right ventricle, in contrast, is pumping under low pressure, so its wall is thin. It takes very little pressure to pump blood through the lungs, because they offer very little resistance to blood flow. The reason for the low resistance is the short length of the pulmonary artery and the rapid dispersion of blood into many pulmonary arterioles (small arteries), which makes pumping blood through the lungs like percolating water through a sponge.

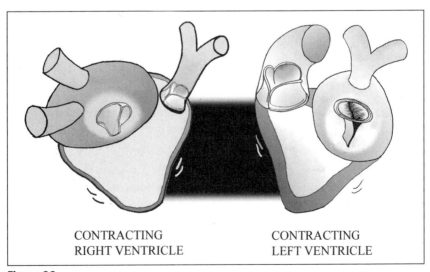

CONTRACTING RIGHT VENTRICLE   CONTRACTING LEFT VENTRICLE

Figure 39

Why does the heart have four chambers if only two are needed to pump the blood?

The two extra chambers, a right and left atrium (an atrium was a large entrance room in ancient Rome), permit faster filling of the right and left ventricles. Each atrium fills with blood while the ventricles are emptying, and when the intake valves open, blood is dumped into the ventricles. Like the ventricles, the left and right atria are separated by a septum.

Why is the pulmonary artery, which is carrying venous blood, called an artery?

Even though blood in the pulmonary artery is deoxygenated and dark red, the pulmonary artery is still an artery, because it's carrying blood away from the heart. Color of the blood is irrelevant to whether the vessel carrying the blood is an artery or a vein. (See chapter 10 for an explanation of why veins carrying deoxygenated blood look blue, not dark red.)

What happens to blood after it leaves the right ventricle?

Once in the lungs, blood percolates through capillaries within the delicate alveolar walls, picking up oxygen and dumping off carbon dioxide. The now oxygenated, bright red blood returns via the pulmonary vein to the left atrium, then passes through the mitral valve into the left ventricle, and out the left ventricle past the aortic valve into the aorta.

What is the "lub-dub" a doctor hears through a stethoscope?

The first sound, the "lub," is the shutting of the mitral valve just before blood is ejected out of the left ventricle. The second sound, the "dub," is the shutting of the aortic valve after blood has been ejected from the left ventricle. Systole is the period of ventricular contraction, which begins with closure of the mitral valve and ends with closure of the aortic valve. Diastole is the period of ventricular filling, which begins when the mitral valve opens to allow fresh blood into the left ventricle from the left atrium and ends when the mitral valve closes.

Why does a doctor listen to the heart with a stethoscope?

The doctor is listening to blood flowing through the heart. Normally, blood flows like a smooth river. What sound does a smooth river make? None. What happens to the sound of the river when the water flows over rocks? You can hear river rapids far away because turbulent water is noisy. Same for the heart. When blood tumbles, it makes a brief whishing sound, or murmur, audible with each heartbeat.

One common cause of a heart murmur is a defective heart valve, but not every murmur is abnormal. A young heart can pump so vigorously that blood literally tumbles out of the heart. This functional murmur is of no significance. So, when a doctor hears a heart murmur, she has to decide whether the blood flow is turbulent because the heart is strong or because the blood is tumbling over a defective heart valve or swirling through a hole in the atrial septum or ventricular septum.

Turbulence of the blood within an artery is audible as a bruit (pronounced "broo-ee") and is due to narrowing of the artery, usually by atherosclerosis.

What happens if one of the heart valves is defective?

Two things: the heart has to pump harder and, sometimes, the defective heart valve becomes infected.

There are two ways a defective valve makes the heart pump harder, depending on whether the valve is stiff and difficult to open (i.e., stenotic) or unable to close properly (i.e., insufficient, or regurgitant). If, for example, the pulmonic valve becomes stenotic, the right ventricle has to exert a lot more pressure to force open the pulmonic valve. The thin-walled right ventricle is not prepared for such hard work and before long will begin to fail.

When the aortic valve becomes stenotic, the thick-walled left ventricle is a little better prepared and generally takes longer to fail. Another thing happens, however: all the extra work causes the left ventricular muscle to thicken (as work does for any muscle). A thick left ventricular wall is dangerous because the coronary arteries feeding the left ventricle from its outer surface now have a more difficult time reaching across the entire thickness of the left ventricular myocardium (heart muscle). As the patient exercises and his heart speeds up and pumps more vigorously, the myocardial demand for oxygen outstrips the ability of the coronary arteries to deliver oxygen to the thickened left ventricular wall. If those muscle cells don't get enough blood soon, they'll die. That's a heart attack.

When a valve is regurgitant, or insufficient, it does not shut tightly and blood leaks backward after the valve closes. When this happens to the pulmonic valve, the right ventricle ends up pumping the same blood twice. That's a lot of extra work for the right ventricle, and eventually it fails. When this happens to the mitral valve, some of the left ventricular blood is pumped backward into the left atrium and has to be pumped again. In aortic insufficiency (or regurgitation), blood pumped into the aorta falls back into the left ventricle, which now has to pump it back out again. All this extra work leads to left ventricular failure.

What is heart failure?

Heart failure is what happens to the heart when it cannot keep up with the body's need for blood. One of the first things that happens is enlargement of the ventricles as the heart tries to pump more blood with each contraction. An enlarged heart, therefore, is often an early sign of heart failure. As the ventricles fail, blood returning to the right and left ventricles begins to back up into the right and left atria. Cardiologists can confirm the elevated pressures by sliding a tube from a peripheral vein into the heart to measure right and left atrial pressures.

As blood continues to back up behind the right ventricle, veins begin to dilate and leak fluid (edema) into the tissues. Because people stand all day, the edema collects in the feet and lower legs. The legs can become so swollen that pressing the skin leaves an indentation, a condition called pitting edema. Blood backing up behind the left ventricle leaks edema into the lungs—pulmonary edema—causing shortness of breath because wet lungs cannot breathe. The pulmonary edema accumulates at the lung bases during the day when the patient is upright, leaving the upper lungs dry enough to breathe. At night, however, the edema redistributes throughout the lungs and the patient suddenly awakens short of breath. The solution patients usually stumble upon is to prop themselves up with an extra pillow or two at night.

Why do defective heart valves get infected more than normal valves?

A normal valve is smooth and glistening, leaving no crevices on its surface for bacteria to adhere to. A defective valve, in contrast, has lumps, bumps, and crevices, ideal for bacteria to latch onto and hide in. Also, bacteria love to infect anything that does not have a blood supply because they can flourish beyond the reach of an organized attack of white blood cells. Heart valves are made of cartilage. No cartilaginous structure in the body—not the tip of the nose, the ears, or the intervertebral discs—has a blood supply within the cartilage itself. Nutrients get to the center of cartilaginous structures by diffusing from capillaries running along the surface of the cartilage. If bacteria gain a toehold in a cartilaginous structure such as a heart valve, white blood cells can only organize an inflammatory response from the surface of the valve.

What happens if the aortic heart valve gets infected?

Bacteria can eat a hole in the valve, making it regurgitant and leaky, or the body's inflammatory response mounted from the surface of the valve can leave scarring in its wake. A scarred valve is stiff and stenotic, and it does not open readily.

The term for an infected heart valve is subacute bacterial endocarditis. Subacute means the infection has been going on for weeks or months; bacterial is the nature of the offending agent; and endocarditis means inflammation of the endocardium—the inner lining of the heart, in this case the heart valve.

Why don't people with defective heart valves just take antibiotics all the time so the valve doesn't become infected?

The risk of taking an antibiotic all the time is that the antibiotic will not kill all the bacteria it is supposed to kill. If surviving bacteria do infect a heart valve, by definition, those bacteria will be resistant to that antibiotic, thus leaving fewer drugs available to treat the infection. This situation is called a superinfection.

To avoid this situation, people with defective heart valves take antibiotics only when they know bacteria are likely to be entering the bloodstream. The most common example is extensive dental work—more than just having a cavity filled—when bacteria in the mouth are shed into the bloodstream. Before performing such dental work, the dentist will begin the patient on an antibiotic for a day or two.

How does a doctor know when a heart valve is infected?

Fever and a heart murmur are the two most important signs, particularly if the murmur is new or has changed. The new or changed murmur is due to blood tumbling over clumps of bacteria, called vegetations, growing on the heart valve. The diagnosis of subacute bacterial endocarditis is confirmed by taking a sample of blood and incubating it for a few days. If bacteria grow from what would normally be sterile blood ("sterile" means there's no bacteria living in it), and the patient has a new or changed heart murmur, the presumption is that the bacteria are coming from an infected heart valve.

What's a blue baby?

A blue baby is an infant whose blood is not fully oxygenated. (The medical term for blue deoxygenated blood is cyanosis, because cyan is blue-green.) The causes of cyanosis are many, including lung disease, heart disease, and brain disease (affecting the control of breathing). When the heart is the culprit, the deoxygenated venous blood is mixing with oxygenated arterial blood, usually because of some serious malformation of the heart.

One of the more easily cured causes of cyanosis in a baby is failure of the ductus arteriosus to close off shortly after birth, as it normally does. (The ductus arteriosus is open during fetal development.) The purpose of the ductus arteriosus is to connect the pulmonary artery with the aorta (see figure 40). This shunt detours blood leaving the right ventricle around the lungs and diverts it directly into the general, or systemic, circulation. One reason for such a shunt is that there is no need for blood to flow to the lungs, because the placenta oxygenates a fetus's blood and the lungs are not breathing yet (remember, the fetus is submerged in a bath of amniotic fluid). The second reason for the shunt is that a fetus's lungs are still collapsed.

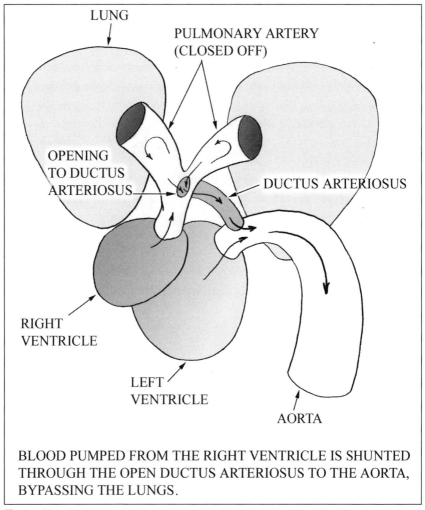

LUNG

PULMONARY ARTERY
(CLOSED OFF)

OPENING
TO DUCTUS
ARTERIOSUS

DUCTUS ARTERIOSUS

RIGHT
VENTRICLE

LEFT
VENTRICLE

AORTA

BLOOD PUMPED FROM THE RIGHT VENTRICLE IS SHUNTED
THROUGH THE OPEN DUCTUS ARTERIOSUS TO THE AORTA,
BYPASSING THE LUNGS.

Figure 40

Collapsed fetal lungs offer high resistance to blood flow. Forcing blood to flow through collapsed lungs would put too great a strain on the right ventricle.

Are holes in the heart the cause of blue babies?

Generally not, and here's why. During fetal development, the heart uses another route besides the ductus arteriosus to bypass the lungs, namely, a hole in the atrial septum (separating the left and right atria). This allows right atrial blood to flow directly into the left atrium without first flowing through the lungs. If the hole fails to close after birth, it rarely allows blue venous blood to flow into the arterial system, because left atrial pressure is higher than right atrial pressure. While an atrial septal defect does allow left atrial blood entry to the right atrium, which forces the right ventricle to pump oxygenated blood to the lungs—a complete waste of effort—the blood exiting the left ventricle is still fully oxygenated, and hence no cyanosis.

The same reasoning applies to a hole in the ventricular septum (which should never have a hole in it, even during fetal development). In the presence of a ventricular septal defect, some left ventricular blood is ejected through the defect into the right ventricle, only to be pumped through the lungs and left ventricle again.

Why are fancy people called "blue bloods?"

The expression "blue blood" originated hundreds of years ago in Spain, where the aristocrats, who were white, pointed to the prominent blue veins in their white skin to avoid any suggestion of inbreeding with the darker-skinned African Moors. The term now refers to a country's nobility and royalty.

Why do athletes have slow heart rates?

Athletic hearts beat slower because they are able to pump more blood with each contraction than sedentary hearts. This is accomplished by enlarging the size of the left ventricle to accommodate the extra blood, and by thickening the wall of the left ventricle to provide the necessary muscle to pump the extra blood.

How does the body make energy for muscle contraction?

Almost all chemical reactions in the body, including muscle contraction, need energy, which is provided by a high-energy molecule called adenosine triphospate, or ATP (phosphorus packs quite a punch, as evidenced by its extensive use in explosives). When a phosphate molecule is released from ATP to form ADP (adenosine *di*phosphate), energy is released to drive chemical reactions (see figure 41). The synthesis of ATP begins with the breakdown of either glucose or fat. Here's how. Glucose molecules are sliced off long chains of glucose, called glycogen, and broken down into 3-carbon fragments of pyruvic acid, releasing 2 ATP energy

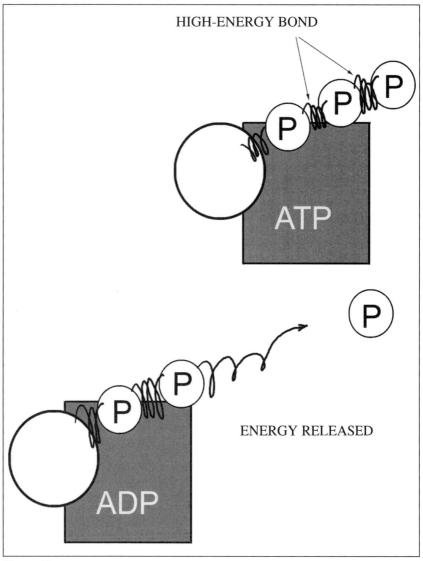

Figure 41

molecules in the process. No oxygen is needed to do this. If there's not enough oxygen in the cell (anerobic condition), pyruvate is converted to lactic acid without making any more ATP (see figure 42A). If there is sufficient oxygen in the cell (aerobic condition), pyruvate is converted into a 2-carbon fragment and escorted into a special chamber, called a mitochondrion, within the cell to make 36 additional ATP molecules (see

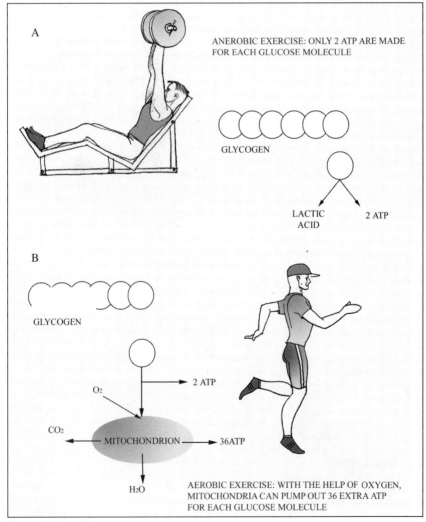

Figure 42A and B

figure 42B). In this process, hydrogen ions are made as a byproduct, and oxygen combines with it to make water (H_2O).

Mitochondria can also use 2-carbon fragments sliced from fat molecules, thus, the beauty of mitochondria is their flexibility. They can use 2-carbon fragments from glucose or 2-carbon fragments from fat. Fat is lightweight and ounce for ounce contains far more calories than glycogen. At 9 calories per gram, a full day's energy requirement of 2,100 calories can be packed into 233 grams—half a pound—of fat. Unfortunately, muscle is much less efficient at slicing up fat than it is at slicing up glucose, which helps explain why the ability to sustain muscular activity for long periods depends on muscle glycogen stores, not fat stores. Whether mitochondria use 2-carbon fragments from glucose or fat, mitochondria must have a steady supply of oxygen to run their machinery.

Why don't all muscle cells use mitochondria to make ATP, since so much more ATP can be made from a single molecule of glucose?

The huge difference in ATP production between aerobic and anaerobic metabolism may make anaerobic metabolism of glucose look inferior, but it isn't. The breakdown of glucose to pyruvate is extremely efficient because it takes place in the cytoplasm of the cell, where it's used immediately for muscle contraction, while mitochondrial production of ATP takes place in isolated chambers and involves a lot of enzymes passing 2-carbon fragments along a disassembly line. So while 36 ATP is great, it takes time to make them, and after they *are* made, they have to be transported out of the mitochondria and across the cytoplasm to the sites where they're needed. The problem with anaerobic metabolism is lactic acid buildup. Rapidly contracting muscles can only keep up anaerobic metabolism for a few minutes before the buildup of lactic acid is too much for the muscle to bear, which you feel as an intense burning in the muscles.

What is the difference between white and dark meat in a chicken?

Dark meat, such as in the legs and thighs, is used for slow, steady work (chickens do a lot of milling around) and therefore depends on mitochondria to provide a slow, steady supply of ATP. Dark meat is specially built to handle the oxygen and fat necessary for mitochondrial function.

First, dark meat derives its color from a dark-colored protein called myoglobin, a cousin of hemoglobin, which holds onto oxygen in muscles. Second, dark meat stores fat inside the muscle as triglycerides. White meat is quite different, as breasts only periodically flap the wings for liftoff. For this, the breast meat needs a sudden, short burst of energy, perfect for anaerobic metabolism, because anaerobic metabolism can last only a few minutes before lactic acid buildup shuts it off. With no need for oxygen, there's no need for myoglobin, hence the white color of breast meat. Ducks, by contrast, use their breast muscles aerobically for long stretches of flying, so even their breast meat is dark.

Aerobic metabolism uses both glycogen and fat for its energy supplies, while anaerobic metabolism uses only glycogen. So not only is aerobic muscle dark, it's greasy (and to many, it is tastier than white meat) because of the fat it uses for energy, while white meat, without the fat, is dry. The absence of fat in white meat is also why it's considered healthier than dark meat.

Humans don't have this bulk separation of white and dark meat, but some people are born with more aerobic fibers than others, and they may end up as long-distance runners. By contrast, the muscles of a cheetah are mostly anaerobic fibers for quick pursuit. Likewise, fish meat is mostly white, anaerobic meat that allows for short bursts of power to escape a predator or capture a meal. Fish have only a small amount of dark aerobic meat, for meandering through the water. Since seals and whales can't breathe underwater, their muscles contain tons of myoglobin to store plenty of oxygen for deep sojourns into the sea.

What is the difference between aerobic exercise and anaerobic exercise?

Weight lifting and other isometric exercises ("iso" means same and "meter" means length) create an anaerobic environment because the muscles are contracting continuously and building up very high pressure. The pressure is high enough to slow blood flow—and therefore oxygen delivery—to the muscles at a time when the continually contracting muscles are demanding more and more oxygen. Anaerobic situations can occur in any sport that requires intense muscular contractions, such as sprinting, wrestling, and weight lifting. In these sports, the demand for ATP outstrips the ability of the heart and blood vessels to deliver sufficient oxygen to the mitochondria.

In aerobic, or dynamic, exercise such as long-distance running, cross-country skiing, swimming, and bicycling, the muscles contract and relax. Each time the muscles relax, blood flows through them to deliver oxygen. With an adequate oxygen supply, the mitochondria are able to make sufficient ATP without the serious buildup of lactic acid, so aerobic exercise can continue for hours.

Another difference between aerobic and anaerobic exercise is the effect on a person's blood pressure. The blood pressure during isometric exercise rises considerably as muscular compression of arteries increases arterial resistance and the production of lactic acid stimulates the brain to raise the blood pressure to deliver more blood to oxygen-starved muscles. In dynamic exercise, the blood pressure remains constant or falls, because without continuous compression of arteries by contracting muscles, there is no increase in arterial resistance.

Is carbon dioxide made during aerobic ATP production or during anerobic ATP production?

Carbon dioxide is a byproduct of aerobic ATP production only. No carbon dioxide is made during anaerobic metabolism. However, the lactic acid made during anaerobic exercise does break apart into hydrogen ions (H^+) and lactate. The lactate is remade into glucose in the liver, while the H^+ combines with bicarbonate in the bloodstream to make water and carbon dioxide. The carbon dioxide is then exhaled by the lungs. So, directly or indirectly, carbon dioxide is a byproduct of both aerobic and anaerobic ATP production.

How does regular exercise improve exercise tolerance?

There are two major factors that determine exercise endurance: one is the ability of the heart and lungs to deliver oxygen to the muscles, and the second is the ability of the muscles to use the oxygen. Lungs that have not been damaged by cigarette or marijuana smoke are extremely good at delivering oxygen to the bloodstream and regular exercise cannot improve on that.

Aerobic exercise improves endurance primarily by improving the heart's ability to deliver oxygen. By thickening the wall of the left ventricle and making it contract more vigorously, exercise is able to make the heart pump more blood per heartbeat, which, as mentioned, is why an athlete's heart beats slower than a nonathlete's heart.

Aerobic exercise does not convert aerobic muscle fibers into aerobic ones, but it does improve the ability of anerobic muscles to use oxygen and fat by increasing the number of mitrochondria in muscle cells, increasing the enzymes that metabolize fat, and increasing the number of muscle capillaries. To increase the size of muscle fibers, you need to perform anerobic, or resistance, exercise, such as weight lifting.

Why do some athletes take creatine?

Contracting muscles use a number of tricks to satisfy their need for a steady, robust supply of ATP. One is to store their own glycogen instead of depending on glycogen stored in the liver. Another is to bank their own oxygen in large stores of myoglobin. The third is to rapidly replenish ATP as soon as the high-energy phosphate molecules are released from ATP to form ADP. Muscles do this by storing high-energy phosphate molecules on a molecule called creatine in the form of creatine phosphate. As soon as ATP releases its phosphate and becomes ADP, creatine phosphate transfers its phosphate to the ADP to make ATP again. Extra creatine in the diet increases the supply of ATP, making athletes able to exercise a little longer and faster. For unclear reasons, muscle mass also increases. Unfortunately, very few scientific studies of creatine supplementation have been done to confirm that creatine is safe in the long run.

What is the "second wind" many athletes get?

When exercising vigorously, the unpleasant and distressful shortness of breath we all experience can suddenly dissipate, a phenomenon called second wind. No one knows for sure what causes second wind. Some think that second wind occurs as the liver clears the bloodstream of lactic acid and converts it to glucose. Some believe second wind is due to more efficient oxygen consumption, so less lactic acid is made or, possibly, the diaphragm overcomes its fatigue. Another thought is that the spleen contracts and pumps extra blood into circulation. Some authorities don't even believe second wind exists at all.

When a person begins to exercise, the heart rate rises and breathing increases to deliver more oxygen to our muscles. How do the heart and lungs know to speed up?

At the same time the brain sends a message to our legs to start running, it sends messages to the heart to speed up and to the lungs to breathe harder. Another reason the heart and lungs speed up is that exercising muscles release lactic acid into the blood, which stimulates the brain to increase the heart and respiratory rate. Also, as exercising muscles use up oxygen and produce carbon dioxide, these chemical changes are detected by a small pad of tissue, called the carotid body, attached inside the left and right carotid artery on either side of the trachea. (Each carotid artery carries blood to one side of the brain.) When stimulated by low oxygen and rising carbon dioxide, the carotid bodies send signals to the brain to stimulate faster, deeper breathing and faster, more forceful heartbeats.

How can you get more oxygen to the muscles?

Think about what's necessary: lungs to breathe in oxygen, blood to pick it up from the lungs, a heart to pump the blood, and arteries to deliver the blood to the muscles. If you don't smoke (so you have a normal number of alveoli without a lot of mucus and inflammation in the bronchial tubes), there is not much you can do to improve lung function, because the lungs are very efficient at absorbing oxygen from the air. If your hemoglobin level in the blood is normal, there's not much you can do to raise it further unless, as some athletes have done, you donate a unit of blood several weeks before the athletic event, allow your body time to restore the hemoglobin level, and then transfuse the blood back into your veins the day before the event. Another trick is to inject erythropoietin, the protein synthesized by the kidney to stimulate the bone marrow to make blood. (Of all the organs in the body, you would not expect the kidney to monitor the blood count, but it does.) Donating blood to yourself and using erythropoietin are of course outlawed by athletic associations.

Arteries rarely pose a problem in delivering oxygen because an artery has to be narrowed by 70% before blood flow significantly decreases. This leaves the heart as the limiting factor on your ability to deliver oxygen to muscles, and thus how long and how hard your muscles can exercise before having to stop.

Why do some people have an irregular pulse?

While there are lots of reasons for an irregular heartbeat, or arrhythmia, there are only a couple of mechanisms by which they occur. The pace of the heartbeat is controlled by two pacemakers, one located in the right atrium, which stimulates the second pacemaker, situated between the left and right ventricles. The atrial pacemaker is called the sinoatrial, or SA, node, and the ventricular pacemaker is called the atrioventricular, or AV, node (see figure 43). The SA node begins by spreading an electrical discharge out across the two atria to stimulate the atria to contract. When the electrical discharge reaches the AV node, the AV node then sends another electrical discharge through two bundles of electrically excitable heart tissue, called the bundle of His, to stimulate the right and left ventricles.

So far so good, but sometimes another spot in the right or left atrium decides to become the SA node. The new atrial node may fire before the legitimate SA node has a chance to fire. If the new discharge reaches the AV node first, it will trigger a premature beat. A similar situation can develop in the ventricles. Some other spot besides the real AV node can decide it wants to be the AV node. Premature atrial contractions are not very serious, because most of the pumping is done by the ventricles. Premature ventricular beats are more serious, because a renegade AV node is never in the right place to give a coordinated signal to both ventricles. As a result, the premature ventricular contraction is never as strong as it should be. If the patient is having a lot of premature ventricular contractions, the heart becomes a much less effective pump.

Another mechanism for arrhythmias occurs when the electrical signal doubles back and reenters the SA or AV node. Thus, after sending off a normal discharge, the SA or AV node may find itself on the receiving end of another reentry signal. The SA node can end up being stimulated up to 300 times a minute; the AV node, 180 times a minute. Once the ventricles are contracting more than about 180 times a minute, there is not enough time between contractions for the ventricles to fill with blood, resulting in essentially no blood being pumped. This serious arrhythmia is called ventricular tachycardia ("tachy" means rapid).

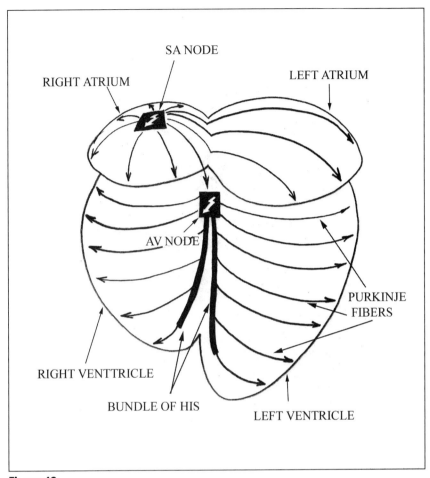

Figure 43

A third mechanism occurs in hearts that take too long to recharge after a normal contraction. The next electrical impulse, finding sections of ventricular muscle unresponsive, may try to detour around the sleepy ventricular muscle and end up in a reentry pathway, precipitating a bout of ventricular tachycardia. This is not an uncommon cause of fainting or even sudden death in young people during exercise. On an EKG, the T wave represents ventricular repolarization, so a prolonged duration between the QRS complex (ventricular contraction) and T wave—

known as a long QT interval—should alert the doctor to this cause of her patient's fainting.

When the SA node is being stimulated 250 to 300 times a minute, the atria don't have time to contract before the next impulse arrives, so they just stand there quivering, or fibrillating. This has relatively little effect on cardiac output, because atrial contractions don't contribute very much to ventricular filling. However, when the atrial walls are not contracting, blood tends to stagnate and form clots in little pockets of the left atrium. Bits of those blood clots may break off and float through the left ventricle, into the aorta, and out to the periphery. If the periphery happens to be a small artery in the brain, the person may suffer a stroke.

Another mechanism for an irregular heartbeat is the failure of the SA node to send out an electrical signal. The heart may stall for 15 seconds or more, causing the patient to faint. The solution for this sick sinus syndrome is to thread a pacemaker wire through a vein into the right atrium to stimulate the heart to contract whenever the SA node fails to fire after 2 seconds or so.

Worse yet, if the signal from the renegade AV node collides at just the right moment with the signal from the legitimate AV node, the signals can wipe each other out, causing the heart to stop beating in the electrical chaos, a phenomenon called ventricular fibrillation. It takes only a few seconds for a person with a nonbeating heart to become unconscious, and if cardiac resuscitation or spontaneous recovery of a heartbeat doesn't happen within a few minutes, the person will likely die or be left seriously brain damaged.

What's a cardiac arrest?

A cardiac arrest is a sudden failure of the ventricles to pump, usually because of ventricular tachycardia or ventricular fibrillation. Ventricular tachycardia can spontaneously revert to normal, but fibrillation rarely does unless something is done to reset the electrical rhythm of the heart. One way to reset the electrical rhythm is to thump hard on the sternum with the base of your fist. A more effective way is to zap the heart with a jolt of electricity from defribrillator paddles held against the chest wall. Just make sure you're not touching the bed when you press the button on the defribrillator paddles. The electrical surge traveling through the patient is also conducted through the bed and can wipe out the rhythm of *your* heart and send you into ventricular fibrillation. To prevent this from happening, the doctor yells "clear" before pressing the defibrillator button to get everyone back from the bed.

Wouldn't it be nice if people with ventricular premature beats carried around their own defibrillator?

They can. A wire threaded through a large arm vein into the heart is attached to a battery implanted in the chest wall under the skin. If the heart goes into the ventricular tachycardia or fibrillation, the battery sends a small electrical jolt to the heart to reset the SA and AV nodes.

What do you do if someone suddenly keels over unconscious?

If there's no pulse, you have to assume the person's heart is in ventricular fibrillation. No defibrillator paddles, now what? If a hard thump on the sternum doesn't get the heart pumping, you'll have to externally pump the heart until you can get the patient to a facility that has a defibrillator. External compression is performed by forcefully pushing down on the sternum with the heel of your palm. Compressing the ventricles like this 30 to 40 times a minute will pump enough blood from the heart to keep the patient alive. Generally, another person does the mouth-to-mouth breathing between compressions.

How do you do mouth-to-mouth resuscitation?

To ensure that air does not come out the nose, pinch the nostrils shut. To ensure that air goes into the trachea and not the esophagus, open the epiglottis by pulling the jaw forward. Now cover the victim's mouth with yours and blow.

What's an EKG?

An EKG, or electrocardiogram, is a paper display of the electrical activity of the heart (see figure 44). Atrial contraction is represented as a "P"

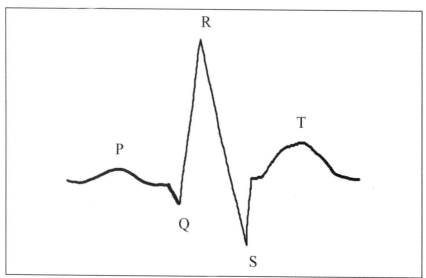

Figure 44

wave; ventricular contraction, as a "QRS" complex. The final wave is the "T" wave, representing repolarization, or recharging, of the left ventricle. (There is a wave for repolarization of the atria, but it's buried in the QRS complex.)

The heart is encased in a sac called the pericardium ("peri" means around, "cardium" is the heart). What risk does the heart run by beating inside a closed sac?

If for some reason the pericardium begins to fill up with fluid—say a virus infects the pericardium—the ventricles will be squeezed and won't have room to fill with blood between pumps. As the heart begins to beat less and less effectively, the blood pressure drops, and eventually the patient dies. This condition is called cardiac tamponade. ("Tamponade" comes from the same root as "tampon"—to stop up.)

How do you get rid of fluid in the pericardium?

In an emergency situation, the fastest way to get fluid out of the pericardium is to stick a needle up under the sternum, pass it upward through the diaphragm into the bottom of the pericardial sac, and suck out the fluid with a large syringe (see figure 45). You have to advance the needle slowly so as not to puncture the heart, but it's really not too difficult. There are no big arteries between the skin over the upper stomach and the pericardial sac, and it's difficult to miss the pericardial fluid, because the fluid-filled pericardial sac is very wide and the layer of fluid around the heart is quite thick. I would let a doctor do it, though.

What's a heart attack?

The heart needs oxygen like any other organ, but it doesn't get its oxygen from blood inside its ventricles. Like every other organ, oxygen is brought

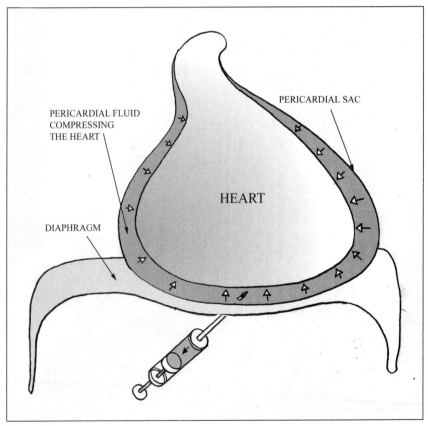

Figure 45

to it by arteries, in this case, the coronary arteries (see figure 46). If one of the coronary arteries should become occluded, the section of heart muscle dependent on that coronary artery will die. Death of any tissue in the body due to sudden lack of a blood supply is called an infarction, or infarct. In the case of the heart, it's called a myocardial infarction, or heart attack. (In the case of the brain, it's called a cerebral infarction, or stroke.)

Why do the coronary arteries get blocked off?

The blockage is almost always due to buildup of cholesterol, fatty acids, blood clots, and calcium inside the lumen of the coronary arteries. The

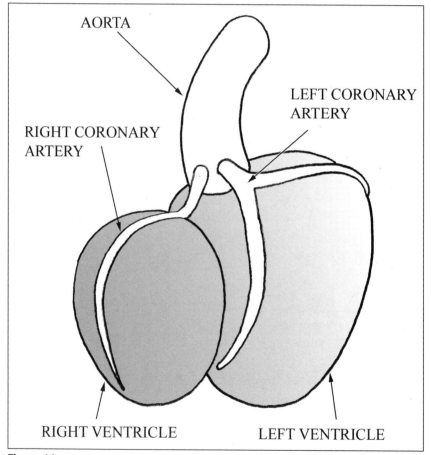

Figure 46

general term for buildup of cholesterol, fatty acids, blood clot, and calcium in an artery is atherosclerosis, and the term for the gunk accumulating within the artery is plaque.

Why are heart attacks (myocardial infarctions) dangerous?

Three reasons. The first is the occurrence of potentially fatal arrhythmias because the electrical system of the heart may be damaged in the heart attack. Also, immediately after a heart attack, irritating chemicals are released from the dead and damaged heart tissue and also from inflammatory white blood cells migrating in to repair the damaged heart tissue. These chemicals irritate the electrical system of the heart.

Second, after a section of heart muscle dies, the body repairs the damage with scar tissue. A scar is great because it's tough and won't tear apart. Unfortunately, a scar doesn't do anything—such as contract to help the heart pump blood. So after a heart attack the heart is a less effective pump.

Third, heart attacks can impair the function of the mitral valve by damaging small papillary muscles in the heart that help the mitral valve stay shut when it closes. Normally, the papillary muscles insert on the forward surface of the mitral valve as small tendons called chorda tendineae (see figure 47). When the left ventricle contracts, so do the papillary muscles to prevent the mitral valve from bulging backward and leaking blood back into the left atrium.

What is mitral valve prolapse?

Upward of 5% of the normal population has mitral valve prolapse, a benign condition in which the mitral valve bulges backward into the left atrium with each ventricular contraction causing very mild mitral regurgitation. Some of these patients also suffer unexplained bouts of unusual chest discomfort, excessive fatigue, anxiety, and panic attacks.

What's angina?

Angina is chest pain coming from the heart when it is not receiving adequate blood. When an organ other than the heart cries out for more

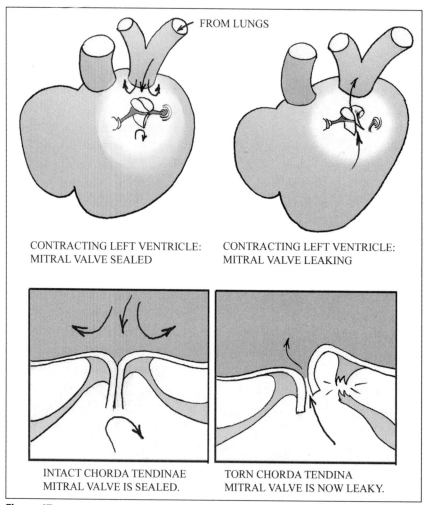

FROM LUNGS

CONTRACTING LEFT VENTRICLE:
MITRAL VALVE SEALED

CONTRACTING LEFT VENTRICLE:
MITRAL VALVE LEAKING

INTACT CHORDA TENDINAE
MITRAL VALVE IS SEALED.

TORN CHORDA TENDINA
MITRAL VALVE IS NOW LEAKY.

Figure 47

blood, it's called claudication. For example, that pain in your side when you run for a long time is probably claudication of the gut as blood is diverted to muscles. Angina is typically brought on by exercise or any stressful activity that speeds up the heart and increases the heart's demand for more oxygen. The reason for the pain is probably lactic acid buildup in heart muscle contracting under anaerobic conditions.

The usual reason the heart is not getting enough blood is that one or more of the coronary arteries is partially blocked by atherosclerotic plaque (see figure 48). Since the artery someday is probably going to close off completely and cause a myocardial infarction, the doctor has to either enlarge the lumen of the artery or surgically bypass the partially blocked artery. In coronary bypass surgery, a vein is taken from the leg and sewn into the aorta. The other end of the vein is sewn into the coronary artery downstream from the partial blockage, detouring blood around the obstruction (see figure 49). The terms double, triple, and quadruple bypass refer to how many arteries are bypassed.

If the patient is lucky, the site of blockage is located near the origin of the coronary artery where it first enters the heart. In that case, a cardiologist can puncture the femoral artery in the groin (where the femoral artery is carrying blood to the leg) and snake a catheter (tube) upstream

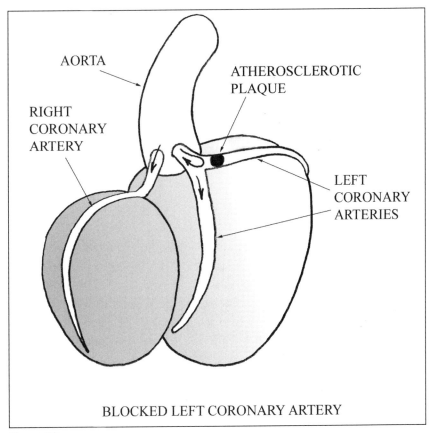

BLOCKED LEFT CORONARY ARTERY

Figure 48

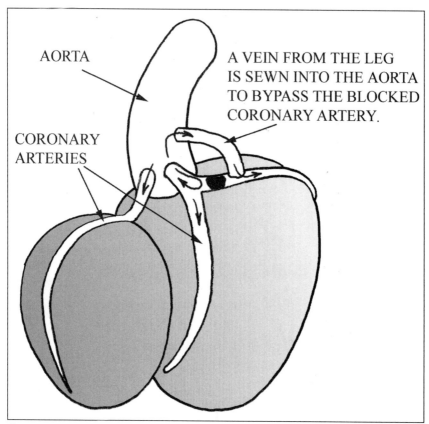

AORTA

A VEIN FROM THE LEG
IS SEWN INTO THE AORTA
TO BYPASS THE BLOCKED
CORONARY ARTERY.

CORONARY
ARTERIES

Figure 49

against the flow of aortic blood being pumped from the heart. Just before the catheter reaches the heart, the cardiologist carefully directs the catheter into the partially occluded coronary artery. At the tip of the catheter is a balloon. Once the catheter is placed into the coronary artery, a syringe full of air is injected into the catheter to blow up the balloon (see figure 50). The expanding balloon smashes the cholesterol plaque into the wall of the coronary artery, opening up the central lumen. This procedure is called an angioplasty. Newer methods of cleaning out the artery via catheterization include blasting the plaque with a laser or even drilling it out. Drilling may be necessary when calcium collecting in the plaque makes the plaque particularly hard.

BALLOON CATHETER

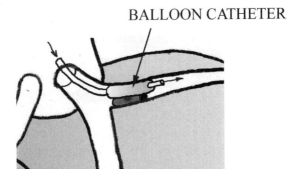

BALLOON CATHETER
INFLATED

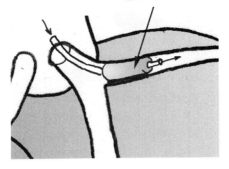

BLOOD CLOT NO LONGER
OBSTRUCTS THE ARTERY

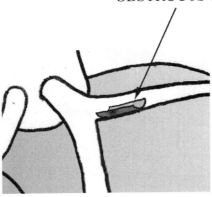

Figure 50

If all the heart does is pump blood, then why have so many philosophers and poets over the years bemoaned that they are heartsick over the loss of a loved one? Why does our heart ache when loved ones are gone? Why do you grab your heart when you fall in love or hear beautiful music? Why do our hearts go out to flood victims? Why do our heartfelt thanks go out to those who help us in times of need? Why is the heart the seat of our emotions?

It's not. Emotions are created in the brain, but their impact on the body is expressed through nerves carrying signals to the heart, blood vessels, gut, and just about every other internal organ. These nerve signals control the body's automatic and reflex functions, such as speeding up the heart, raising and lowering the blood pressure, sweating, and pupillary constriction. These nerves are called the autonomic nerves (which conveniently sounds like automatic). Thus, when you're love struck, you breathe faster and deeper, the heart pumps faster and harder, your pupils dilate, the blood vessels in your cheeks dilate into a blush, and blood flow to your crotch increases.

The section of brain controlling the autonomic nervous system is called the hypothalamus. The hypothalamus lies near the base of the brain, where it receives extensive input from many different regions of the brain, all vying to get the hypothalamus to express the brain's emotions by, for example, blushing or making the heart pound. We feel emotions in brain areas outside the hypothalamus, but we manifest them through the hypothalamus, which serves as the headwaters for the autonomic nervous system (see figure 51).

Can you learn to control the autonomic nerves?

There are some people who, through deep meditation, can raise and lower their own blood pressure or cause their body temperature to change. Biofeedback is sometimes successful in training people to control their own blood pressure by controlling their autonomic nervous system.

How can the autonomic nerves speed up *and* slow the heart?

There are two kinds of autonomic nerves: sympathetic and parasympathetic. The parasympathetic nerves are used when we are relaxed and at peace with ourselves, such as after a big meal. When the parasympathetic nerves rule,

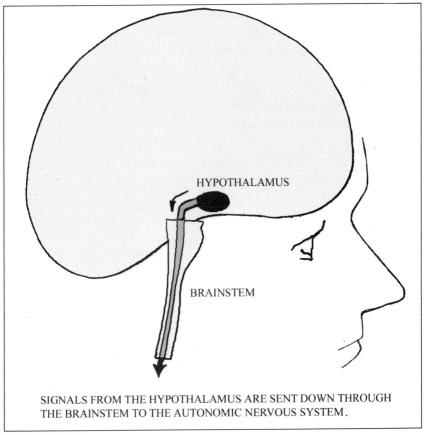

SIGNALS FROM THE HYPOTHALAMUS ARE SENT DOWN THROUGH THE BRAINSTEM TO THE AUTONOMIC NERVOUS SYSTEM.

Figure 51

the heart slows, the salivary glands produce saliva, the tear glands make tears, the gut moves food along the intestines, the bladder contracts, the rectum empties, and arteries and veins relax to lower the blood pressure. The next time you vomit, pay attention to how much extra saliva and tears you're making, as the parasympathetics simultaneously contract the stomach to make you vomit and stimulate the salivary and tear glands.

Sympathetic nerves stimulate things in the body you need to prepare for fight or flight, hence the name sympathetic, stemming from the Greek "syn" (with) and "pathos" (feeling). What would you need in these situations? First, you want to make sure all the internal organs—the heart, the lungs, the brain, the kidneys, the liver, and the muscles—get plenty of blood flow. To ensure a good blood supply, sympathetic nerves raise the blood pressure by speeding up the heart, making it contract more vigorously, and constricting arteries and veins. Constricted arteries raise the blood pressure by narrowing the hose—the same way you increase the water pressure in a hose by holding your thumb over the end of the hose. Besides raising the blood pressure, sympathetics ensure good blood flow to the internal organs by diverting blood from the skin to the internal organs, such as when you're scared, which is why we have the phrase to "turn white as a sheet."

You also want the sympathetics to dilate the bronchial tubes so you can breathe better, dilate the pupils to see better in the dark, and open the eyes wider for an unobstructed view. Under stress or great fear, the eyes open so wide that you can see the white of the eye above the iris. It's a scary look and may function in animals to scare away predators. You also want the sympathetics to stimulate the sweat glands to keep the body cool. The last thing you need in a fight or flight situation is to start peeing or have a bowel movement, so you want the sympathetics to slow the gut and relax the bladder to accommodate more urine. You want the sympathetics to tell the liver to transfer its stores of glucose into the bloodstream to provide plenty of energy. Your mouth dries because you don't need saliva. If you're a dog or cat, you want the sympathetics to stimulate a tiny muscle attached to the hairs on the back of the neck to scare off enemies. (Similarly, humans experience goose bumps during a "hair-raising" experience.) Finally, you want the brain to be vigilant and anxious, ready to spring into action.

Since the sympathetic nervous system doesn't extend into every tissue in the body, it extends its reach through the bloodstream by stimulating the adrenal glands lying atop the kidneys to release adrenaline (a.k.a. epinephrine) into the bloodstream. The rush of adrenaline acts just like the sympathetic nervous system and heightens the body's preparedness for fight or flight.

The one time the heart slows under sudden stress is when you dive into cold water. This is called the diving reflex. Seals and whales use the diving reflex to slow the heart during deep dives to preserve energy. Between the diving reflex and muscles loaded with myoglobin, some sea mammals can remain underwater for 30 minutes. Because the diving reflex also shifts blood away from the skin to the brain and other vital internal organs, and because the brain can withstand periods of low oxygen so long as there is no disturbance of blood flow to the brain, people have been successfully resuscitated after falling into icy lakes and remaining submerged for up to 20 minutes or more. Also, a chilled brain requires less oxygen.

How does a lie detector work?

A lie detector, or polygraph, works by measuring the changes in heart rate, blood pressure, respiratory rate and depth, and sweating that accompany your answers to questions, the assumptions being that you get nervous when you lie and that your nervousness stimulates the sympathetic nervous system.

What is ephedrine?

Ephedrine is a chemical that acts like adrenaline, stimulating the sympathetic nervous system and thereby helping athletes perform better. The risk of ephedrine and other sympathetic stimulants such as cocaine and amphetamines is that stimulating the sympathetic nervous system shuts down the blood supply to the skin, blocking an important method of ridding the body of excess heat during heavy exercise. Normally, the extra heat generated by vigorously contracting muscles is dissipated in two ways: by sweating and by opening up arteries to the skin to carry hot blood to the skin surface. As sweat evaporates off the skin, it cools the body. Sweating is so effective at keeping your body cool that, so long as you can keep drinking, you can chase down any land animal. Even though you're slower than, say, a gazelle, a fur-covered gazelle can't sweat and therefore can't rid its body of excess heat as effectively as humans can. Eventually, the gazelle has to stop running to cool off, giving you plenty of time to catch up.

Excessive sweating during vigorous exercise, however, eventually depletes the bloodstream of its water, a process called dehydration. Now the body has two obstacles to ridding itself of excess heat: not enough volume in the vascular tree to deliver blood to the skin surface and no open arteries to deliver it. As the body's temperature climbs to 106 degrees or more, proteins in the brain and elsewhere start to unravel, causing the athlete or soldier to become confused and delirious, and eventually causing the arterial system to begin to collapse, a deadly condition known as heat stroke. To prevent heat stroke, avoid sympathetic stimulants such as ephedrine and drink plenty of fluids, preferably containing sodium and potassium to replace what's being lost in the sweat.

How are we able to control when we urinate or defecate if bowel and bladder function are under autonomic control?

Not all bowel and bladder functions are under autonomic control. The sphincter muscles at the anus and the neck of the bladder are under voluntary control. (Any muscle that closes a hole is called a sphincter.) Squeezing these sphincters buys some time until you get to a toilet, where you can voluntarily relax them to urinate and defecate. Urination and defecation are also initiated by tightening the abdominal muscles to exert pressure on the bladder and rectum.

If the sympathetics are activated in fight or flight situations, and if the sympathetics slow gut movement, why do you suddenly have to have a bowel movement when you're scared before a big exam, and why do prisoners walking to the electric chair sometimes have bowel movements in their pants?

Movement of the gut is controlled by more than the sympathetic and parasympathetic nervous system. The wall of the gut has its own complex of nerves called the enteric nervous system, which seems to respond to hormones released from the brain under periods of high anxiety, an emotion critical to being scared shitless.

In stressful situations where the specific threat is clear and immediate action is demanded, fear rules. In situations where the specific threat is unclear, anxiety rules. This subtle difference pops up when the doctor suspects cancer. Before the patient knows one way or the other, he experiences tremendous anxiety. If he learns he does have cancer, the anxiety is over and rational fear sets in. Immediate fear elicits a response from the sympathetic nervous system, while anxiety involves more than the sympathetics. Anxiety causes the brain to release stress hormones into the bloodstream, including corticotropin releasing factor, which appears to stimulate the enteric nervous system. Some investigators think this may be the mechanism for the stress-induced abdominal cramping of irritable bowel syndrome.

Why do people faint when they hear bad news or see blood?

It's thought that sudden fear or emotional shock triggers a jolt of sympathetic output from the brain, causing a very forceful ventricular contraction, more forceful than usual. Nerves in the heart and blood vessels sense this sudden demand on the heart and alert the brain, which responds by shutting off the sympathetics and stimulating the parasympathetic nerves. The abrupt termination of sympathetic output allows veins in the legs to dilate while the parasympathetic stimulation slows the heart. The combination of inadequate amounts of blood returning to the heart and a slow heart rate results in a sudden drop in blood pressure. The reflex response of fear or shock followed by a drop in the blood pressure is known as a vasovagal reflex, "vaso" referring to blood vessels and "vagal" to the vagus nerve, which slows the heart.

Is that why some people faint in a barber chair?

Yes, but in this case the vasovagal reflex is triggered by that paper collar the barber wraps around the customer's neck. The collar compresses and thereby stimulates a small secton of the carotid artery called the carotid sinus. The carotid sinus normally monitors blood pressure in the carotid artery and alerts the brain when the blood pressure rises or drops. If the blood pressure rises (or you press on it with your finger or apply too tight a collar), signals from the carotid sinus stimulate the brain to respond with a volley of parasympathetic signals to slow the heart and relax the veins returning blood to the heart, all of which lowers the blood pressure. In some patients, the parasympathetic response is so strong that the blood pressure drops too much and the patient faints. Psychiatrists had postulated at one point that fainting in a barber chair was due to the "Samson complex," a fear of losing one's strength when having one's hair cut.

The carotid artery can be felt by gently holding your fingertips along each side of the trachea and feeling for pulsations. Rubbing the carotid artery will stimulate the carotid sinus and firm pressure will completely compress the carotid artery and cut off blood flow to the brain. The Romans chose the name carotid, which means sleep in Latin, because they knew that if you pressed firmly on both carotid arteries, the victim would become unconscious, a state akin to sleep.

The carotid sinus reflex can be taken advantage of when someone presents with a rapid heart rate due to a cardiac arrhythmia. A doctor can slow the heart by rubbing the carotid sinus, triggering a volley of parasympathetic impulses from the brain. There is a risk in doing this, however, which is why you should never rub the carotid artery in anybody for any reason. Rubbing the carotid artery may dislodge a piece of atherosclerotic plaque attached to the inside of the carotid artery, causing it to float, or embolize, downstream, lodge in a small artery in the brain, and cut off its blood flow, causing a stroke.

Why shouldn't children run around with pencils, lollipop sticks, or popsicle sticks in their mouths?

After coursing alongside the trachea to the top of the neck, the carotid arteries pass through the back of the throat behind each tonsil. They're hard to feel there because of the gag reflex. If a child runs around with a pencil or popsicle stick in his mouth, and then falls on his face, the pencil or popsicle stick can be driven into the back of the throat against the carotid artery (see figure 52). A sharp jab like that may injure the interior lining (endothelium) of the carotid artery and cause a blood clot to form in the lumen (center) of the artery. The clot can either obstruct the carotid or break off and embolize to the brain. Either way, blood flow to a portion of the brain can be interrupted, causing a stroke. Depending on what part of the brain is killed, the child can be blind in one eye, paralyzed on one side, or unable to speak.

Jabbing the carotid is not the only way to damage the wall of the carotid artery. A more common way is to whiplash the neck and stretch the carotid artery enough to tear the wall of the carotid. Bleeding develops in the wall of the artery and either pinches off the lumen or causes a clot to form inside the lumen. Either way, the victim is at serious risk of suffering a stroke. Bleeding into the wall of an artery is called dissection. The only warning you have of carotid dissection is pain in the neck. Big deal, everybody has neck pain after a whiplash injury. Yes, but not everybody with pain in the neck after whiplash has tenderness over the carotid artery. Still, it's a hard diagnosis to make before disaster strikes. The clue to carotid artery damage is in the eye, because the sympathetic nerves get to the eye (to dilate the pupils and pull back the upper eyelid during times of high stress) by snaking up the wall of the carotid arteries. Damage to the wall of a carotid artery also damages the sympathetics traveling along the wall of the artery, causing the eyelid on that side to droop slightly and the pupil to become slightly smaller. The combination of a mildly drooping eyelid and slightly smaller pupil is called Horner's syndrome.

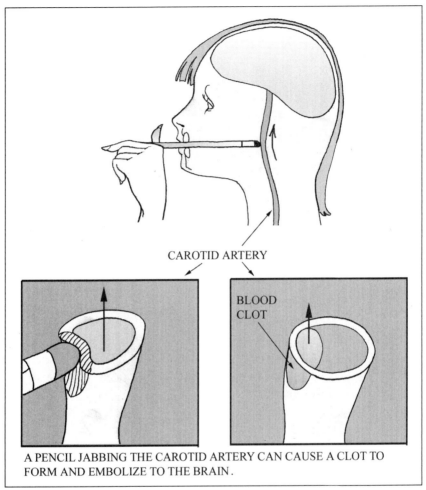

A PENCIL JABBING THE CAROTID ARTERY CAN CAUSE A CLOT TO FORM AND EMBOLIZE TO THE BRAIN.

Figure 52

If damage to the carotid artery occurs before the age of two, the iris on the affected side won't pigment as much, because pigmentation of the iris depends on sympathetic nerve input to the iris. (A person with a slightly droopy eyelid, smaller pupil, and lighter colored eye looks at you a little funny when you ask him what type of neck injury he suffered as an infant.) To take it one step further, before reaching the carotid artery, the sympathetic nerves skirt over the top of the lung. It wouldn't be unusual for a doctor to walk into the examination room, spot the patient's obvious weight loss and fatigued look, note the Horner's syndrome, and within 15 seconds diagnose cancer of the dome of the lung.

8

————∿∿∿∿∿∿∿∿∿————

GASTROINTESTINAL SYSTEM

The gastrointestinal system absorbs and digests food, detoxifies poisons, synthesizes important proteins for the bloodstream, and with the help of the immunologic system, screens out potential infections. Digestion is a big job because proteins, fats, and carbohydrates need different mechanisms to be absorbed and digested. And once they are broken down, the gastrointestinal system has to present them to the bloodstream in a deliverable size and shape for transport to distant organs starving for nutrients. Let's begin in the mouth.

Why are teeth different shapes?

The front teeth are flat for grabbing onto and slicing through food. The two corner teeth, the incisors, stab food and keep it from getting away. The back teeth are flat, just the thing for grinding food into a paste for swallowing.

What are teeth made of?

Calcium, just like our bones. The hardest substance of the body is the enamel of teeth. Underneath the enamel is softer bone called dentin, and in the center of the tooth is the pulp, where the blood vessels and nerves are found (see figure 53).

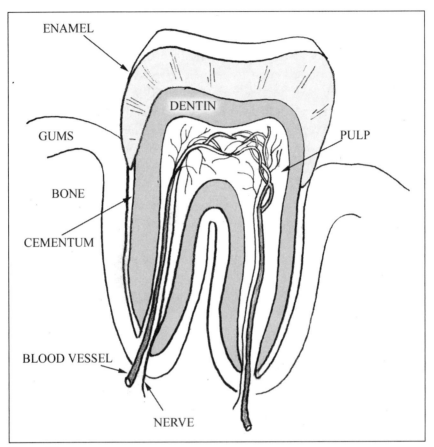

Figure 53

Enamel covers only the top of the tooth. When enamel reaches the gum line, a hard substance (but not as hard as enamel) called cementum covers the roots. Being rather thin, cementum does not provide much protection for the underlying dentin in the roots. It's important, therefore, not to let the vulnerable roots become exposed. Unfortunately, as we age, our gums recede from the edge of the enamel and expose the roots. Scrubbing the gums with a tooth brush and frequent flossing help prevent our gums from receding.

Why do they put fluoride in toothpaste?

About a hundred years ago, Dr. Frederick McKay, a dentist in Colorado Springs, Colorado, noticed that many of the children in town had brownish, pitted teeth. As defective as these teeth appeared, they had surprisingly few cavities. About ten years later in Bauxite, Arkansas, another dentist, Dr. F. L. Robertson, noticed the same mottled appearance in the teeth of children living near a recently dug well. In 1930, high concentrations of fluoride were discovered in the well. McKay had samples of water from Colorado Springs tested and they, too, had elevated fluoride levels. Eventually, the proper concentration of fluoride was arrived at which would prevent tooth decay without staining the teeth. Fluoride is now added to the water supply and toothpaste. How fluoride prevents decay is not exactly clear, but it probably has something to do with hardening the tooth enamel. Some investigators think fluoride inhibits the action of bacteria in the mouth.

Why are there blood vessels in the pulp of teeth?

In order for teeth to grow during childhood, blood vessels in the pulp bring in the necessary nutrients, which they continue to do into adulthood. If the blood supply to a tooth is lost, the tooth eventually turns gray as the dead pulp seeps into the enamel.

What is a cavity?

A cavity is a bacterial infection in the enamel. The medical term for dental decay is caries (Latin for rotten). The only way to clean out the bacterial infection is to drill it out and fill up the hole with metal or some other equally hard material. If the cavity is not fixed, the bacteria will eat their way through the enamel, into the dentin, and then into the pulp.

What happens if the infection gets into the pulp?

First off, the nerves in the pulp will be screaming in pain. Eventually, the infection will kill the pulp by causing it to lose its blood supply. Without a blood supply, the bacteria are free to multiply in the pulp without fear of white blood cells or antibiotics reaching them. If the infection is not taken care of, it can spread into the gums or even into the jawbone. The only way to get rid of a pulp infection is to perform a root canal.

What's a root canal?

This is a procedure in which a hole is drilled through the enamel to enable the dentist to scrape out the pulp. After the pulp space is hollowed out, it is filled in with a sealant so that bacteria can no longer enter the pulp space. While a root canal is necessary to clean out an infected pulp, root canals are also done electively to prevent a tooth that's lost its blood supply from turning gray.

How do bacteria infect a tooth in the first place?

The mouth is full of bacteria. The reason we brush our teeth is not so much to cleanse the surface of the tooth of bacteria but to cleanse the teeth of excess food particles. Those food particles provide a source of food for bacteria that can then multiply and release acids and other potent chemicals that eat away the enamel. You don't have to brush too hard or too long to brush away food particles. In fact, if you do brush too hard and too long, you will wear down the enamel and make it easier for bacteria to invade the tooth. As important as brushing is, flossing is even more important, because it removes food particles hiding between teeth and out of reach of a toothbrush.

All bacteria love sugar. In one recent English study, dental caries quadrupled in children given sugary snacks and drinks before going to bed. Sugary snacks during the night are particularly harmful, because at night when we stop chewing food our mouths have less saliva, and saliva contains natural bacteria-fighting chemicals.

What is plaque?

Bacteria tend to collect on and between teeth in a tenacious film called plaque. Plaque is difficult to brush away, so a dental hygienist usually has to scrape it away with a metal instrument. Smoking enhances plaque formation but it's not clear why. One theory is that the nicotine in tobacco smoke causes small blood vessels in the gums to constrict, which reduces the delivery of oxygen and white blood cells to fight accumulating bacteria.

Plaque becomes particularly dangerous when it creeps below the gum line. In the sliver of space between the tooth and the gum, there are no blood vessels, which allows bacteria free rein to grow and flourish. The inflammation around the developing plaque eats away at the collagen ligaments holding teeth in their bony sockets, and also at the bony sockets themselves, eventually causing teeth to lose their footing and fall out. The problem is compounded by vitamin C deficiency, because collagen, a protein, can be made only with the help of vitamin C. One of the signs of vitamin C deficiency—scurvy—is loosening of the teeth, a common problem among seamen in the 18th century, before people realized that vitamin C–containing lemons and limes (and also oranges and grapefruit) could prevent scurvy. (Another sign of vitamin deficiency—almost any vitamin deficiency—is a smooth, red, burning tongue.)

Why do teeth hurt when the dentist fills a cavity?

There are nerves in the pulp and dentin, but not in the enamel. So long as the cavity remains confined to the enamel, drilling shouldn't hurt.

How does the dentist prevent your teeth from hurting when drilling into dentin?

Before drilling, the dentist injects a local anesthetic in the back of the mouth behind the molars to numb up the nerve.

If the dentist is going to drill on a tooth in the middle of the jaw, why does he put the numbing medicine way in the back of the jaw? (see figure 54).

It's difficult to numb up the nerves to a single tooth, because they enter the pulp from below the tooth. It's a lot easier to block the nerves upstream, where they are still bundled into a single large nerve entering the jaw, even though it means numbing more teeth than necessary.

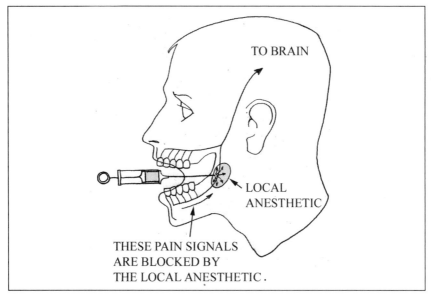

TO BRAIN

LOCAL ANESTHETIC

THESE PAIN SIGNALS ARE BLOCKED BY THE LOCAL ANESTHETIC.

Figure 54

Why are there bacteria in the mouth?

It's hard to keep bacteria out of the mouth, since we continually put bacteria into our mouths when we eat. As a result, the mouth is full of bacteria, some of them pretty nasty. You're better off being bitten by a dog than a human (so long as the dog is not rabid). Human bites are much more likely to become infected with aggressive bacteria or even nastier infectious agents, such as syphilis, hepatitis B, and HIV.

If the mouth is contaminated by bacteria, why don't we become infected when we swallow food?

Because the stomach contains strong hydrochloric acid that kills most bacteria. Some bacteria do survive, though, and cause infections. The government routinely inspects meat, poultry, eggs, and other foodstuffs for evidence of contamination by bacteria that might survive the stomach. An important reason for heating food is to kill any dangerous bacteria. In 1998, a group of people in Washington State died after eating hamburgers that had not been cooked hot enough or long enough to kill an acid-resistant strain of E. coli bacteria that had somehow contaminated the meat.

What is salmonella food poisoning?

Salmonella is another dangerous bacterium that caused serious public health problems prior to the discovery of antibiotics. Salmonella is still a risk if food, especially eggs and chicken, are left out at room temperature. Eating uncooked eggs and raw meat is a no-no because of the risk of salmonella. Reptiles, including turtles, may also carry salmonella.

Salmonella causes typhoid fever. Some patients may suffer only a few days of fever, diarrhea, and abdominal cramps, while others suffer a more prolonged course. In either case, the salmonella may hole up in the gall bladder and be continually shed through the bile into the intestines and eventually the stool. If such carriers of salmonella are not careful about washing their hands after a bowel movement, they can infect other people. Typhoid Mary was one such person. Around the turn of the century, working as a chef no less, she infected a large number of people and yet still refused to stop working as a food preparer. Eventually, she had to be taken into custody and confined against her will, from 1907 until 1910. After being set free and infecting even more people, she was confined again, from 1915 until her death in 1938.

Why does mayonnaise pose a risk of food poisoning at picnics?

Not all food poisoning is caused by live bacteria. The other type of food poisoning is caused by eating a bacterial toxin. Even if the bacteria are killed by the stomach acids, the toxin may survive and disrupt the intestines, usually with vomiting and diarrhea. The most common example of a food poisoning toxin is one made by staphylococcus, a bacteria that loves mayonnaise. That's why tuna salad, coleslaw, and other creamy foods have to be properly chilled before being served at a summer picnic.

Because stomach acids don't destroy all bacterial toxins or kill all strains of salmonella, food should be heated, if at all possible, to a temperature of 160 degrees or more to kill any bacteria and destroy any toxic proteins. This process is called pasteurization, after Louis Pasteur, who first discovered the protective benefit of heating food.

Why do you have to kill the bacteria inside a sealed can? How can bacteria get inside a sealed can? Besides, there's no oxygen in a sealed can for the bacteria to grow.

A sealed can is ideal for anerobic bacteria such as *Clostridium botulinum*, the maker of the deadly botulinus toxin. Botulinus toxin is resistant to digestion by the stomach, and once absorbed through the intestines the toxin is free to paralyze muscles, including the respiratory muscles. Botulinus bacteria get into the can before it's sealed, as tiny spores. Botulinus spores are not uncommon in the environment, especially in dirt. Once inside a sealed can, the botulinus spores spring to life and form into botulinus bacteria. To kill the heat-resistant spores before they have a chance to become botulinus bacteria, sealed cans and home canning jars are heated to 160 and preferably up to 250 degrees. Since water boils at only 212 degrees, home canning jars have to be boiled in a large pressure cooker. The tip-off to anerobic contamination of canned food is bulging of the can—from gas produced by the anerobic bacteria. Such contamination in glass jars may cause them to burst.

The threat of botulism is the reason for not thawing and refreezing frozen food. Here's why. Frozen food contaminated with botulism spores is safe to eat because the spores have not transformed into botulinus bacteria and produced the deadly toxin. (The spores will be killed in the stomach.) When frozen food is thawed, spores of botulism transform into botulinus bacteria, which lie dormant because there's oxygen around. When the food is refrozen, the surface freezes first, leaving an unfrozen center, cut off from any oxygen—a perfect anerobic environment for botulinus bacteria to grow and produce botulinus toxin.

Why shouldn't infants be fed honey?

In ancient Greece, long before tin cans were invented, perishable food was stored in honey because bacteria have a difficult time growing in honey due to its low oxygen and water content. The problem with honey, though, is that bees often brush up against botulinus spores, which then contaminate the honey. Fortunately, the spores don't grow in honey and, when eaten, are killed by stomach acid—in adults. Babies' stomachs don't produce enough acid to kill the spores, so if honey contaminated with botulinus spores is fed to a baby, the spores can revert to toxin-producing bacteria. The botulism toxin that's produced attacks the baby's muscles, causing the baby to become weak, floppy, and unable to suck. For this reason, honey should not be fed to babies until they are a year old—when their stomachs start making enough acid to kill botulinus spores.

What is the tongue made of?

The tongue is an exquisitely controlled muscle for manipulating food, swallowing, and changing sounds generated by the voice box—the larynx—into "th," "l," "s," "d," and so on.

How does the tongue taste food?

The tongue tastes food with rows of taste buds situated around the tongue. Like the olfactory hair cells, taste buds send off an electrical signal when the right molecule fits into a receptor. There are only four receptors on taste buds: one each for salt, sugar, bitter, and sour. A lemon and a pickle are sour, while oversteeped coffee is bitter (try putting some instant coffee on your tongue). Taste buds are more sensitive when they are warm, which is why you shouldn't judge the taste of food cold if it is going to be served hot.

Why do snakes have forked tongues?

Snakes have poor eyesight, so instead of visually chasing mice and rats, snakes rely on their sense of taste. The way a snake tells whether the mouse scurried left or right is by sampling the air with its forked tongue, bringing the tongue back into its mouth, and inserting the two tips of its tongue into two olfactory receptors in the roof of its mouth. Whichever olfactory receptor detects a stronger mouse odor tells the snake which direction the mouse turned. It's amazing that the inch of space between the two tips of a snake's tongue contains that much difference in a mouse's odor, and that a biological structure could have evolved to detect that infinitesimal difference.

Where does saliva come from?

Saliva is made in the parotid gland, situated alongside the mandible of the jaw and in the submandibular gland under the jaw (see figure 55). The parotid and submandibular glands can readily be felt (palpated) through the skin. Salivary glands squirt saliva into the mouth via salivary ducts under the tongue and along the cheeks. If you lift your tongue in front of a mirror, you may find a tiny opening on the floor of the mouth through which saliva is squirted. Some talented people can squirt their saliva quite forcefully from these ducts and strike a target several feet away. In 6th grade, this trick always worked well to disrupt music class as the front-row students below were hit by a wet spray on the back of their necks.

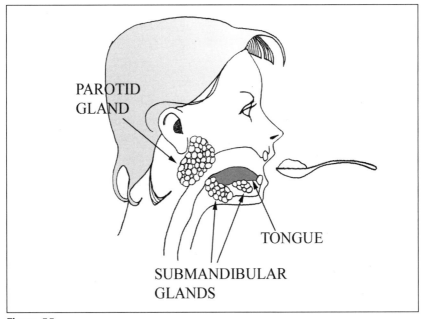

Figure 55

Can the salivary gland become obstructed?

Yes indeed. Once in a great while someone will come to the emergency room with horrible pain in the side of his jaw because of a tiny grain of calcium lodged in the salivary gland duct. The obstruction backs up saliva under high pressure into the salivary gland. Sometimes the stone will pass, but if it doesn't, surgery will be required to remove it.

Why do we need saliva (besides to spit)?

We make saliva to moisten our food for easier swallowing. Saliva also contains enzymes that kill bacteria, and enzymes that break down carbohydrates, thereby beginning the digestion of food.

What's that thing hanging down from the roof of the mouth?

It's called the uvula (which means grape in Latin). The roof of the mouth is called the palate. You can feel the hard palate up front and a soft palate further back (you may gag doing this). The uvula hangs off the soft palate. There does not seem to be any real purpose to the uvula, because it can be cut off without any problem.

Do we need a soft palate?

Yes, most definitely. The soft palate moves up and down to shut off the nasal chambers so that when we drink a glass of water, none of the water washes up into the nose. One of the ways a doctor knows that the soft palate is paralyzed is when a patient complains of liquids coming out his nose while drinking. Another reason we need to shut off the nasal chambers is to say certain sounds, such as "ng," as in "finger" or "string." Sometimes you don't want to block off the nasal chamber, such as when you breathe through your nose or blow smoke out your nose.

What is heartburn?

First of all, heartburn has nothing to do with the heart. The reason it's called heartburn is that the pain of heartburn is felt right behind the sternum, where the heart lies. As you recall, food is propelled down the esophagus, which passes through the diaphragm to connect to the stomach. Once food reaches the stomach, it must be broken down into a liquid slush in order to be absorbed and used by the body. The stomach secretes juices to moisten the food, and along with these juices it secretes two molecules to continue the digestive process begun by saliva. One of the molecules is hydrochloric acid and the other is a powerful protein, an enzyme called pepsin, that tears apart large protein molecules into amino acids. Pepsin and hydrochloric acid are prevented from eating a hole in the stomach wall by a layer of bicarbonate-containing mucus. Unfortunately, the esophagus does not have the stomach's protective mucus coating, so any hydrochloric acid that washes back up into the esophagus will burn the esophagus.

At the juncture of the esophagus and stomach is a sphincter muscle that is supposed to close off the esophagus. If the esophageal sphincter is weak, however, hydrochloric acid may wash back up into the esophagus, which you feel as heartburn. One common cause of a weak esophageal sphincter is a hiatal hernia, in which the stomach pushes upward through the diaphragm. The esophageal sphincter is also weakened by smoking.

Persistent and longstanding reflux of hydrochloric acid into the esophagus may allow fumes of hydrochloric acid to waft up the esophagus and then down the trachea, stimulating the vagus nerve and irritating the tracheal and bronchial mucosa, all of which may lead to bronchial constriction and asthma.

What do you take for heartburn?

Most people take antacids—medications that neutralize stomach acid. The opposite of an acid is a base, a solution that has too few free hydrogen ions. Tums, Maalox, Aludrox, Gaviscon, and bicarbonate work by sopping up free hydrogen atoms. A more effective approach than antacids, which after all only treat the symptoms, is something that prevents excess acid in the first place—drugs such as Zantac, Tagamet, Prilosec, and Nexium, which prevent the stomach from making hydrochloric acid.

What would happen if something interfered with the stomach's mucous lining?

The stomach's hydrochloric acid would eat a hole in the stomach wall and cause an ulcer.

What things interfere with the mucous lining the stomach wall?

Aspirin, Motrin, Prednisone, and most other anti-inflammatory medications disrupt the mucous lining of the stomach by interfering with COX-1 synthesis of mucus. Only recently have chemists been able to invent anti-inflammatory medications, such as Vioxx and Celebrex, that don't.

Helicobacter pylori, one of the few bacteria that survives in the stomach, damages the stomach's mucosal lining directly. *Helicobacter pylori* in the stomach is actually quite common, but only a few people harboring it develop gastric (stomach) ulcers. Antibiotics are very effective in curing gastric and duodenal ulcers caused by *Helicobacter pylori* (the stomach empties into the duodenum).

What's an acid?

An acid is any liquid that has free hydrogen ions floating around. Free hydrogen ions are nothing more than the positively charged nucleus of a hydrogen atom, so any time the nucleus of a hydrogen atom, symbolized by H^+, breaks free from a molecule and floats free in a liquid, that liquid is now acidic. If only a few positive hydrogen atoms are present, the acid is mild and tastes tart or sour. A good example is lemon juice. If a lot of positive hydrogen atoms are present, the acid is strong and will burn your skin. An acid is named by whatever atom or molecule the hydrogen atom is attached to, for example, hydrochloric acid (HCl; attached to a chlorine atom) or sulfuric acid (H_2SO_4; a sulfate molecule).

What's a protein?

A protein is a very large molecule made up of a long string of amino acids. Some of these amino acids have positive and negative electrical charges on them that attract or repel other charged amino acids in the protein. The result of all this electrical pushing and pulling is a folding of the protein into a specific shape. The various shapes and their ability to attach to other molecules are what make proteins so useful.

Each cell in the body is busily taking molecules into the cell, building molecules, tearing other molecules apart, moving molecules around the cell, and kicking other molecules out of the cell. Proteins help with all these functions. For example, some proteins grab on to a complicated sugar molecule and break it apart into individual glucose molecules, while another protein takes those individual glucose molecules and makes a different sugar molecule. Some proteins break apart the proteins we eat into individual amino acids, after which other proteins assemble them into still other proteins.

Proteins that speed up chemical reactions are called enzymes. Each enzymatic protein can do only one thing because each protein has only one shape designed for a specific purpose. For this reason, there have to be thousands of different enzymatic proteins for the thousands of different chemical reactions in the body.

A protein that remains stationary, say, as part of a cell wall, is a structural protein. Proteins that latch onto foreign antigens are antibodies.

What foods have lots of protein?

Meat, of course, but also nuts and many vegetables and cereals. A good liquid protein is egg white, which is loaded with a protein called albumin.

What if you don't eat any protein: can the body make protein from sugar and fat?

Not totally. Fat and sugar can only be converted into some amino acids. The amino acids the body cannot synthesize, and that therefore have to be eaten, are called the essential amino acids. Of the 20 different amino acids, we can synthesize only 12 from fat and carbohydrates, leaving 8 essential amino acids.

How do you inactivate a protein?

Proteins can be inactivated by unraveling, or denaturing, them. The easiest way to do this is to heat them or whip them. You've all seen this happen when you fry an egg or whip egg white. In either case, the albumin in egg white slowly denatures from a colorless jelly into something white and firm. Another protein denatured by heat is collagen, a major component of cartilage. Cartilage forms the flexible tip of your nose, your ear, and the gristle in joints between bones. By boiling collagen in a mild acid solution, collagen is denatured to gelatin, which is used in all sorts of food.

What are amino acids?

Each amino acid is about the size of a glucose molecule, but all amino acids have one thing sugar molecules don't: a nitrogen atom. One of the reasons fertilizer is so nutritious is that it contains nitrogen for plants to make amino acids and, from them, proteins. During World War I, the Allies blockaded Germany's sources of nitrogen, which was doubly crippling, as nitrogen was also used to make explosives. The German chemist Fritz Haber developed a now famous process for extracting nitrogen from the air (which is 80% nitrogen), allowing Germany to continue its war efforts with adequate supplies of explosives and fertilizer.

Some plants don't need fertilizer to get their nitrogen; they harbor clumps of bacteria around their roots, which pick nitrogen out of the air. These clever plants are called legumes and include peas, beans, and soybeans.

In the normal, everyday chemical activity of the body, proteins are continually being synthesized and disassembled. If a protein is disassembled and the amino acids are not going to be reused to make another protein, the amino acids are broken apart for other uses. The nitrogen atoms in the amino acids are discarded by hooking them to carbon atoms to form a new molecule, urea, which the kidneys excrete through the urine. Bacterial breakdown of urea is what gives old urine its distinctive odor.

What happens to food after it leaves the stomach?

After an hour or so of churning, the stomach pumps its mixture of food and digestive juices through the pyloric sphincter (pyloris means gate keeper) into the first part of the small intestine, the duodenum. Into the duodenum are added fluids from the pancreas and liver (see figure 56). Pancreatic juice contains sodium bicarbonate to stop the action of pepsin (which needs an acid environment such as the stomach to remain active) and three ferocious digestive enzymes, one for breaking apart carbohydrates, one for fats, and one for proteins.

When fat first enters the intestines, most of it is in the form of large globs of water-insoluble triglycerides. The "tri" in triglyceride refers to three long chains of carbon atoms called fatty acids. The "glyceride" refers to glycerol, a small molecule to which the three fatty acids are attached. To get at the energy stored in fatty acids, fatty acids first have to be separated from glycerol. The intestines begin pulling fatty acids off glycerol while triglycerides are still inside the intestines, because fatty acids are a lot more soluble in water than triglycerides and because blood is mostly water.

The pancreatic enzyme that breaks apart triglycerides is lipase. Unfortunately, lipase is a water-soluble enzyme and can only nibble at the edges of large globs of triglycerides. To break up the globs of triglycerides into tiny droplets for easier attack by lipase, bile is released into the duodenum from the gallbladder, which is tucked up under the liver. Bile is only stored in the gallbladder; it is synthesized in the liver by mixing a metabolite (breakdown product) of heme (part of hemoglobin) with a metabolite of cholesterol into a greenish slurry. The liver discharges bile down the hepatic duct to the gallbladder for storage. When we eat a fatty meal, bile is released from the gallbladder via the cystic duct and then down the common bile duct into the duodenum (see figure 56). Before entering the duodenum, the common bile duct joins the pancreatic duct so that bile and pancreatic juices enter the duodenum together.

The clumps of triglycerides that are not broken apart by bile and lipase are too big and too water insoluble to be absorbed into the tiny capillaries lining the intestines. Instead, the clumps of triglycerides are absorbed into small lymphatic vessels called lacteals lining the intestinal walls. Lacteals transport the triglycerides (and cholesterol) as chylomicrons to the main lymphatic duct—the thoracic duct—which travels up the chest to connect to the left subclavian vein, a large vein in the upper chest (see figure 57). Triglycerides in the bloodstream are further broken down by lipase also circulating in the bloodstream. Whatever triglycerides remain

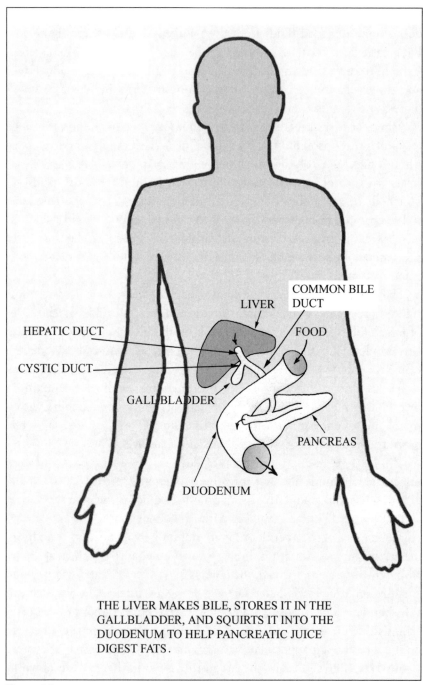

THE LIVER MAKES BILE, STORES IT IN THE
GALLBLADDER, AND SQUIRTS IT INTO THE
DUODENUM TO HELP PANCREATIC JUICE
DIGEST FATS.

Figure 56

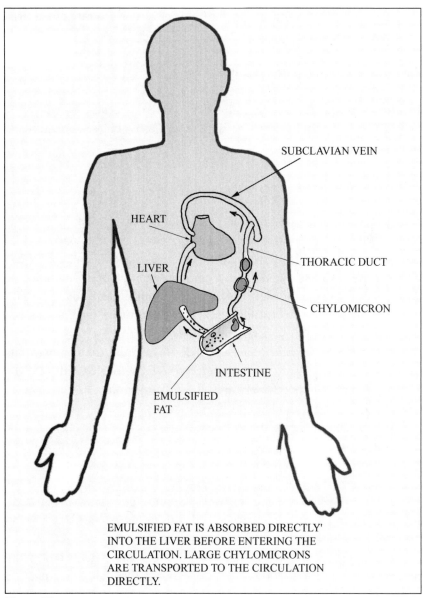

SUBCLAVIAN VEIN

HEART

LIVER

THORACIC DUCT

CHYLOMICRON

INTESTINE

EMULSIFIED
FAT

EMULSIFIED FAT IS ABSORBED DIRECTLY'
INTO THE LIVER BEFORE ENTERING THE
CIRCULATION. LARGE CHYLOMICRONS
ARE TRANSPORTED TO THE CIRCULATION
DIRECTLY.

Figure 57

are taken up by the liver and muscles for digestion or deposited in arterial walls and fat cells.

Do you need your gallbladder?

No, lots of people have their gallbladder removed because of gallstones, and they seem to handle fatty foods quite well using bile secreted directly from the liver.

What's a gallstone?

Sometimes, the cholesterol in bile precipitates out of solution, forming balls of bile ranging in size from small grains up to large marbles, in a process called cholelithiasis. Exiting the gallbladder, gallstones can obstruct the cystic duct and cause a painful damming up of bile into the gallbladder. If enough pressure builds up for a long enough time, the gall-bladder may lose its blood supply and die. Dead tissue such as this is a perfect site for a deadly gangrenous infection.

Obstruction of the bile duct further downstream in the common bile duct causes back pressure on the liver, too, causing bile to spill into the bloodstream as jaundice (see figure 58). Yellow jaundice is best seen in the whites of the eyes and also as brownish, tea-colored urine.

If obstruction of the common bile duct takes place after it has joined the pancreatic duct, back pressure also builds up into the pancreas. If the pressure gets too high and remains too long, the pancreas can be damaged, permitting its digestive enzymes to escape into pancreatic tissue. The free pancreatic enzymes begin digesting the pancreas, releasing more pancreatic enzymes and causing more autodigestion, an intensely painful condition called pancreatitis.

Because the common bile duct courses through the head of the pancreas, tumors in the head of the pancreas can also obstruct the common bile duct and cause jaundice.

What is the grumbling in your stomach when you're hungry?

From the duodenum to the large intestine—about 20 feet—food is nudged along the small intestine by slow contractions called peristalsis.

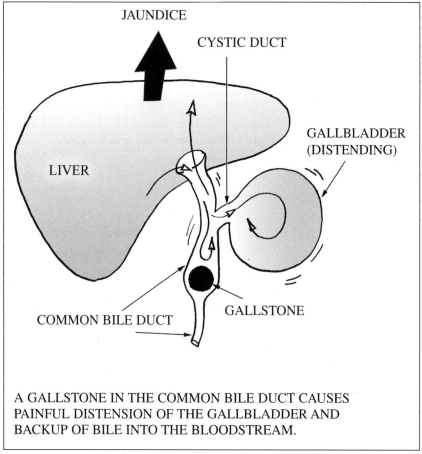

JAUNDICE

CYSTIC DUCT

LIVER

GALLBLADDER
(DISTENDING)

COMMON BILE DUCT

GALLSTONE

A GALLSTONE IN THE COMMON BILE DUCT CAUSES
PAINFUL DISTENSION OF THE GALLBLADDER AND
BACKUP OF BILE INTO THE BLOODSTREAM.

Figure 58

The doctor can hear these slow peristaltic movements with a stethoscope. Sometimes, when the intestines are really rolling, you can hear them yourself without a stethoscope. Peristaltic contractions are controlled by the parasympathetic side of the autonomic nervous system. Parasympathetic nerves stimulate the gut to move by releasing a chemical called acetylcholine. Any drug that increases the amount of acetylcholine will increase the speed of peristalsis, and conversely, any drug, such as atropine, that blocks acetylcholine will slow peristalsis. The belladonna plant, which is loaded with atropine, has been used for hundreds and hundreds of years to treat abdominal cramping and diarrhea. Made into eyedrops, belladonna was also used to block parasympathetic nerves from constricting the pupil. The dilated pupils gave women an alluring look, hence the name belladonna (beautiful woman). Unfortunately, anyone who inadvertently ate too many of the tasty berries or roots on wild belladonna plants would also block acetylcholine in the brain, resulting in delirium and even death. As you might expect, belladonna has been a favorite poison throughout the ages.

What happens to food as it travels down the intestines?

As food meanders down the small intestine, enzymes break down the proteins, carbohydrates, and clumps of fats for easier absorption through the intestinal wall and into the bloodstream (see figure 59). The first place freshly absorbed food goes is the liver, which removes the carbohydrates, amino acids, and fatty acids. The carbohydrates are stored as glycogen. Later, when the blood sugar falls, the liver slices individual sugar molecules—glucose—off the glycogen and secretes glucose into the bloodstream. The liver uses the amino acids to synthesize a large variety of proteins for the body, including most of the proteins floating around the bloodstream, such as albumin. Proteins in the bloodstream absorb water from peripheral tissues. When the liver is severely damaged and can no longer make proteins for the bloodstream, water in the bloodstream leaks into the peripheral tissues, especially the abdomen, which becomes distended with ascites, giving these patients an odd, almost pregnant, look. For such a multipurpose organ it's amazing that you only need 10% of your liver to survive, and if for some reason a surgeon has to remove part of your liver, it will grow back.

Venous blood carrying digested food from the intestines drains directly to the liver, so that the liver can also detoxify the blood before allowing it into the systemic circulation. A chemical considered toxic by the liver may be something as simple as an aspirin tablet, which is why you have to take medications every 4 to 6 hours to keep up with their destruction by the liver. After a few weeks or months, the liver becomes more effective at destroying the medication. The resulting lower blood levels of the medication make it appear as if the medication has lost its effectiveness or that you've somehow gotten used to it, when in fact all that's happened is that the liver has smartened up and figured out how to detoxify the medication more effectively.

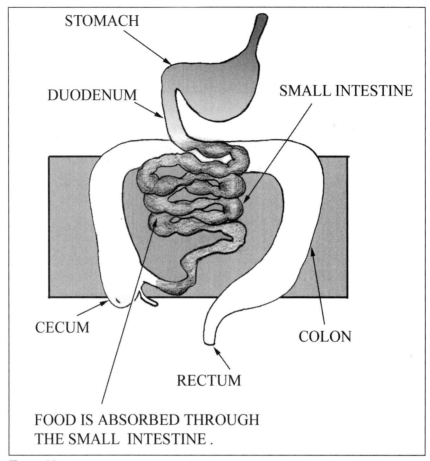

STOMACH

DUODENUM

SMALL INTESTINE

CECUM

COLON

RECTUM

FOOD IS ABSORBED THROUGH
THE SMALL INTESTINE .

Figure 59

While the liver is busy detoxifying the blood, millions of white blood cells scattered throughout the liver are simultaneously checking the absorbed food for dangerous foreign proteins, just as the tonsils and Peyer's patches already have. So, for a dangerous foreign protein to gain access through the intestines, it has to get by the tonsils and adenoids, the destructive acids and digestive enzymes of the stomach, Peyer's patches lining the intestinal wall, and the white cells clustered throughout the liver.

Not all toxins can be detoxified by the liver. In fact, some toxins damage the liver. What is the most common toxin to damage the liver?

Alcohol. Too much alcohol over too long a period damages liver cells. The inflammatory response to repair the liver damage leaves in its wake scar tissue that, being scar tissue, cannot function like the liver. As the scar tissue builds up, there's less and less room for normal liver cells. All this scarring is called cirrhosis. There's no cure for cirrhosis except to stop drinking.

Mushroom poisoning is a more deadly poison than alcohol. Ingestion of even small amounts of amanita, which accounts for 90% of mushroom poisonings, can rot out the liver, and there's no treatment once the damage begins. Mushroom hunting is a little tricky for amateurs, as the deadly mushrooms are difficult to identify. A helpful reminder of this is the old adage, "There are old mushroom hunters, and there are bold mushroom hunters, but there are no old, bold mushroom hunters." If you are going to chance it, save a few mushrooms for the doctors to identify in case you do get sick.

What is hepatitis?

Hepatitis is inflammation of the liver—from any cause. The type of hepatitis that most concerns us is viral hepatitis, because drugs are not very effective against hepatitis viruses and the resulting chronic inflammation ends up as liver cirrhosis. The three avoidable viruses are hepatitis A, hepatitis B, and hepatitis C. Be careful around people infected with hepatitis A, because it's pretty contagious. Hepatitis A is transmitted by fecal contamination of food, which is one of the reasons they have those signs in restaurant bathrooms telling employees to wash their hands. Hepatitis B is a particularly bad actor: it attacks the liver with a vengeance and can turn the liver to mush within weeks. You get hepatitis B from the body fluids of someone infected with it: a blood transfusion, sexual contact, sticking yourself with an infected needle, intravenous drug use with a needle used by an infected person, and mixing of an infected mother's blood with the baby's blood during childbirth. Hepatitis C is a huge problem in the United States. It infects around 1% of the population with chronic liver inflammation, and about a quarter of those end up with cirrhosis. Like hepatitis B, hepatitis C is transmitted by mixing body fluids. Vaccines exist to help prevent contracting hepatitis A and B, but we are still waiting for a vaccine for hepatitis C.

What are carbohydrates?

Carbohydrates are sugars—rings of carbon with oxygen and hydrogen attached. Glucose, fructose, and galactose are single sugars, or monosaccharides. Glucose is the main source of energy for the body. Honey is a superdense solution of glucose, fructose, and a few other things with very little water. Disaccharides—two monosaccharides linked together—include table sugar (sucrose, i.e., glucose-fructose) and the sugar in milk (lactose, i.e., glucose-galactose). Long chains of glucose, fructose, and galactose are called polysaccharides. Examples of polysaccharides are mucus, starch (mix a little water with cornstarch and see if it doesn't feel sticky like mucus), cellulose, and glycogen.

Carbohydrates form the backbone of DNA, and when a phosphorous atom is attached to adenosine (a stripped-down glucose molecule) to make ATP, carbohydrates become *the* energy molecule driving the body's chemical reactions.

Vertebrates (animals with backbones) are incapable of digesting plants, because they cannot digest the carbohydrate cellulose. Cows and other ruminants that chew their cud (and termites, too) rely on bacteria living in their intestines to digest cellulose. Because these intestinal bacteria can synthesize *all* the amino acids, cows can survive eating practically anything. In fact, the bacteria can even make amino acids using nitrogen from urea, allowing cows to be fed urine to rev up their protein production. Great.

One interesting story behind cellulose began when a chemist mixed cotton (which is almost pure cellulose) with nitric acid. The resulting cellulose nitrate was soon discovered to be quite explosive—just in time for World War I. When formed into hard balls, cellulose nitrate was also found to bounce well without losing its shape, making the perfect substitute for ivory billiard balls. The only problem was—you guessed it—they would occasionally explode when the cue ball slammed into them.

The DNA for making cellulose has recently been discovered in some of the most ancient of all bacteria, meaning we can let bacteria make cellulose. Someday, we may not have to cut down trees or grow cotton to get cellulose for such products as paper, explosives, rope, plastics, and film. Even more exciting is that these bacteria, called cyanobacteria, grow in saltwater—seawater! Scientists are also isolating from *modern* plants the DNA to make cellulose. This DNA may someday be transplanted into saltwater cyanobacteria, or other bacteria, to synthesize cellulose.

Why can't a lot of old people drink milk?

The older a lot of people get, the less they are able to absorb lactose from the intestinal tract, because their gut walls make less of the enzyme lactase to break apart lactose for absorption (lactose alone cannot be absorbed). Consequently, lactose remains in the gut to be digested by bacteria in the colon, releasing gas in the process, which is why old people are called "old farts."

What's the difference between carbohydrates and fat?

Carbohydrates dissolve in water. Fats and oils—lipids—do not. Lipids that remain liquid at room temperature are called oils. Lipids that solidify at room temperature are fats. Fats and oils are greasy or waxy, and being lighter than water they float on water. Next time you make chicken soup, look for the oil on the surface of the soup. When soup is placed in a refrigerator overnight, the oil hardens and can be scooped off as fat.

Just as carbohydrates are linked together into long chains, fats are also linked into long chains, called fatty acids, for energy storage. Three fatty acid chains hooked to a small glycerol molecule are known as a triglyceride. Fatty acids pack a lot more energy than chains of carbohydrates. Fat generates 9 calories per gram, while carbohydrates generate only 4 calories per gram. The advantage of high-energy, compact, lightweight, flexible fats such as triglycerides is that they give animals mobility. Trees and plants use starch in their sap, roots, and tubers to store energy, but so much starch is needed to store a tree's energy that the sheer weight of the starch, along with its stiff structural polysaccharide, cellulose, prevents trees and plants from moving about. The only oils plants use to provide compact sources of energy are for their seeds and fruits, such as corn oil, peanut oil, palm oil, canola oil, and sunflower oil.

Where are carbohydrates and fat stored in the body?

Carbohydrates are stored in liver and muscles as long chains of glucose molecules called glycogen. Fat is stored all around the body, carried there as triglycerides in the bloodstream. At 9 calories per gram, a person carrying 30 pounds of extra fat stores carries more than 120,000 calories, or about two months' worth of caloric needs. Jogging could easily burn up about 500 calories an hour, so in a mere 240 hours—half an hour a day for a year and a half—a person could jog away the entire 120,000 calories, and that's without any change in diet.

A plain potato has almost no fat in it, so why are potatoes supposed to be so fattening?

Potatoes are almost all carbohydrate, specifically, starch (a polysaccharide). Liver and muscles store about one day's supply of glycogen, but once the liver and muscles are filled up with glycogen, any extra carbohydrates, such as those from potatoes, are converted to fat for long-term storage. That's why potatoes are fattening. Daily exercise uses up the muscles' stores of glycogen and prevents the carbohydrates you eat from being converted to fat. In fact, however, the vast majority of the fat we accumulate comes from the fat we eat, not from carbohydrates being converted to fat. It's not the potato so much as what you put on the potato (butter, sour cream, cheese) that makes potatoes so fattening.

Is excess protein also turned into fat?

Excess protein can be converted to fat or carbohydrates to make ATP in times of starvation, but in everyday life high-protein meals are not converted to fat. Conversely, fat and carbohydrates can be converted back into amino acids—all amino acids except the essential amino acids—to make protein.

How does glucose become the main energy source for the body?

Glucose is carried to every part of the body, where it is converted to adenosine triphosphate (ATP), which the body uses for virtually all its energy needs. Without ATP, we would have no energy to do anything. In synthesizing ATP, two byproducts are released: CO_2 (carbon dioxide) and hydrogen atoms. Carbon dioxide is easy to get rid of: just breathe it into the air. The lungs also come to the rescue for the hydrogen atoms by breathing in oxygen. Oxygen mops up those hydrogen atoms by combining two hydrogen atoms and one oxygen atom to form H_2O—water—which is easily discarded through the urine (see figure 60).

What happens if you run out of glucose? Is there anything left for the body to use as a source of energy?

In times of starvation, muscle protein is broken down into amino acids and converted into glucose, while long-chain fatty acids are snipped apart into two-carbon fragments called ketones to make ATP.

What are vitamins?

Vitamins are relatively small molecules that insert themselves into enzymes to allow the enzymes to function properly. Some vitamins are water soluble and some are fat soluble. Water-soluble vitamins such as thiamine (B1), riboflavin (B2), niacin (B3), pyridoxine (B6), folic acid, and vitamin C (ascorbic acid) are easy to absorb, but fat-soluble vitamins (vitamins A, D, E, and K) need to be dissolved in fat. Once in a while, an extremely low-fat diet or an intestinal disease that prevents fat absorption (for example, insufficient lipase secretion by the pancreas) can get someone into trouble with fat-soluble vitamin deficiency. (There are no vitamins F, G, H, or I. After vitamin E was discovered, the next vitamin to be discovered was shown by Dr. Henrik Dam to cure a hemorrhagic condition in chickens raised on a fat-free diet. The "koagulation" vitamin—Dam was Danish—became vitamin K.)

The discovery of vitamins began in the 1890s, when Christiaan Eijkman, a Dutch physician, was sent to Indonesia to figure out why so many inhabitants were contracting a disease called beriberi, an Indonesian term meaning "I can't, I can't," derived from beriberi's damage to the heart and to the nerves controlling the arms and legs. Eijkman was observant enough to notice that a similar lameness in the local chickens had developed when their rice diet was switched from

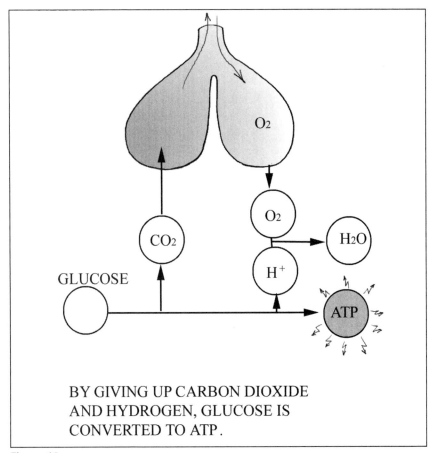

BY GIVING UP CARBON DIOXIDE
AND HYDROGEN, GLUCOSE IS
CONVERTED TO ATP.

Figure 60

whole husk rice to polished rice. Eijkman showed that replacement of the outer husk could cure the chickens. He then matched these observations in local prisoners suffering from beriberi and concluded that something in the rice husks was vital for normal nerve function. Meanwhile, in England, Frederick Hopkins was tripping to the idea of vital dietary molecules by showing that rats could not grow on an artificial concoction of fat, carbohydrates, and amino acids until they got some real food.

A few years later, around 1912, Casimir Funk, a Polish chemist working in France, isolated the chemical from rice husks that cured beriberi. Because the chemical was an amine, Funk postulated that the vital food substances that cured beriberi (vitamin B1, or thiamine), scurvy (vitamin C, or ascorbic acid), pellagra (vitamin B3, or niacin), and rickets (vitamin D) were also amines—vital amines. Hence the term "vitamines," which was shortened to "vitamins" when it was later shown that, in fact, not all vitamins were amines.

When the Nobel Prize was handed out in 1927 to Eijkman and Hopkins, Funk was unfortunately left out. Little did the Nobel committee know that when Funk isolated thiamine, he had also isolated niacin from rice husks, but ignored it when niacin couldn't cure beriberi. It took another 25 years for niacin to be rediscovered as the missing vitamin in pellagra, a prevalent disease among the poor of the American South that caused a horrible skin rash, intellectual changes, and diarrhea and that often resulted in death. It was already known that pellagra was due to a vitamin deficiency, owing to the courage of Joseph Goldberg during years around World War I. To overcome the prevailing certainty among the medical community that pellagra was an infectious disease, and battling for the cause of people too poor to eat an adequate diet, Goldberg injected blood and ingested skin and excretions from pellagra victims into himself, his family, and other supporters. Even when nothing happened to Goldberg and his covolunteers, people remained skeptical— until the 1930s, when niacin was finally accepted as the cure for pellagra.

What is vitamin B12?

Vitamin B12 is vital for the production of blood and for normal function of the brain, spinal cord, and peripheral nerves. Before vitamin B12 was discovered, patients suffering vitamin B12 deficiency became anemic (meaning they had a low blood count), paralyzed (because of damage to the spinal cord), and demented (from damage to the brain). Luckily, in the 1920s, three doctors, George Whipple, George Minot, and William Murphy, made a fortuitous mistake. They tried to treat the anemia in these patients with the one thing they knew was good for anemia: iron. Since the liver stores lots of iron, Whipple, Minot, and Murphy made the patients eat raw or lightly cooked liver. Lo and behold, the patients got out of their wheelchairs and started balancing their checkbooks again. It was not until the 1940s that vitamin B12 was finally isolated and the real reason for raw liver's success was sorted out.

Vitamin B12 works in synchrony with folate, another vitamin, which is why they should be taken together. Taking folate without vitamin B12 can mop up any free vitamin B12 and, as happened in the 1930s and 1940s, worsen the neurologic damage from vitamin B12 deficiency.

Vitamin B12 is present in a lot of foods. How do you become deficient in vitamin B12 if so much of it is around?

Vitamin B12 is different from other vitamins in that it is absorbed only through the very last part of the small intestine—the ileum. For example, suppose someone has a tumor in the terminal ileum and to remove the tumor the surgeon has to take the terminal ileum with it. Goodbye vitamin B12. The odd thing about vitamin B12 is that, to be absorbed through the terminal ileum, it must be attached to a specific protein. That protein, called intrinsic factor, is made by the wall of the stomach (see figure 61). So if part or all of the stomach is removed for, say, cancer or as treatment for massive obesity, intrinsic factor won't be made in sufficient quantities to allow vitamin B12 to be absorbed downstream. The only way to get B12 into such patients is to give them a shot of vitamin B12 every month, bypassing intestinal absorption altogether.

How do you make stool?

Once food reaches the end of the ileum, it is ready to be sent into the large intestine—the colon. Almost all the goodies have been removed, save some complex carbohydrates to be digested by colonic bacteria. Any fluids that have not already been absorbed through the small intestines are extracted by the large intestine, after which the colon periodically dumps what's left into the toilet. The colon is shaped like an inverted U, beginning in the right lower abdomen as the cecum (see figure 62). The colon ascends up the right side of the abdomen to the diaphragm, turns left, and passes over to the left side of the abdomen, where it descends, does a little S-shaped twist through the sigmoid colon (sigma is the letter S in Greek), and terminates in the rectum (which means straight in Greek).

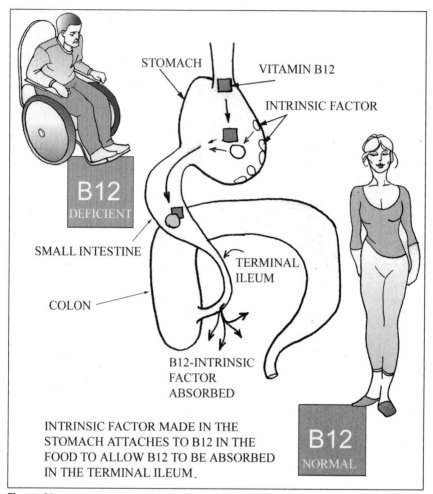

STOMACH   VITAMIN B12

INTRINSIC FACTOR

B12
DEFICIENT

SMALL INTESTINE

COLON

TERMINAL
ILEUM

B12-INTRINSIC
FACTOR
ABSORBED

INTRINSIC FACTOR MADE IN THE
STOMACH ATTACHES TO B12 IN THE
FOOD TO ALLOW B12 TO BE ABSORBED
IN THE TERMINAL ILEUM.

B12
NORMAL

Figure 61

Why do we get diarrhea?

If intestinal peristalsis propels food down the intestinal tract too fast for
the colon to remove the remaining water from the intestinal slush, stool
becomes watery diarrhea. Sometimes diarrhea is caused by a virus interrupting the water-extracting machinery of the colon.

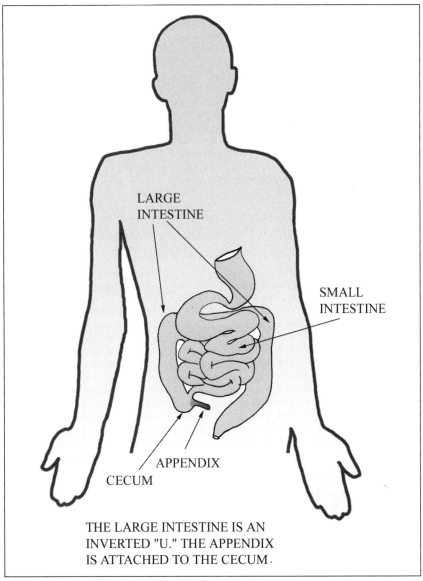

LARGE
INTESTINE

SMALL
INTESTINE

APPENDIX

CECUM

THE LARGE INTESTINE IS AN
INVERTED "U." THE APPENDIX
IS ATTACHED TO THE CECUM.

Figure 62

Why is stool brown?

Bile, which is green, is excreted into the intestines to emulsify fat. When
the bile reaches the colon, bacteria in the intestines and colon change it
to a more aesthetic brown.

What is a hemorrhoid?

A hemorrhoid is a dilated vein at the anus. Hemorrhoids are often painful and sometimes bleed. The cause of hemorrhoids is prolonged abdominal pressure, which creates back pressure on the anal veins trying to send blood north to the heart. Things that cause prolonged abdominal pressure include pregnancy, a big fat stomach, frequent lifting of heavy objects, and lots of straining on the toilet.

Why is fiber good for you?

Fiber is not broken down very well by intestinal enzymes, so it remains in the gut all the way to the colon. Because fiber tends to hold onto water, all that wet fiber adds bulk to the stool and keeps the stool light and fluffy, making it easier to crap out. Hence, there's less straining, fewer hemorrhoids, and less chance of diverticulosis. Many laxatives, such as bran, Metamucil, and milk of magnesia, work by retaining water in the colon, lending bulk and softness to the stool.

What's diverticulosis?

Dried out poop has to be forced out, which people do by bearing down. Over the years, all that bearing down causes, besides hemorrhoids, little out-pouches, or diverticuli, in the wall of the colon. This condition is called diverticulosis. Once in a while, stool blocks off the opening of a diverticulum and mucus trapped in the diverticulum becomes infected, causing diverticulitis. If the infection erodes through the wall of the diverticulum, it can spread throughout the abdominal cavity, a life-threatening event. If the infected diverticulum erodes instead against a loop of small intestine or the bladder, the infection can burn a hole in that other organ and establish a tunnel, or fistula, between it and the colon.

What's a fissure?

A fissure is a tear in the skin that communicates with a natural orifice such as the mouth or anus.

Where does the gas come from in a fart?

Fart gas is made in the colon by bacteria. While your intestines may have a hard time digesting certain carbohydrates found in beans, broccoli, cabbage, and cauliflower, colonic bacteria seem to relish them, making hydrogen and smelly methane, hydrogen sulfide, and other gases in the process. Hydrogen and methane, of course, are flammable, and there have been messy explosions in the operating room when an electric cautery knife has been used to make incisions into the colon, especially an obstructed colon.

Don't the intestines ever get twisted up?

There are 20 feet of intestines inside your abdomen, and with that much tubing constantly in motion, there's bound to be problems. The intestines may get twisted on themselves, a condition called torsion, or a short stretch may telescope on itself, called intussusception (see figure 63). Torsion and intussusception block any food from getting through. They can also cut off the blood supply to that section of intestines, and any bacteria living in the area will attack the infarcted intestines and cause a dangerous gangrenous infection.

Intussusception is not uncommonly seen during the first year of life. The child will suddenly stop playing, cry with abdominal pain, and often vomit. Surgery is needed for those intussusceptions that fail to resolve spontaneously.

What's a hernia?

A hernia is the protrusion of intestines through a hole anywhere in the abdominal wall, typically near the umbilicus or in the inguinal region (groin). Inguinal hernias are more common in men because during fetal development, the testicles descend from the abdomen into the scrotum, leaving a small hole in the lower abdomen (see figure 64). Most of the time the hole seals up, but if not, the intestines can wiggle through the inguinal hole into the scrotal sac. Usually, the intestines slip back out but if they don't, they can become strangulated and lose their blood supply. Bacteria will attack the incarcerated intestine and cause a gangrenous infection.

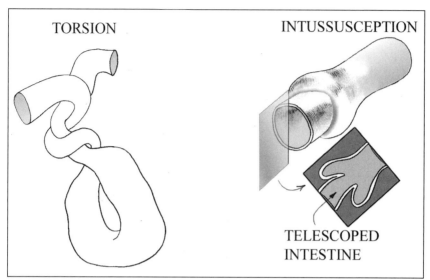

Figure 63

Where do bacteria in the intestines come from? Doesn't the stomach kill almost all bacteria carried in by food?

Yes, and the stomach and small intestines are relatively, but not completely, free of bacteria. The large intestine, however, is chock full of bacteria. The most common one is *E. coli*. Colonic bacteria complete the process of digestion by breaking down fiber-laden food such as beans that cannot be digested by the stomach and small intestines. Antibiotics taken for any infection may kill some of the intestinal bacteria, but the new bacteria that replace the killed bacteria are often irritating to the colon, resulting in loose bowels or even diarrhea.

What's a prolapse?

A prolapse is a sagging of an internal organ through a normal opening of the body, such as the anus or vagina, due to a laxity of surrounding supporting structures.

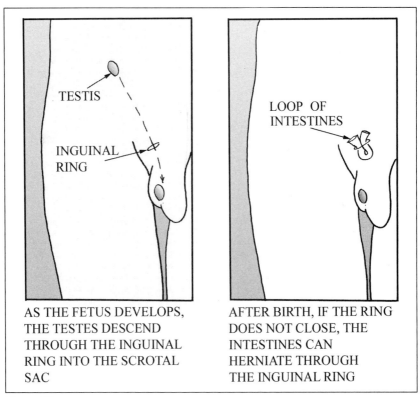

AS THE FETUS DEVELOPS, THE TESTES DESCEND THROUGH THE INGUINAL RING INTO THE SCROTAL SAC

AFTER BIRTH, IF THE RING DOES NOT CLOSE, THE INTESTINES CAN HERNIATE THROUGH THE INGUINAL RING

Figure 64

What is appendicitis?

The appendix is just that—an appendage, a tiny one about the size of your little finger hanging onto the cecum in the right lower abdomen. The appendix is just like the adenoids or the tonsils. Its walls are filled with white blood cells checking out bacteria and other proteins entering the colon. We don't really need an appendix, because there are similar collections of white blood cells within the walls of the small intestines, and if the appendix is removed, we don't suffer any adverse consequences.

Once in a while something floating in the gut gets stuck in the opening of the appendix. Mucus trapped in the appendix gets infected, causing the whole appendix to become inflamed—swollen, hot, red, and tender. The inflammation stops the gut from moving, which is why appendicitis patients vomit any food they try to eat. The best way to deal with appendicitis is to cut the appendix out before it bursts and spreads the infection throughout the abdominal cavity. Appendicitis used to be very common before the advent of antibiotics, but it's thought that with everybody taking antibiotics for one thing or another, the appendix is periodically sterilized.

What's a colostomy?

Recall that "otomy" means to make a hole, "ostomy" means to make a hole in an internal organ and bring that hole to the skin surface, and "ectomy" means to remove from the body. A colostomy, then, is a procedure by which a hole is made in the colon and the hole is brought to the skin surface. Colonic slush is then dumped into a bag attached to the colostomy hole. A colostomy is done in many situations, for example, when the rectum has been removed because of cancer.

Why do doctors check the stool for microscopic amounts of blood?

Cancers anywhere along the gut wall often leak microscopic amounts of blood that doctors can detect in the stool. Larger amounts of bleeding—6 tablespoons or more—turns the stool black, as the hemorrhaged blood is digested by the stomach and small intestines, freeing up the iron in hemoglobin. Iron stains the stool black.

9

ENDOCRINE SYSTEM

The endocrine system is a collection of glands that control distant organs by secreting hormones into the bloodstream. The power of the endocrine system is that, by secreting hormones, it can control the function of many organs at one time. The endocrine glands include the pituitary, thyroid, parathyroid, islets of Langerhans, adrenal, ovaries, and testes (see figure 65).

What is the pituitary gland?

The pituitary gland is really two different glands—an anterior and a posterior pituitary gland tucked up underneath the middle of the brain directly behind the bridge of the nose. ("Posterior" means behind, in this case behind the anterior pituitary gland; "anterior" means in front of.) The posterior pituitary is a teardrop-shaped peninsula of the hypothalamus dangling from the bottom of the brain. Hypothalamic axons extend into the posterior pituitary gland to release either antidiuretic hormone (ADH), to tell the kidneys to retain water, or oxytocin, to stimulate the uterus to contract when it's time to deliver ("oxytocin" means rapid birth in Greek). Oxytocin is also released from the posterior pituitary when a mother nurses in order to stimulate muscle cells in the

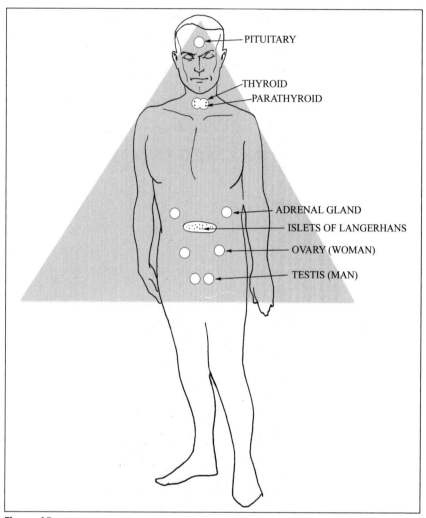

Figure 65

breast to squeeze milk from the breasts (the breast is actually a modified
sweat gland) (see figure 66).

The anterior pituitary controls the thyroid, adrenal gland, ovaries, and
testes, while the parathyroid and islets of Langerhans function on their
own. Because the pituitary controls so many endocrine glands, it's known
as the master gland, but it's really more of a middle management gland,
since it only does what the hypothalamus tells it to do. The hypo-

thalamus releases potent chemicals called releasing hormones into tiny veins that carry the hormones immediately south to the anterior pituitary gland. These hypothalamic releasing hormones direct the pituitary to secrete six different hormones named according to the acronym FAT PIG: Follicle-stimulating hormone, Adrenal-stimulating hormone, Thyroid-stimulating hormone, Prolactin, Interstitial cell–stimulating hormone (in men; luteinizing hormone in women), and Growth hormone (see figure 66).

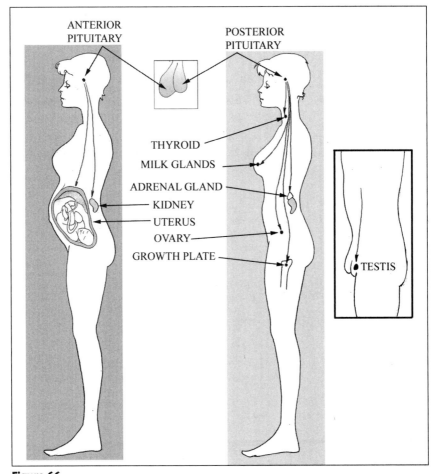

Figure 66

How do the ovaries know when to release their eggs?

Each month, one or the other ovary releases a single egg under directions from two pituitary hormones: follicle-stimulating hormone (FSH) and luteinizing hormone (LH) (see figure 67). A woman's cycle begins after her menstrual period with the release of FSH from the pituitary. FSH signals a single egg in the ovaries to slim down from 46 to 23 chromosomes. It also signals the ovaries to increase their estrogen production in order to prepare the uterus endometrium for implantation. After about 14 days of this, the pituitary suddenly releases a burst of luteinizing hormone, which precipitates the release of the 23-chromosome egg from the ovary.

How do birth control pills work?

Since estrogen and progesterone are elevated during pregnancy, birth control pills, which are a combination of estrogen and progesterone, fool the pituitary into thinking the woman is pregnant. This suppresses the release of FSH and LH, hence no ovulation.

What do follicle-stimulating hormone and interstitial cell-stimulating hormone (luteinizing hormone) do in men?

Follicle-stimulating hormone stimulates the testes to make sperm. Interstitial cell-stimulating hormone stimulates the testes to make testosterone. Testosterone makes a boy into a man by causing his beard to grow, his muscles to develop, his voice to deepen, his Adam's apple to enlarge, his penis to enlarge, and in some cases, his head to grow bald.

Are birth control pills the only way to prevent ovulation?

No, the other way is to nurse a baby. When a baby sucks on its mother's breast, nerves in the breast signal the brain to instruct the pituitary to release oxytocin and prolactin. Prolactin stimulates the breast to make the milk and oxytocin stimulates the breast to deliver the milk to the nipple. Prolactin also inhibits ovulation. This ensures that a mother can devote full attention to her baby without having to contend with a pregnancy and the birth of another child. Unfortunately, ovulation can

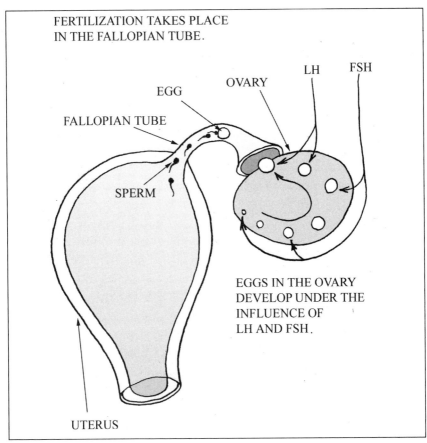

FERTILIZATION TAKES PLACE
IN THE FALLOPIAN TUBE.

LH FSH

OVARY

EGG

FALLOPIAN TUBE

SPERM

EGGS IN THE OVARY
DEVELOP UNDER THE
INFLUENCE OF
LH AND FSH.

UTERUS

Figure 67

still occur, despite the presence of prolactin, as many a nursing pregnant woman will attest to.

Where is the thyroid gland in the body?

Locate the prominent tip of the Adam's apple and slide your finger down the cartilage to a tiny notch at the base. Now slide your fingers around to either side of the trachea and swallow. You should feel a firm, flat structure slide by your fingers. That's the thyroid gland. If you feel a little "pea" in your thyroid or a friend's, notify a doctor, because it could be a small tumor.

Incidentally, that little notch at the base of the Adam's apple is a thin section of the tracheal wall that a doctor (not you) can cut through in an about-to-die choking victim after the Heimlich maneuver, pounding on the chest, and reaching into the victim's mouth have all failed to dislodge a piece of aspirated food.

What does thyroid-stimulating hormone do?

Thyroid-stimulating hormone (thyroxine) tells the thyroid gland to secrete thyroid hormone. Thyroid hormone is a molecule that regulates how fast our internal organs work. Too much thyroid—hyperthyroidism—causes the heart to speed up, the blood pressure to rise, the intestines to speed up (diarrhea), the brain to race, and the muscles to generate more heat. Everything is working so fast that fat stores burn away like crazy. Wouldn't that be a great way to lose weight—just taking thyroid hormone? This was tried in the 1920s but the excess thyroid hormone exhausted the heart and other muscles, killing scores of people before it was stopped.

The pituitary secretes thyroid-stimulating hormone whenever the thyroid gland starts to slow down. Thyroid-stimulating hormone whips the thyroid gland into enlarging and making more thyroid hormone. If the thyroid continues to have trouble producing thyroid hormone, pretty soon the thyroid becomes so large that it sticks out from the neck as a goiter. One of the reasons the thyroid gland might have trouble making hormones is that it can't get its hands on enough iodine, a vital ingredient in thyroid hormone. Today, that's rarely a problem because table salt is often supplemented with iodine. Nowadays, the most common cause of thyroid failure is Hashimoto's thyroiditis—unexplained inflammation of the thyroid gland that interferes with its production of thyroid hormone.

Once the thyroid begins to fail, either because there's no thyroid-stimulating hormone being released by the pituitary or because the thyroid has been damaged in some way, the whole body slows down. These hypothyroid patients ("hypo" means there's too little of something, "hyper" means there's too much) become sluggish: their thinking is sluggish, their gut is sluggish (constipation), their metabolism is sluggish (they feel cold all the time and gain weight), even their voice is affected, becoming lower pitched as the vocal cords accumulate edema. When I was a medical student, a husband and wife were getting a divorce over fights about how high to set the thermostat in their house. It turned out that the husband was becoming hyperthyroid while his wife was becoming hypothyroid. But after their respective conditions were treated, they still got divorced.

What does adrenal-stimulating hormone do?

Adrenal-stimulating hormone, or more accurately, adrenocorticotropic hormone (ACTH), stimulates the outer part of the adrenal gland (the adrenal cortex) to release cortisone and aldosterone—two hormones that prepare us for fight or flight. Cortisone prepares us for fight or flight by tightening up blood vessels and preventing them from leaking, stimulating the liver to make glucose, inhibiting muscles and fat cells from taking up glucose, stimulating the breakdown of fat for additional energy, and stopping inflammation.

Aldosterone prepares us for fight or flight by telling the kidneys to conserve salt. The extra salt in the bloodstream attracts water, keeping the vascular tree at full volume.

Most of a man's testosterone is made in the testes, but some is also made in the adrenal cortex; most of a woman's testosterone is made in the adrenal cortex, with a little made in the ovaries. Testosterone makes us all a little aggressive, which is also useful in fight or flight situations, but whether ACTH causes the release of testosterone from the adrenal cortex is unclear.

If ACTH stimulates the adrenal cortex, what stimulates the inner core of the adrenal gland—the adrenal medulla?

The adrenal glands look like Napoleon's hat atop each kidney (why they are situated atop the kidneys is unclear), and when cut open, the outer adrenal cortex is readily distinguishable from the inner adrenal medulla. While the adrenal cortex is responsive to ACTH, the adrenal medulla is only responsive to stimulation by sympathetic nerves. When stimulated by sympathetic nerves, the adrenal medulla releases epinephrine, which produces the same effects as prolonged sympathetic nerve stimulation:

the heart rate increases, the heart beats with more force, blood vessels constrict, the blood pressure rises, bronchioles dilate, blood is shunted from the skin and gut to the heart, muscles, and brain, the liver pumps glucose into the bloodstream, fat cells break down fatty acids to provide a rapid source of energy, the pupils dilate, your mouth dries, the gut slows, and the brain becomes more vigilant. The only detrimental thing epinephrine does is cause the hands to shake.

What are endorphins?

Besides stimulating the release of ACTH from the pituitary and epinephrine from the adrenal glands, fight, flight, and stress stimulate the release of two other hormones—both from the pituitary gland. To make ACTH, the pituitary splits apart a very large protein, one part becoming ACTH and the other endorphins and enkephalins, two proteins that inhibit pain and provide a feeling of euphoria—perfect for going into battle.

What are steroids?

All three chemicals released from the adrenal cortex—cortisol, aldosterone, and testosterone—are variations of a four-ringed compound known as a steroid, but of the three, only testosterone is an anabolic steroid, meaning it is capable of building up muscles. Cortisol (hydrocortisone) and its corticosteroid cousins, in contrast, catabolize—break down—muscle protein and convert the amino acids into glucose for immediate energy needs. (The names of many, if not most, steroids end in "one.")

Are there any other bad effects from corticosteroids besides breaking down your muscles?

If cortisone levels remain elevated for a long time—for example, if you take daily cortisone, if a pituitary tumor oversecretes ACTH, or if an adrenal tumor pours out cortisone—more serious problems may develop. First, excess corticosteroids redistribute fat from the arms and legs into the face and trunk (the fat accumulating in the upper back is known as a buffalo hump). Since they also cause the muscles to atrophy (shrink), taking corticosteroids long term makes patients look like a robin red breast with a big stomach and chest and skinny little arms and legs. By causing people to retain salt, corticosteroids also raise the blood pressure, and in its effort to keep the blood sugar elevated, corticosteroids tend to make people diabetic. Corticosteroids try to keep calcium in the bloodstream instead of storing it in bones. The result is osteoporosis—the bones become soft, thin, and brittle. Sometimes, corticosteroids cause a mysterious rise in pressure within the head of the femur and humerus bone. The pressure rises so high that blood cannot get into the bone to supply it with nutrients, infarcting the head of the femur in the hip joint or infarcting the head of the humerus in the shoulder joint, a condition called aseptic necrosis of the head of the femur or humerus ("aseptic" means not infected). The dead heads have to be replaced with metallic prostheses. Finally, corticosteroids cause stomach ulcers because they inhibit the synthesis of the stomach's mucous coating. Corticosteroids are wonderful drugs, but they do carry risks.

Why do we undergo a growth spurt in our teenage years?

Growth is governed by a special pituitary hormone, called, not surprisingly, growth hormone. While the hypothalamus tells the pituitary to secrete growth hormone, at the time of puberty the hypothalamus appears to receive its instructions from a small gland in the dead center of the brain called the pineal gland. No one knows how the pineal gland realizes after 12 or 13 years of being asleep that it's time to wake up and start puberty.

Most growth hormone is released from the pituitary at night, and the highest blood levels of growth hormone occur soon after the onset of deep sleep, which is why a good night's sleep is necessary for growth. By the time puberty is over, the bones have doubled in size. The denser the bone, the better, but it requires a steady and robust supply of calcium. Later in life, especially in women, the bones start losing their calcium and become brittle and squishy, like styrofoam, a condition called osteoporosis. Starting out with dense bones gives a person a leg up when their bones begin to lose their calcium.

Why are 12-year-old girls often taller than boys that age?

In other words, why does the growth spurt of puberty begin a few years earlier in girls than in boys? Growth hormone lengthens bones in conjunction with estrogen for both girls and boys. Estrogen lengthens bones by stimulating the growth plate, a thin section of the bone located at either end from which new bone is continuously added (see figure 68). Presumably, girls launch their growth spurt by producing estrogen in quantity beginning in their preteen years. In boys, the estrogen necessary to lengthen bones is derived from the conversion of testosterone by enzymes at the growth plate. Thus, in girls born with a genetic defect that makes their bones insensitive to testosterone, the growth spurt is normal. However, in boys born with a genetic defect of estrogen synthesis or a genetic defect that makes their bones insensitive to estrogen, there is no growth spurt at all. A delayed growth spurt for boys may therefore reflect a lag in the secretion of growth hormone or a lag in the production of estrogen at the growth plate.

It turns out that estrogen also turns off the growth plate after several years of intense stimulation, causing the bones on either side of the growth plate to fuse together, which of course stops further growth. In boys with the genetic defects of estrogen production and estrogen sensitivity, the growth plates fail to close on time and the boys end up being quite tall.

What's the problem with taking anabolic steroids?

Anabolic steroids, being a variant of testosterone, are converted to estrogen in the bones. Since estrogens normally close the growth plate,

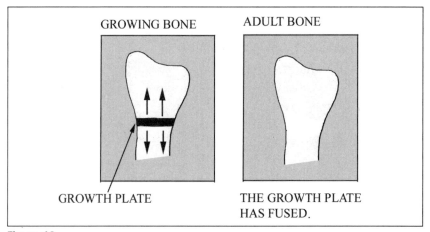

Figure 68

taking anabolic steroids during the teenage years may cause premature closure of the growth plate, causing a young person to end up shorter than he or she might have been.

Also, because anabolic steroids mimic testosterone, when the pituitary gland in a young man senses all the testosterone-type steroids in the bloodstream, it lowers its output of FSH and interstitial cell-stimulating hormone (ICSH), and sperm production drops as the testicles shrink. When the anabolic steroids are stopped, though, the testicles should return to normal. A more permanent change occurs to a man's breasts when taking anabolic steroids. Normally, a man disposes of anabolic steroids by converting them to estrogen, so the more anabolic steroids he takes, the more estrogen he makes and the more his breasts grow, a condition called gynecomastia. Gynecomastia often remains as a permanent fixture.

One of the more popular anabolic steroids, androstenedione, is a precursor to testosterone (a precursor is a molecule that changes into something, in this case, testosterone). Unfortunately, androstenedione is also a precursor to estrogen, the female sex hormone. Estrogen makes girls curvy by widening the hips, accumulating fat in the breasts and around the hips, and hastening closure of the growth plate, but it's unclear yet if androstenedione has these estrogenic effects in men.

What would happen if a young person developed a pituitary tumor composed of cells making growth hormone?

The excessive amounts of growth hormone produced by the tumor would make the child grow rapidly, reaching seven to eight feet. If the tumor develops after the bony growth plates have already fused shut, the person would not grow vertically. Instead, their bones and soft tissues would thicken: the brow would become prominent, the jaw would enlarge, the hands and feet would enlarge, and even the skin would thicken. This condition is called acromegaly. While there is a hormone called somatostatin that inhibits the release of growth hormone from the pituitary, in most cases acromegaly is treated by surgery on the pituitary gland to remove the tumor.

Goliath is thought to have harbored a growth hormone–secreting pituitary tumor. The tumor would certainly explain his great height, and the location of the tumor in the pituitary would explain why he allowed a nimble fellow such as David to strike him in the temple with a rock. The pituitary gland sits directly below the optic chiasm, where the two optic nerves join (see figure 69). As a pituitary tumor enlarges, it rises up out of the pituitary to compress the center of the optic chiasm. In the center of the optic chiasm are the nerve fibers from the nasal part of each retina. Since the nasal part of each retina sees the peripheral visual fields, the growing pituitary tumor causes blindness there. Without peripheral side vision, Goliath would have been unable to see David sneaking up from the side to fling his fateful rock (see p. 302, optic chiasm).

What is diabetes?

Diabetes, full name diabetes mellitus, is known on the streets as sugar diabetes because of high blood-sugar levels associated with it. Carbohydrates are absorbed through the intestines and eventually converted into individual glucose molecules. As glucose levels rise in the bloodstream, special clusters of cells called the islets of Langerhans, embedded in and scattered throughout the pancreas, sense this rise and squirt out a protein called insulin into the bloodstream. Insulin lowers the blood glucose by instructing the liver to stop pouring glucose into the bloodstream and by escorting glucose into all the cells of the body except in the brain. If the body's cells are already stuffed with glucose (in the form of glycogen), insulin escorts the glucose into fat cells, where it is converted to fat. In addition, insulin prevents fat from being broken down into free fatty acids.

The brain was designed to absorb glucose without the help of insulin because it would be too risky for the brain to depend on insulin for its energy supply. The brain uses glucose, and only glucose, for its enormous energy needs—20% of the body's energy for an organ making up only 2% of body weight. To make matters more precarious, the brain does not store glucose as muscles do.

Lacking insulin, as happens in childhood diabetes, glucose cannot get into cells and is instead peed out in the urine, hence the Latin name mellitus, or sweet—don't ask. Since there's no insulin around to escort glucose into fat cells, and no insulin to prevent fat from being broken down, these children are generally thin.

Adult onset diabetes differs from childhood diabetes in that there is plenty of insulin around but the cells are insensitive to it and ignore

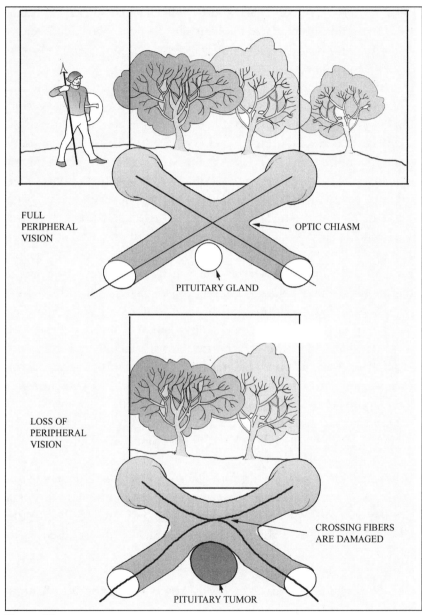

FULL
PERIPHERAL
VISION

OPTIC CHIASM

PITUITARY GLAND

LOSS OF
PERIPHERAL
VISION

CROSSING FIBERS
ARE DAMAGED

PITUITARY TUMOR

Figure 69

insulin's efforts to escort glucose into cells. The reason cells become insensitive to insulin is related to obesity. It's thought that fat cells release free fatty acids plus a number of special hormones into the bloodstream that somehow make the body resistant to insulin.

The discovery of insulin around 1922 was one of the greatest medical breakthroughs ever. When insulin was discovered, the only medications around were aspirin, digitalis (to stimulate a failing heart), phenobarbital (a sedative to control seizures), codeine, and morphine—no vitamins, no antibiotics, no Motrin, no Tylenol. It was known that insulin was manufactured in the islets of Langerhans, but how to isolate them from the rest of the pancreas? In 1920, Dr. Frederick Banting happened upon a paper describing a man who had died of pancreatitis when a stone obstructed the pancreatic duct. At autopsy, the pancreas was destroyed, but the islets of Langerhans were still intact because they had their own blood supply. From this, Banting conceived the idea of tying off the pancreatic duct in dogs to obtain a pure collection of islet cells. Once they had the islets of Langerhans isolated, Banting and his partner Charles Best (a medical student) teamed up with a biochemist, James Collip, to extract the insulin. Oddly enough, the Nobel Prize was awarded only to Banting and Dr. John Macleod, in whose lab much of the work was performed while Macleod was out of town. As good and decent Canadians, they generously shared their prize money with Best and Collip.

Injecting yourself with insulin is a little tricky. If you inject too much, the blood glucose will fall below normal. Since the brain uses only glucose for its energy supply, a low blood glucose causes a person to drift into a coma. Every time a child with diabetes takes an afternoon nap, the parents may reasonably fear that the child is lapsing into a coma. Someday, when researchers figure out how to grow stem cells into islet cells, diabetes will be a thing of the past. (Stem cells are discussed in chapter 12, on the genital system.)

How does the body raise the blood sugar when the blood sugar falls?

During stress, adrenalin raises the blood sugar to keep our bodies primed for action, but for everyday activities, a downward drift of the blood sugar stimulates the islets of Langerhans to release glucagon, a hormone that stimulates the liver to slice off glucose molecules from its stores of glycogen and release the glucose into the bloodstream.

What is hypoglycemia?

Hypoglycemia is low blood sugar. One of the more common types of hypoglycemia occurs in early diabetics after a carbohydrate meal. Normally, when carbohydrates are eaten, insulin is released to escort the sugar into the body's cells. Even without insulin, however, the body is still able to lower the blood sugar somewhat. The brain, for example, absorbs 20% of the blood sugar without insulin at all. In early diabetes, the release of insulin is a little sluggish. After a sugary meal, even before insulin is released, the blood sugar is already beginning to fall on its own. When the insulin is released, it drives down the blood sugar even further and the patient develops reactive hypoglycemia, with symptoms of headache, dizziness, fatigue, lightheadedness, and as the sympathetic nerves respond to the falling blood sugar, heart pounding, tremor of the hands, sweating, and anxiety.

What are the parathyroid glands?

The islets of Langerhans are one of two endocrine glands not controlled by the pituitary. The other endocrine gland not controlled by the pituitary is the parathyroid gland, which actually consists of four parathyroid glands, two buried in each lobe of the thyroid gland ("para" means next to). The parathyroid's job is to maintain a stable supply of calcium in the bloodstream, because calcium is used everywhere in the body—for blood clotting, muscle contraction, enzymatic reactions, and plenty more. Fortunately, the bones provide a huge pool of calcium for the parathyroid glands to utilize. When the blood concentration of calcium falls, parathyroid hormone (parathormone), along with vitamin D, raises the calcium level by extracting calcium from bones, improving the absorption of calcium from the intestines, and reducing the excretion of calcium from the kidneys.

10

~~~~~~~~~~~~~~~~~

VASCULAR SYSTEM

The reason blood flows is the same reason any liquid flows. Liquids flow from a region of high pressure toward a region of low pressure. This chapter reviews how blood is delivered and the things that prevent it from being delivered.

What is the difference between an artery and a vein?

An artery carries blood away from the heart while a vein carries it back. Blood is ejected from the left ventricle under high pressure and carried under high pressure to distant sites by thick-walled arteries. Once blood passes through (perfuses) the organs, it is carried back to the heart by thin-walled veins under low pressure (see figure 70).

Why do arteries pulsate?

With each heartbeat, a wave of blood is propelled throughout the arterial tree. You can feel the wave as a pulsating artery. The easiest artery to feel is the radial artery at the wrist. Feel the radius bone at the very outside of your wrist an inch or so up from the base of the thumb. Now roll your finger a smidgen toward the center of the wrist. The pulse you feel at the wrist is the surge of blood being pumped from the heart to the radial

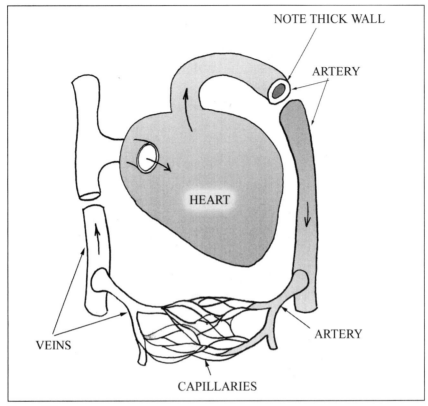

NOTE THICK WALL

ARTERY

HEART

ARTERY

VEINS

CAPILLARIES

Figure 70

artery. Don't press too hard on the radial artery, or you will pinch it closed and it won't pulsate.

By feeling the pulse, can you prove the heart is a pump?

Yes, by crossing your right leg and gently feeling with your left hand the ankle pulse just below and a little behind the inside right ankle. Using the fingertips of your right hand, feel your heart tapping against the left side of your chest. If you can't feel your heart tapping against your chest, gently feel the carotid artery pulsating alongside the trachea (on either side). Now close your eyes and concentrate. The heart (or the carotid artery) taps first and then a split second later you feel the pulse arrive at the ankle. What you're feeling is the wave of blood starting out in the heart and arriving a split second later in a small artery below the ankle, proving that the heart pumps blood. The idea that blood circulates around the body and returns to the heart wasn't postulated until 1628— by William Harvey. Until then, it was thought that the peripheral tissues devoured the blood and new blood was made with each pump of the heart. (William Harvey was also the first one to propose that the creation of a fetus involved the union of a sperm and an egg.)

Why do those squiggly veins in the temples pulsate?

Because those squiggly veins aren't veins—they're arteries, and very important arteries in one particular circumstance. Old people (over the age of 60) sometimes contract an illness called temporal arteritis, inflammation of their midsized arteries, including the temporal artery and its neighbor, the ophthalmic artery, which supplies the optic nerve. Left untreated, the inflammation can thrombose (clot off) these arteries and cause instantaneous blindness. (A blood clot inside an artery or vein is known as a thrombus; outside an artery or vein, it is a hematoma.) Fortunately, before they thrombose, the inflamed arteries in the scalp present with headaches. So, if you hear an old person complaining of headaches, you could be a hero by discovering enlargement and tenderness of one or both temporal arteries (or a hard cord, indicating that the temporal artery has already thrombosed). Quickly notify a doctor, because if steroids are started immediately, blindness can be prevented.

Which is more dangerous, accidentally cutting an artery or a vein?

Cutting an artery. Blood coming out of an artery is shooting out at high pressure, and you have to squeeze that artery shut with great force to stop the bleeding. Blood coming out of a vein oozes out under low pressure and requires little pressure to stop the bleeding. Arterial bleeding is sometimes so profuse that the only way to compress the artery is to apply a tourniquet like you would a blood pressure cuff: you keep twisting the tourniquet until the bleeding stops. A tourniquet can be pretty dangerous, though, because it cuts off all the circulation to a limb, and if left on for too long the limb will die and have to be amputated. It's always better to compress just the bleeding artery alone. This allows blood to detour around the compressed artery into smaller alternative arteries and veins.

What's an aneurysm?

An aneurysm is a dilation of any artery in the body. The entire artery can swell out (causing a fusiform aneurysm), or just one part of the wall can form a bubble (a saccular aneurysm) (see figure 71). Aneurysms are caused by anything that weakens the wall of an artery, including bad genes, trauma, infections, and atherosclerosis. Over a period of years, or even decades, the aneurysm enlarges and its wall thins out. The larger the aneurysm becomes, the thinner the wall and the more likely it is to hemorrhage.

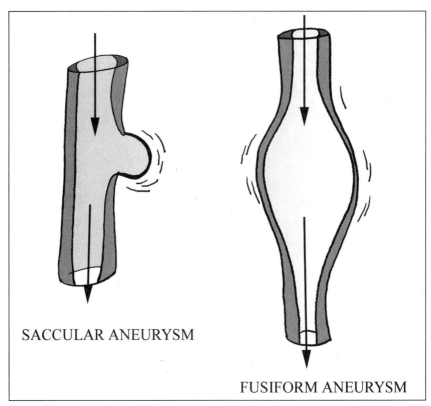

SACCULAR ANEURYSM

FUSIFORM ANEURYSM

Figure 71

Where are capillaries?

Capillaries are the very terminal twigs of arteries, where oxygen, glucose, vitamins, protein, and fluid leak out of the vascular tree into the peripheral tissues. The easiest way to demonstrate capillaries is to squeeze the blood out of them by pressing the pad of one of your fingers. Within a second, blood flooding back into the capillaries turns the blanched finger pad pink again. Without capillaries, high-pressure arteries would be connected directly to low-pressure veins. Pretty soon, the thin-walled veins would enlarge and, being unable to withstand high arterial pressure, would hemorrhage. Malformations like this, called arteriovenous malformations, can occur throughout the body, especially the brain. Once a cerebral arteriovenous malformation is discovered, it is either removed surgically or obliterated by radiation or injection of something to make it clot off.

Why are veins blue but when you cut yourself, the blood is red?

Veins are blue, but not because deoxygenated venous blood is blue. When you cut yourself, you're cutting a vein and the blood in that vein is red. Cutting an artery is quite different than cutting a vein because oxygenated arterial blood is really red, electric red, scary red, and shoots out in spurts with each heartbeat.

If you cut open the skin and look at a vein (not advisable), the vein is no longer blue but dark red. Why isn't the vein red when covered with skin? Light shining onto skin penetrates the skin a short distance and is reflected back. Red light waves are absorbed by the blood vessel, leaving only blue light to be reflected back.

How do you prove that veins are carrying blood back to the heart?

You need someone with large hand veins to show this. Hold the arm down at your side until the veins fill up. Find a vein on the back of the hand that forms a "Y." Now with two fingers press down on one arm of the "Y" and slide one finger up the vein toward the heart. The vein remains flat until you come to the dividing point. As soon as you go beyond the crotch of the "Y," the flattened vein will suddenly pop up as blood from the other arm of the "Y" flows into the flattened arm.

Another clue is found in the veins on the back of your hand. With your hand at your side, the veins bulge. As you raise your hand to the level of the heart, the veins collapse because venous blood is now running downhill toward the heart.

Why do the veins in your face and neck bulge when you get angry?

When people clench their jaw in anger, they also valsalva—bear down against a closed epiglottis—and as pressure in the chest rises, it presses against veins returning blood from the head and neck. Blood backs up into the now distended veins of the face and neck, turning the face red.

What force drives venous blood back to the heart?

Muscle contraction. Each time a muscle contracts, it squeezes veins traveling within the muscle. Blood flows toward the heart because one-way valves inside the veins prevent blood from settling back into the legs (see figure 72).

What happens if you don't pump your muscles? Does venous blood continue to flow?

The two most common situations where failure to pump our legs gets us into trouble is standing at attention and sitting on airplanes. It's not uncommon, especially on a hot day, to see a soldier faint because he doesn't squeeze his leg muscles while standing for a long time at attention. With prolonged standing, venous blood pools in the legs, leaving the heart with inadequate blood to pump to maintain the blood pressure. If the blood pressure falls low enough, no blood gets to the brain and the soldier faints. A hot day makes things worse by causing the soldier to sweat, become dehydrated, and by dilating arteries to the skin to dissipate heat, sacrifice blood flow to the internal organs, including the brain—hence the faint.

Sitting on a long airplane trip limits leg exercise. Venous blood in the legs becomes stagnant, and stagnant blood clots. Blood clots in the legs

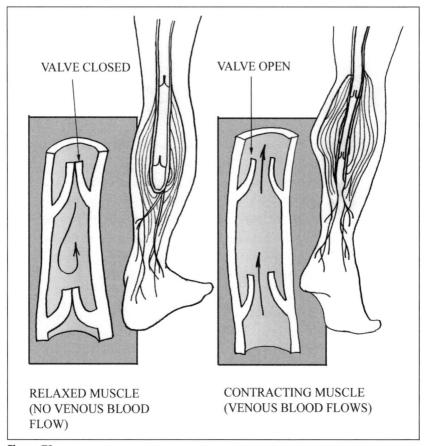

VALVE CLOSED   VALVE OPEN

RELAXED MUSCLE   CONTRACTING MUSCLE
(NO VENOUS BLOOD   (VENOUS BLOOD FLOWS)
FLOW)

Figure 72

can dislodge and be carried upward (embolize) toward the heart. The clot
continues through the right ventricle until it finally lodges as a pulmonary embolus in a small artery in the lung (see figure 73). In this way,
the lungs filter emboli traveling in the venous circulation, preventing
them from reaching the arterial circulation and causing dangerous
infarctions of the internal organs.

A single small pulmonary embolus is not too dangerous, but multiple
pulmonary emboli, or one large one, can obstruct most of the blood
supply to the lungs. With no blood flowing through the lungs, no blood
gets oxygenated and all the body's tissues suffer. Also, the right ventricle
is placed under great strain, as it tries to force blood through obstructed

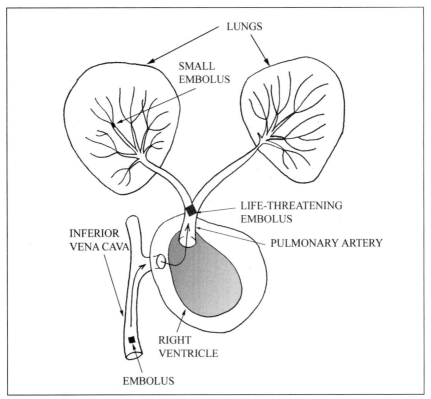

Figure 73

pulmonary arteries. Very soon, the right ventricle fails, which only compounds the problem of pumping blood through the lungs. It's not uncommon for people to die of pulmonary emboli (or one large pulmonary embolus). The treatment for recurrent pulmonary emboli is anticoagulation.

What are varicose veins?

Varicose veins are bulging, dilated veins visible on the surface of the skin, usually in the legs. There are two venous systems draining blood from the legs: one that's superficial (near the surface of the leg), and another that's larger and deep in the center of the leg. The superficial system feeds into the deep system, and where they connect is a valve to prevent blood from flowing back into the superficial system. When these valves don't close properly, blood leaks backward into the thin-walled superficial veins and dilates them. The superficial veins can be surgically removed—stripped—without impairing venous return from the legs, because blood can still find its way into the deep venous system.

What causes varicose veins?

As we age, veins in our legs tend to dilate. If they dilate too much, the valves can't close and blood pools in the superficial veins, dilating them into varicose veins.

Another reason for varicose veins is venous obstruction upstream, causing venous blood to bulge out the deep and superficial veins. The most common cause of venous obstruction upstream is pregnancy, when the pregnant uterus rests against the inferior vena cava, the main pipe in the abdomen and chest transporting venous blood up from the legs, pelvis, and abdomen to the heart. Pregnancy also tremendously expands the mother's blood volume, and the extra blood dilates up the veins. Also during pregnancy, large amounts of estrogen circulating in the blood-stream relax veins in the legs.

What is deep venous thrombosis?

A deep venous thrombosis is a blood clot in the deep venous system of the leg, usually in the calf. Because it obstructs the main vein draining blood from the lower leg, the calf swells. The body fran-tically tries to dissolve and remove the clot with inflammatory cells, causing the calf to become hot, tender, red, and swollen. The thrombus is now a thrombophlebitis ("phlebo" is Greek for vein). Deep venous thrombus and deep venous thrombophlebitis are very dangerous because of their high likelihood of dislodging and embolizing to the lungs. The treatment is immediate anticoagulation with intravenous heparin and then oral anticoagulation for the long term. If, for some reason, the patient cannot take these medications, a surgeon may insert a small porous umbrella into the inferior vena cava to trap emboli before they reach the lungs.

Why is the blood pressure reported as a fraction?

A normal blood pressure is 120/80 or less. The systolic blood pressure is the numerator and the diastolic blood pressure is the denominator. Blood is ejected out of the left ventricle with terrific force. The peak of that force is the systolic blood pressure. As blood runs out of the aorta, into its tributaries, and then into the veins, pressure in the arterial system drops. The blood pressure would plummet if the aorta and the rest of the arterial pipes were constructed of rigid steel. Because the aorta and the arteries have muscular walls, as the blood pressure falls, the walls are able to constrict in order to maintain adequate pressure in the arterial system at all times. The level the arterial pressure falls to is the diastolic pressure (see figure 74).

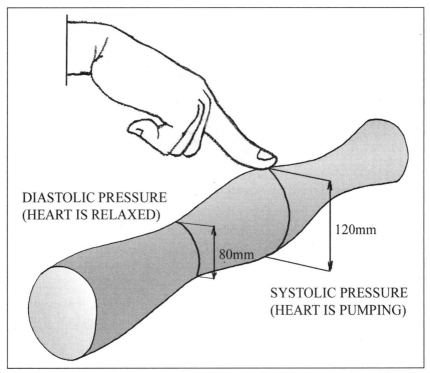

Figure 74

How is blood pressure measured?

First, a blood pressure cuff is wrapped around the upper arm encasing the axillary artery. You can feel the axillary artery pulsating under the biceps muscle along the inside of the upper arm. The cuff is then inflated by a hand pump. Pressure inside the cuff is measured by a little dial on the cuff, or in some blood pressure cuffs by a column of mercury. While the cuff is being inflated, the doctor is listening with a stethoscope to the axillary arterial pulsations over the brachial artery slightly downstream in front of the elbow (see figure 75). As the cuff pressure, measured in millimeters of mercury, is increased, pressure is applied to the axillary artery. When cuff pressure rises high enough to squeeze shut the axillary artery, blood flow through the axillary artery ceases. Now, as air is released from the squeeze bulb, pressure in the cuff drifts downward until it eventually reaches a point where the peak of the arterial pressure is able to open the axillary artery for a split second before the blood pressure cuff squeezes it back shut. This is the systolic blood pressure. As the cuff pressure continues to drift downward, the opening and closing of the axillary artery is audible with the stethoscope, until finally the pressure in the cuff is so low that the pressure inside the artery is able to keep the arterial lumen open all the time and the pulsations are no longer audible. That's the diastolic pressure.

How do you raise the blood pressure?

Three ways: make the heart pump faster and more vigorously, increase the volume of blood being pumped, or narrow the arteries. Conversely, if you slow or weaken the heart, if you become dehydrated or anemic, or if you dilate up the arteries, the blood pressure will fall.

Why is salt bad for you?

In some people, dietary salt raises their blood pressure. The mechanism by which table salt raises the blood pressure in those people is unclear. Part of the reason may well be that people who eat a lot of salt through a diet of potato chips and other junk food have diets that fail to include healthy, low-fat, calcium-rich milk products and nutritious fruits and vegetables. Nevertheless, until it's clear which people can tolerate salty food,

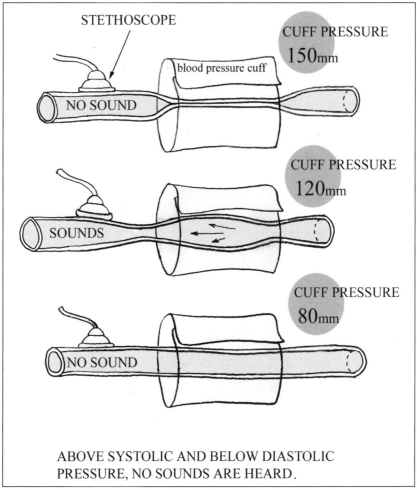

Figure 75

it's probably best to avoid excessive salt intake. The daily recommendation is around 6 grams of table salt, which is about a teaspoon per day. It's difficult to judge how much salt we eat because most of our salt intake is hidden in prepared foods. A regular diet easily reaches 6 grams of salt per day, so try seasoning food with something other than salt. Experimenting with spices and seasonings is challenging and fun for both men and women, and of course, it makes food a lot tastier.

What's the danger of getting into hot bathtubs?

When you get into a hot bathtub, heat from the water enters the body. The body tries to get rid of that heat by dilating the arteries to the skin. A heck of a lot of blood can be sent to the skin, so much so that if you're dehydrated and get into a hot bathtub, enough blood can be diverted to the skin to drop the blood pressure. One way to get dehydrated is to drink too much alcohol, because alcohol makes you pee a lot by inhibiting the release of antidiuretic hormone from the posterior pituitary. Also, alcohol dilates arteries and veins, which by itself lowers the blood pressure, meaning if you're drunk, don't take too hot a bath.

How do arteries constrict?

There are muscle cells in the walls of arteries. These muscle cells are special because they are constantly contracting to maintain pressure in the vascular tree. Muscles that contract continually, slowly, and without a great deal of force, such as the muscles in arterial walls and the intestinal walls, are called smooth muscle cells, because they are slender and smooth under the microscope.

What controls how much arterial smooth muscles constrict?

Arterial smooth muscles constrict in response to cold, sympathetic nerve stimulation, epinephrine, and another potent hormone called angiotensin. Sympathetic nerves innervate almost all arteries, so anything that stimulates the sympathetic nervous system—exercise, fear, excitement, anger, anxiety, nicotine, cocaine, amphetamines—will raise your blood pressure by constricting arteries. Likewise, any stressful event that excites the adrenal glands to release epinephrine will also raise the blood pressure. In Raynaud's disease, overly active sympathetic nerves constrict arteries feeding the fingers, turning the fingers white and then blue as oxygen is leeched from the available blood.

Angiotensin is a vasoconstrictor ("vaso" refers to any blood vessel—artery or vein) released when the kidney senses that it is not receiving enough blood. Angiotensin improves blood flow to the kidney by raising the blood pressure in three ways (see figure 76): by telling the brain to

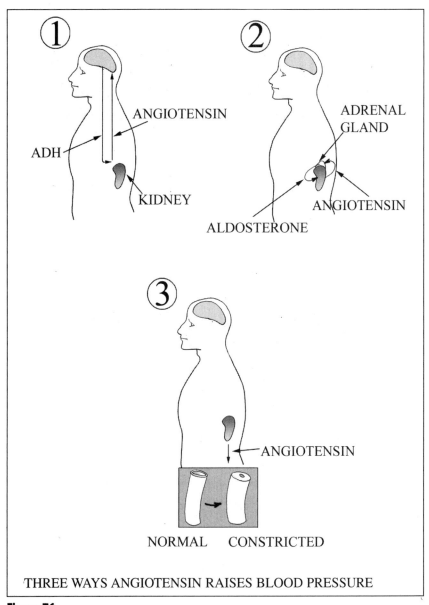

THREE WAYS ANGIOTENSIN RAISES BLOOD PRESSURE

Figure 76

release a hormone called antidiuretic hormone (ADH), which tells the kidneys to retain water; by telling the adrenal glands to release a hormone called aldosterone, which then tells the kidneys to retain salt; and by causing smooth muscle cells in arterial walls to constrict. More ominously, angiotensin stimulates smooth muscle cells in arterial walls to thicken and multiply, and it also initiates an inflammatory response in arterial walls, all of which hastens atherosclerosis.

Angiotensin itself is not released by the kidney. The kidney releases renin, an enzyme that converts angiotensinogen, a protein released by the liver, to angiotensin I. Angiotensin I is then converted in the bloodstream to angiotensin II by angiotensin-converting enzyme, or ACE. Drugs that block angiotensin-converting enzyme, called ACE inhibitors, are effective antihypertensive agents and are particularly useful in reversing the angiotensin II–induced proliferation of smooth muscles in arterial walls. Statins—drugs that block the synthesis of cholesterol—also appear to block the bad effects of angiotensin II.

Is high blood pressure dangerous?

High blood pressure, or hypertension, defined as a blood pressure higher than 120/80, is one of the most dangerous illnesses, in large part because it's silent. Most of the time, you never know your blood pressure is elevated until someone actually measures it with a blood pressure cuff.

There are lots of reasons high blood pressure is dangerous. First, it makes the heart pump more forcefully. Each time the left ventricle contracts, in order for the aortic valve to open, pressure inside the left ventricle has to rise higher than pressure in the aorta. The higher the blood pressure, the harder it is for the left ventricle to open the aortic valve. As with any muscle doing extra work, the left ventricle eventually thickens, making it more difficult for the coronary arteries to supply the inner part of the ventricular wall. Under conditions of vigorous physical activity, heart muscle cells along the inner layer are in real danger of dying from lack of blood supply, especially if the coronary arteries are already compromised by atherosclerosis.

Hypertension also damages the endothelial lining of arterial walls, hastening atherosclerosis. In the kidneys, hypertension damages the small arteries and eventually wrecks the kidneys beyond repair. Hypertensive damage to small arteries and capillaries in the brain can weaken their walls enough to cause a brain hemorrhage.

What do antihypertensive medications do?

Antihypertensives lower blood pressure by making the heart relax, lessening the amount of blood the heart needs to pump, dilating peripheral arteries, and blocking angiotensin.

What happens if the blood pressure falls too low?

Low blood pressure, or hypotension, occurs when there is inadequate pressure to pump enough blood to the internal organs to meet their needs. This usually occurs when the systolic pressure drops below about 80–85 mm. Whenever we stand up, the blood pressure dips for a few seconds as gravity pulls blood toward the legs. If the blood pressure is already borderline when lying down, patients will feel woozy when standing up because of inadequate blood flow to the brain. When the blood pressure falls low enough to threaten a person's life, the patient is in shock.

What is atherosclerosis?

Atherosclerosis is the buildup of cholesterol, triglycerides, blood clot, and calcium along the walls of arteries. A patch of atherosclerosis is called a plaque. Eventually, atherosclerotic plaques enlarge enough to clog the artery. Blood clots forming in atherosclerotic plaques can also break off, embolize, and obstruct an artery downstream (see figure 77).

What's cholesterol?

Cholesterol is a fat widely used throughout the body. It forms a vital component of every cell membrane in the body, and it also forms the chemical skeleton for estrogen, testosterone, cortisone, vitamin D, and bile. Cholesterol is so valuable that virtually every cell in the body can synthesize it. The body cannot afford to depend on diet alone to satisfy its need for cholesterol, so 75% or more of our cholesterol is synthesized

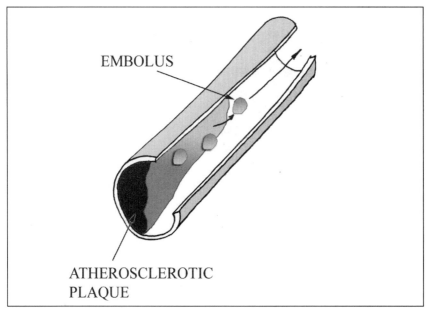

EMBOLUS

ATHEROSCLEROTIC
PLAQUE

Figure 77

by the body itself (much of it by the liver) while only about 25% of our cholesterol comes from the diet. For this reason, lowering the daily cholesterol intake does not have as important an impact on blood cholesterol as we'd like. How cholesterol is *not* used is as a source of energy.

What's a fatty acid, and what's the difference between a saturated and an unsaturated fatty acid?

A fatty acid is simply a long chain of carbon atoms. How they are attached to each other determines their saturation. Each carbon atom has four arms extending from it. Only two of the arms are needed to attach to a carbon atom on either side of it, leaving two arms free. If those two free arms are attached to hydrogen, the fatty acid is saturated with hydrogen. If one of the two free arms is instead used to reinforce the bond (double bond) to an adjacent carbon atom, the fatty acid is unsaturated.

In general, saturated fats such as butter and animal fat are solid at room temperature, while unsaturated fats are liquid oils at room temperature.

When fats combine with oxygen in the air, the free-fatty acids are released and fats become rancid, smelling a lot like baby vomit. Saturated fats don't combine with oxygen in the air as readily as unsaturated fats do, and for this reason, saturated fats have a longer shelf life than unsaturated fats. In fact, manufacturers will often add hydrogen to unsaturated fats to lengthen their shelf life.

What's the difference between a monounsaturated and a polyunsaturated fatty acid?

When only one double bond exists in a fatty acid, the molecule is monounsaturated. When more than one double bond exists, the fatty acid is polyunsaturated. Mono- and polyunsaturated fatty acids are further divided into omega-3 and omega-6, depending on where the first double bond is in relation to the terminal—or omega—carbon atom of the fatty acid. Omega-3 and omega-6 polyunsaturated fatty acids are necessary to synthesize many important chemicals in the body controlling blood clotting, gut function, kidney function, and birth. Since we cannot make omega-3 and omega-6 fatty acids, we have to eat them.

What kinds of foods contain monounsaturated and polyunsaturated fats?

Monounsaturated fats are readily found in olive oil, peanut oil, and canola oil.

Omega-6 polyunsaturated fats are in plentiful supply in a typical diet. Omega-3 polyunsaturated fatty acids are a little more difficult to come by than omega-6 fatty acids. Omega-3 fatty acids are found in plants— walnuts, soybeans, canola oil—and in seafood, especially cold-ocean fish such as salmon, sardines, cod, haddock, and anchovies and oysters, scallops, lobsters, and shrimp. Because big fish eaters such as the Japanese and Greenland Eskimos have low rates of heart attacks and strokes, many authorities advocate diets high in omega-3 fatty acids. Surprisingly, you need to eat fish only once a month to begin seeing its vascular benefits.

What's so bad about saturated fatty acids?

Saturated fats raise the blood cholesterol level in two ways. First, saturated fatty acids are used by the liver to synthesize cholesterol. Diets rich in saturated fatty acids—potato chips, butter, fatty meat, chicken skin, and lard—push the synthesis of cholesterol and drive up the blood cholesterol level. Unsaturated fats and oils—found in vegetable oils, most nuts, olives, avocados, and fish—are used much less by the liver to synthesize cholesterol.

The second way saturated fatty acids raise the blood cholesterol level is by stimulating the release of bile from the gallbladder. Any time we eat a fatty meal, bile is released to break up the fat for absorption. The liver makes additional bile to refill the emptied gallbladder, and since bile is made from cholesterol, the liver has to make more cholesterol, some of which makes its way to the blood and raises the blood cholesterol level.

What is the difference between a "cis" fatty acid and a "trans" fatty acid?

"Cis" and "trans" refer only to unsaturated fatty acids, not saturated ones. At each end of a double bond, the fatty acid bends. If both ends of the unsaturated fatty acid bend in the same direction, the shape is called "cis." If each end of the fatty acid bends in the opposite direction, like a reclining lawn chair, the shape is called "trans."

Almost all plant and fish oils (unsaturated fatty acids) are cis. When cows eat cis fatty acids in plants, bacteria in their stomachs convert many of the cis double bonds to trans, and the trans fatty acids then get incorporated into the cow's milk and fat. The other major source of trans fatty acids is man made: food companies often want to convert liquid unsaturated oils into partially saturated solid fats for easier use at room temperature and to lengthen the fat's shelf life. In the process of adding hydrogen atoms to unsaturated cis fatty acids, many of the cis bonds change to trans bonds. Trans unsaturated fatty acids are commonly used in fried foods, doughnuts, cakes, potato chips, and imitation cheese.

What's so bad about trans fatty acids?

Trans (unsaturated) fatty acids raise the low-density lipoprotein (LDL) cholesterol and lower the high-density lipoprotein (HDL) cholesterol—

a combination that makes trans fatty acids even more harmful than saturated fatty acids.

What are high- and low-density lipoproteins?

Fats are insoluble in water, and more than half of blood is water. For lipids to reach distant sites via the bloodstream, they must be carried there by special proteins in the blood, called lipoproteins. Whether a lipoprotein is high density or low density depends on how fast it sinks when blood is centrifuged. High-density lipoproteins sink fast; low-density lipoproteins sink slowly.

HDLs have a different function than LDLs. LDLs carry cholesterol from the liver (where cholesterol is made) to distant sites in the body, while HDLs carry cholesterol from distant sites back to the liver (see figure 78). HDLs are good because they remove cholesterol from arterial walls; conversely, low-density lipoproteins are bad because they deposit cholesterol into arterial walls. So simply knowing your cholesterol is less useful than knowing how much of your cholesterol is attached to high-

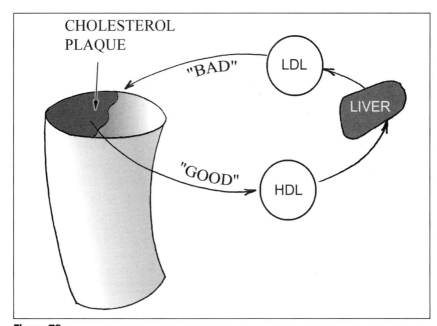

Figure 78

density lipoproteins (good cholesterol) and how much is attached to low-density lipoproteins (bad cholesterol).

Another lipid-carrying protein in the blood, called very low-density lipoprotein (VLDL), carries most of the triglycerides and a little cholesterol. VLDL is also a bad actor, because enzymes in the bloodstream exchange triglycerides on VLDL for cholesterol on HDL, in essence snatching good cholesterol on its way to the liver.

What causes cholesterol, fatty acids, blood clot, and calcium to deposit along arterial walls?

The walls of arteries are normally slick and smooth so that blood can flow without turbulence. Lining the walls likes tiles on a swimming pool is a thin layer of cells called endothelial cells (see figure 79). Being only one cell layer thick, the endothelium is easy to overlook, but because there are so many blood vessels in the body, endothelial tissue weighs as much as the brain. The endothelium helps control the constriction of smooth muscle cells in arterial walls, helps keep blood clots from forming along the walls of arteries, and dissolves the clots when they do form. Another very important function of the endothelium is to prevent LDL cholesterol in the blood from getting into the walls of arteries. The endothelium does all this primarily by releasing a critical molecule called nitric oxide.

If, for any reason, the endothelium is injured, LDLs attach to the arterial wall and deposit their cholesterol there. If not already oxidized by cigarette smoke (smoking increases the level of oxidized LDLs), the cholesterol becomes immediately oxidized within the arterial wall. The oxidized cholesterol quickly attracts a variety of inflammatory cells, including macrophages, which gobble up the oxidized LDL cholesterol and turn into fat-laden foam cells (see figure 80). Macrophage foam cells, in turn, cause muscle cells in the arterial wall to proliferate, thickening the arterial wall. Thickened arterial walls are stiff, hence the term "hardening of the arteries."

Eventually, the foam cells become overwhelmed by the accumulating cholesterol, and little lakes of cholesterol begin to form amid a thicket of foam cells and proliferating muscle cells within the arterial wall. As this hodgepodge of LDL cholesterol, foam cells, and muscle cells enlarges, it begins to intrude into the lumen of the artery. The endothelium tries to

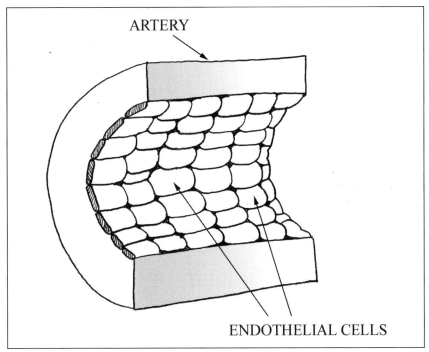

ARTERY

ENDOTHELIAL CELLS

Figure 79

keep a lid on the tip of this growing volcano, but eventually the unstable lid leaks, stimulating blood clots to form at the site of leakage. If you're lucky, the blood clot that forms just sits there and slowly shrivels up, but if you're not, the clot will enlarge and occlude the artery, or else break off, embolize, and occlude a smaller artery downstream, hence the term thromboembolism. Investigators have started measuring C-reactive protein, a protein released during inflammation, to predict the instability of atherosclerotic plaques.

What injures the arterial endothelium in the first place?

The big-ticket items are LDL cholesterol, high blood pressure, smoking, and diabetes.

LDL cholesterol is readily susceptible to oxidation in the bloodstream, and oxidized LDL cholesterol damages the endothelium.

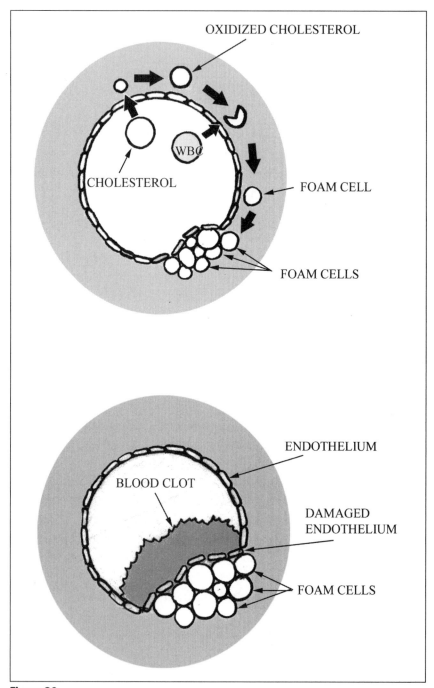

Figure 80

High blood pressure physically damages the endothelium by hammering away at it. High blood pressure also damages the endothelium by causing LDL cholesterol to become oxidized, and then oxidized LDL cholesterol damages the endothelium. Finally, high blood pressure damages the endothelium when hypertension is due to elevated angiotensin II, because angiotensin II itself disrupts the endothelium. In other words, if angiotensin II is elevated, lowering the blood pressure alone—without also lowering the angiotensin II level—won't fully protect the endothelium. To make matters worse, angiotensin II is also made by macrophages chasing down oxidized cholesterol within arterial walls.

How does smoking damage the endothelium?

Toxic chemicals in smoke damage the endothelial lining of arterial walls, as evidenced by the fact that after a person smokes cigarettes, the number of endothelial cells found in the person's bloodstream doubles. In animals, microscopic studies have shown nicks and abrasions in the endothelium from tobacco smoke. Hundreds of studies have demonstrated rapid acceleration of atherosclerosis in smokers' arteries. Smoking also makes the blood "sticky"—more likely to clot. Smoking raises the LDL levels and lowers the HDL levels. Smoking stimulates the sympathetic nerves to increase the heart rate and raise the blood pressure. The nicotine in smoke constricts arteries, restricting blood flow. If only smoking didn't wrinkle your skin, dull your senses of smell and taste, stain your teeth, promote dental plaque, cause bad breath, cause a chronic cough, destroy the alveoli, cause lung and mouth cancer, promote hiatal hernias, greatly hasten atherosclerosis, and cost so much, it wouldn't be such a bad habit.

How does diabetes hasten atherosclerosis?

Without insulin, or in the case of adult onset diabetes, without cells responsive to insulin, extra glucose in the bloodstream has difficulty getting into fat and muscle cells. In response, fat tissue mobilizes its fat stores and releases fatty acids into the bloodstream, where they are brought to the liver for synthesis into very low-density lipoproteins (VLDLs). Elevated levels of VLDL lower the level of HDL in the bloodstream and help deposit fat in arterial walls, an easy job in diabetes because diabetes also impairs endothelial function by interfering with nitric oxide. Meanwhile, free-fatty acids raise the blood pressure by damaging vascular endothelium and stimulating the sympathetic nervous system. Diabetes ravages arteries everywhere in the body. It is not uncommon for diabetics to end up with blindness, kidney failure, amputations, strokes, and heart attacks.

Is being fat a risk factor for atherosclerosis?

Yes. Fat cells release into the bloodstream free-fatty acids, tumor necrosis factor, leptin, and resistin. In obese people, fat cells are inhibited from releasing adiponectin, a protein that is thought to inhibit atherosclerosis. The combined effect of all this is to make cells resistant to insulin. The islets of Langerhans respond by releasing more insulin. Here's where the trouble begins, because insulin stimulates the sympathetic nervous system (as part of the fight or flight reaction), which causes the blood pressure to rise. Insulin also raises the blood pressure by instructing the kidney to retain salt and water. Meanwhile, the free-fatty acids being released by fat cells are taken up by the liver, converted to triglycerides, and released alone or as part of an LDL cholesterol mix back into the bloodstream to damage the endothelial lining of arteries. To make matters worse, the level of HDL cholesterol drops. In addition, all the extra insulin damages arteries directly. It's been known for many years that infusing insulin into the artery of a dog's leg causes atherosclerosis in that leg. Part of the explanation for this is thought to be insulin's role as an agent for the fight or flight response: insulin makes the blood clot more easily and inhibits clots from being dissolved naturally by the body.

Can insulin resistance be reversed?

While there are drugs that increase a body's sensitivity to insulin and drugs that stimulate the release of insulin from islet cells, the first steps— before drugs—are exercise and weight loss. Weight loss is clearly the most important step, because extra body fat is the primary reason for insulin resistance in the first place. Exercise uses up free-fatty acids, one of the culprits in insulin resistance. The more you use your muscles, the better they become at taking up glucose from the bloodstream. Since muscles absorb more glucose from the bloodstream than any other organ in the body, considerably less insulin is needed to escort glucose into muscle cells, and less of a burden is placed on islet cells to produce insulin.

What are healthy levels of cholesterol, low-density lipoprotein, high-density lipoprotein, and triglycerides?

Total blood cholesterol should be less than 200 mg per 100 cc of blood, LDLs should be less than 130, HDLs more than 35 (ideally, more than 60), and triglycerides less than 200. Many doctors use the cardiac risk ratio: total cholesterol divided by the HDL. A value over 7.0 indicates that steps need to be taken to lower LDLs and raise the HDLs.

How do you lower the levels of low-density lipoproteins and raise the levels of high-density lipoproteins?

Six ways: lower the amount of cholesterol you eat, switch from saturated fats and trans polyunsaturated fats to monounsaturated fats and polyunsaturated cis fats, go on drugs that block the synthesis of cholesterol in the liver, eat lots of fiber, exercise, and stop smoking.

Lowering the amount of cholesterol you eat is important, but more important is lowering the amount of saturated fats you eat, because saturated fats in the diet are more effective at driving up the blood cholesterol than eating cholesterol is. When checking the grams of saturated fat on a food label, a useful guide is that eating 5 grams of saturated fat is the equivalent of eating a teaspoon of pure butter. Monounsaturated fats from olive oil, peanut oil, and canola oil are better than polyunsaturated cis oils, because polyunsaturated fatty acids from corn oil, sunflower oil, and safflower oil reduce low- *and* high-density lipoproteins. Monounsaturated fatty acids reduce only the LDLs without reducing HDLs.

Drugs that block the synthesis of intracellular cholesterol are called statins ("intra" means within; "inter" means between). In response to the drop in intracellular cholesterol, cells respond by absorbing cholesterol from the bloodstream, leaving less cholesterol in the blood to cause atherosclerosis.

Fiber lowers cholesterol by trapping it in the intestines. A great deal of cholesterol synthesized by the liver is made into bile, which is squirted into the intestines to help digest fats. Most of the cholesterol-filled bile is reabsorbed further down the intestines (some remains in the large intestine and stains the stool brown). Fiber in the diet binds and traps cholesterol in the gut, preventing it from being reabsorbed. The cholesterol is then dispensed with in the stool. Soluble fiber is better at this than insoluble fiber. Soluble fiber is found in oatmeal, citrus fruits, beans, peas, and barley. Insoluble fiber is found in wheat bran, whole wheat bread, carrots, cauliflower, beets, brussel sprouts, and cabbage. Insoluble fiber is better, however, at preventing constipation.

Regular exercise, even walking, lowers the blood pressure, lowers VLDL, raises the HDL cholesterol, and improves LDL cholesterol—so long as you exercise long enough, the equivalent of walking about 2 miles a day. Admittedly, some of the improvement in lipid profile may be due to weight loss from exercise. In any case, whether you're normal or already have bad coronary artery atherosclerosis, probably the best predictor of risk of death from heart disease is your peak exercise capacity, better than a history of high cholesterol, smoking, high blood pressure, or diabetes.

Can antioxidants help keep low-density lipoproteins from being oxidized and damaging the endothelium?

Some antioxidants seem to promise protection from atherosclerosis. One such antioxidant is lutein, which is found in dark green plants such as spinach, broccoli, kale, and collard greens and also in corn. Besides its beneficial effect in preventing atherosclerosis, lutein also seems to protect the eyes against degeneration in old age, protects the lungs from aging, and even protects against cancer. Other antioxidants with beneficial effects on atherosclerosis and cancer are allicin in garlic; lycopene in tomatoes, ketchup, salsa, and watermelon; polyphenols in cranberry juice; and flavonoids in red grapes, blueberries, apples, soy, onions, grapefruits, and green tea. As a general rule, the more colorful and smellier the fruit or vegetable, the higher its antioxidant value.

What does homocysteine have to do with atherosclerosis?

Homocysteine is an amino acid. People born with a genetic defect that allows homocysteine to accumulate suffer early atherosclerosis. Even in people without this defect, elevated homocysteine levels are associated with atherosclerosis. Smoking raises homocysteine levels, while folic acid lowers homocysteine levels by helping metabolize homocysteine to methionine. It's unclear yet whether lowering homocysteine levels with folic acid lowers the risk of atherosclerosis.

Why don't women have atherosclerosis as often as men?

Estrogen protects arteries from atherosclerosis, probably by increasing the amount of nitric oxide in the endothelium. Unfortunately, estrogen given to women after menopause does not seem to have the same antiathero-sclerosis effect as estrogen before menopause.

How much cholesterol and saturated fatty acid is safe to eat each day?

Nutritionists have concluded that, of your daily intake of calories, 30% should come from fat, 20% from protein, and 60% from carbohydrates. If an average adult eats about 2,000 calories per day, this translates into 600 calories from fat, 1,200 calories from carbohydrates (preferably fruits and vegetables rather than breads and pasta), and 400 calories from protein. Another way to look at it is, per day, you should consume about 1 to 1.5 grams of protein per kilogram of body weight. If you weigh 175 pounds, or 80 kg, that translates into 80 to 120 grams of protein. A quarter pound hamburger is about 25 grams of protein.

Only one-third of our daily intake of fat should be in the form of saturated fats—about 20 grams. Unfortunately, saturated fat is pretty prevalent in the diet. A small 3-ounce hamburger has 8 grams of saturated fat; a medium croissant, 7 grams; an ounce of cheese, 6 grams; and a cup of whole milk, 5 grams. As for cholesterol, only 0.3 grams (300 mg) should be eaten per day. One egg yolk contains 0.2 grams (200 mg) of cholesterol.

What do food labels reveal about the foods we eat?

A typical bag of potato chips has about 150 calories per serving (one serving is about 20 chips). Total fat is 9 grams per serving, which at 9 calories per gram is 81 calories. Since 600 calories a day should come from fat, the 81 calories you eat from 20 potato chips is about 13% of the total daily recommended fat. The saturated fat from those 20 potato chips is 2 grams. We should keep our daily saturated fat intake below about 20 grams, so the 20 chips supply 10% of our daily allowance.

Look again at the fat content of the potato chips. By calculating the calories derived from fat and dividing by the total calories, you can determine the percentage of calories coming from fat. Of the 150 total calories, 81 came from fat (9 grams × 9 calories per gram = 81 calories). Dividing 81 by 150 gives you 0.54, so 54% of the calories from potato chips come from fat. A piece of fried dark-meat chicken typically contains 30 grams of fat and 430 calories: 30 × 9 = 270, which divided by 430 is 0.63—63% of calories from fat. The total calories in an order of onion rings is about 175. An order of onion rings contains 16 grams of fat (144 calories), so the percentage of calories from fat is 144/175, or 82%.

Here's a typical soft-drink label: 16 ounces contain 200 calories, all from sugar. Each teaspoon of sugar contains 16 calories. Dividing 200 by 16 gives you 12.5 teaspoons of sugar in a 16-ounce soft drink. This is striking, because if you had an 8-ounce cup of tea instead, you would put in only one teaspoon of sugar, or 2 teaspoons in 16 ounces of tea. That's an extra 10.5 teaspoons of sugar for a 16-ounce soft drink. A cotton candy—virtually pure sugar—contains only 7 teaspoons of sugar.

Is all that sugar in soft drinks the reason they're such picker-uppers during the afternoon doldrums?

The afternoon sinking spell may be due in some people to a drop in blood sugar. If the blood sugar level is low, there's nothing like a jolt of sucrose to improve brain function. Sucrose is quickly split into glucose and fructose, and the glucose immediately enters the brain to revive its energy supply. The only time the brain uses fat for energy is during periods of starvation, when there is no glucose around and fatty acids are broken down into tiny two-carbon fragments called ketones. Under those conditions, the brain will use ketones for energy.

The other reason we droop in the afternoon may have to do with a drop in adrenal hormones. The adrenal glands secrete a number of hormones, with widespread effects, including a feeling of well being and preparedness for action. The adrenal glands tend to secrete less hormone in the afternoon, which may be partially countered by an afternoon sugar buzz.

11

UROLOGIC SYSTEM

You'd think that if we made stool, we wouldn't need to make urine, but stool is just the leftovers the body can't absorb. In order to get rid of waste already inside the body, we have to either breathe it out or pee it out.

Where are the kidneys?

You have two kidneys, a left one and a right one, each about the size of your closed fist. They are located about halfway up the abdomen, pressed up against the back muscles and protected by the rib cage (see figure 81). That's why when the doctor suspects a kidney infection, she thumps the middle of the back looking for tenderness over the kidneys.

What do the kidneys do?

The kidneys do a remarkable number of tasks. First, every organ of the body—the brain, the liver, the heart, the lungs, you name it—makes toxic waste and dumps it into the bloodstream. The kidneys clean up the blood, including many drugs and toxic chemicals not handled by the liver, by dumping all of them into the urine. As part of the process of making urine, the kidneys regulate the acidity of the blood; regulate the level of sodium, potassium, and chloride in the blood; release a hormone

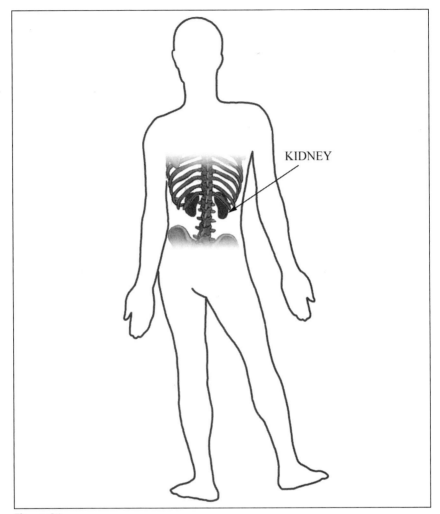

KIDNEY

Figure 81

called erythropoietin, which stimulates the bone marrow to make blood; control the volume of water in the body; and make vitamin D. In addition to all this, the kidneys raise the blood pressure by making an enzyme called renin, which initiates the synthesis of angiotensin, the powerful vasoconstrictor. If you want problems, just ask for kidney failure. Luckily, the most common cause of kidney failure—hypertension—is treatable.

How do the kidneys clean the blood?

First, we have to get blood to the kidneys. Not a problem. As soon as the aorta passes through the diaphragm, it gives off a large artery—the renal artery—to each kidney. The kidneys utilize a method to clean the blood that few of us would have thought of. Each kidney first filters the blood through millions of individual tiny filters, called glomeruli, into tubules (small tubes) (see figure 82). The glomeruli keep all the large proteins and red blood cells carrying hemoglobin in the bloodstream. Everything else is filtered into the kidney's tubules and is now headed for the bladder. As this filtrate slowly drifts through the kidney to be excreted as urine, the kidney selects the substances it wants the body to keep and transports them back into the bloodstream. It may seem like a lot of unnecessary work to filter everything out of the bloodstream and then to select back what's needed—two steps—instead of simply excreting the toxins in one step. However, in that one simple step, glomerular filtration isolates all the blood's filterable toxins into a small, protein-free solution for cleansing by the kidney tubules.

Many of the kidney's decisions about what needs to be transported back into the blood and what needs to stay in the urine are governed by hormones. For example, when the blood gets too salty or the blood pressure drops, the posterior pituitary gland secretes antidiuretic hormone, which stimulates the kidney to retain water in order to expand the volume of blood. When the blood pressure drops, the adrenal glands secrete aldosterone, which instructs the kidneys to reabsorb sodium from the kidney tubules. Wherever sodium goes, so goes water, thereby increasing the blood volume. When the blood pressure rises, both the heart and the kidney release natriuretic hormone ("natrium" means sodium; "uresis" means urinate) instructing the kidney not to reabsorb sodium from the kidney tubules. As sodium floats through the kidney tubules on its way to the bladder, it drags water with it into the urine.

What's a diuretic?

A diuretic is a pill that makes you urinate. It works by preventing the kidneys from transporting sodium from the kidney tubules back into the blood.

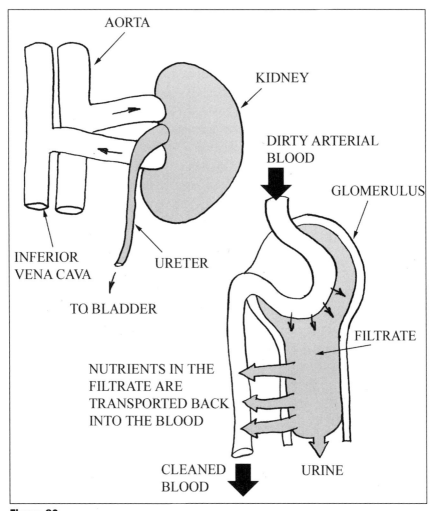

AORTA

KIDNEY

DIRTY ARTERIAL
BLOOD

GLOMERULUS

INFERIOR
VENA CAVA

URETER

TO BLADDER

FILTRATE

NUTRIENTS IN THE
FILTRATE ARE
TRANSPORTED BACK
INTO THE BLOOD

CLEANED
BLOOD

URINE

Figure 82

Why do doctors insist that you take penicillin for a full ten days to properly treat strep throat?

The good thing about the kidney is that it's effective. The bad thing about the kidney is that being so complicated and delicate, it's vulnerable to lots of diseases. One good example is strep throat when it is caused by the strain of streptococcus known as Group A beta hemolytic strep. In the days before antibiotics, the body's only defense against Group A beta hemolytic strep was its own immune system. But when white blood cells made antibodies against the streptococcus, there was something in the streptococcus that resembled the kidney glomerulus, so the antibodies would attack the glomeruli. To add insult to injury, after latching on to the strep antigen, the antigen–antibody complex would clog up the glomeruli. In some patients, the streptococcus altered the antistrep antibody, enough to make it look foreign to the body, triggering a new antibody response. This antigen–antibody complex would also lodge in the glomeruli. All three of these mechanisms would trigger an inflammatory response in the glomeruli that sometimes led to scarring, rendering the kidneys functionless. Without kidneys to clean the blood, the patient's days were numbered. The incidence of this condition, called poststreptococcal glomerulonephritis ("nephritis" means inflammation in the nephrons, an old term for the kidneys), has been greatly reduced since the advent of penicillin, but the penicillin has to be taken for its full course to ensure that all the strep has been killed.

How does urine get from the kidneys to the bladder?

The bladder is situated at the base of the abdomen, just behind the symphysis pubis, the union of two bones you can feel at the bottom of your abdomen. You can't feel the bladder unless it gets so filled with urine that it balloons up over the rim of the symphysis pubis. A thin tube called the ureter carries urine from the kidneys down to the bladder a full foot away (see figure 83).

What happens to urine in the bladder?

Nothing. It just sits there accumulating. We make about 50 cc of urine an hour, more at a bar, because alcohol inhibits the release of antidiuretic hormone from the posterior pituitary. When the bladder fills up, it sends a signal to the brain and the brain sends a signal back through the parasympathetic nerves to contract the bladder. As we voluntarily relax the urinary sphincter muscle, urine is squeezed out of the bladder through a small tube called the urethra.

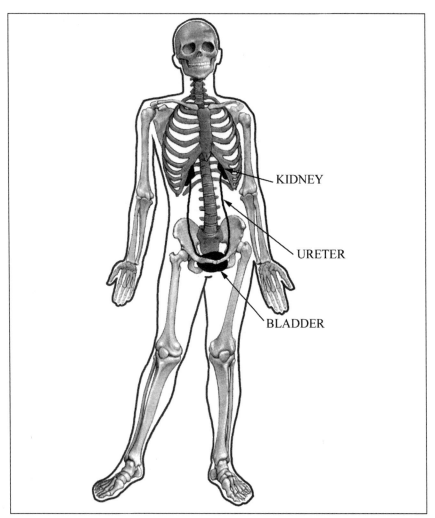

KIDNEY

URETER

BLADDER

Figure 83

What's a kidney stone?

A kidney stone is just that, a stone in the kidney, ranging from the size of a tiny grain of sand to the size of a marble or larger. The stone can be made of calcium, oxalate, uric acid, the amino acid cystine, and other insoluble molecules. Proper treatment depends on the type of stone, so it's important to capture the stone for analysis in the laboratory. The stone is captured by peeing through a filter for a week or more until the stone passes.

How do you know when a kidney stone forms?

Believe me, you'll know. The pain is terrible. It's felt in the back, along the sides of the abdomen (the loins), and in the lower abdomen down into the groin, and it is accompanied by intense urges to urinate frequently. As the ureter balloons up, the pain often comes in waves that build to a crescendo over a period of seconds up to a minute. In fact, colicky pain such as this is a clue that one of the hollow organs—the esophagus, stomach, small intestines, gallbladder, colon, ureter, or bladder—is obstructed.

How do you get rid of a kidney stone?

Depending on where the stone is stuck, drinking lots of water will usually wash the stone down into the bladder and eventually out the urethra. Sometimes, though, a urologist has to fish the stone out with the help of a thin telescope that's slipped slowly through the urethra into the bladder. After doing this, the urologist looks around the bladder for the opening into the ureter and slides the telescope up the ureter until he sees the stone. Alongside the shaft of the telescope is a tiny tube. Through that tube, the urologist threads a very small wire basket and with considerable skill nabs the stone and pulls it out of the ureter (see figure 84).

What's lithotripsy?

Lithotripsy is used when the stone is so big that the urologist cannot capture it with a wire basket. Lithotripsy shatters the large stone with a blast of intense sound waves. A good blast will shatter the stone into such small pieces that the patient just pees them out over a few days.

What's a urinary tract infection?

Urine is normally sterile, meaning there's no bacteria in urine, which is why it's permissible to drink urine—if you're into that kind of thing. The

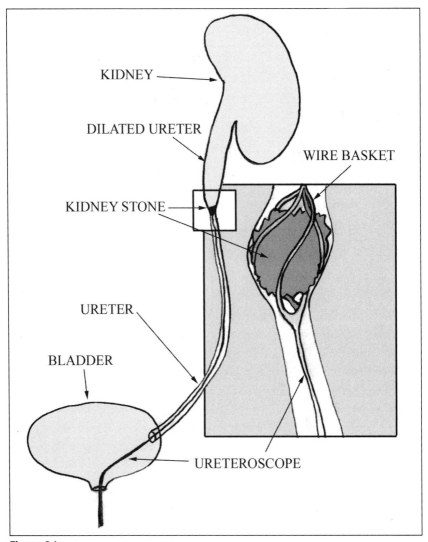

KIDNEY

DILATED URETER

WIRE BASKET

KIDNEY STONE

URETER

BLADDER

URETEROSCOPE

Figure 84

smell of urine is from urea being broken down by bacteria outside the bladder. Sometimes, though, bacteria do gain access to the kidneys or bladder. There are lots of nutrients in urine for the bacteria to enjoy, and the bacteria are beyond the reach of white blood cells. One way to clear the urine of bacteria is to drink lots of water to wash them out of the kidney and bladder—as they say, "the solution to pollution is dilution." Another way is antibiotics. The one thing you don't want a bladder infection to do is travel up the ureters into the kidneys, a condition called pyelonephritis, because repeated bouts of pyelonephritis can damage the kidneys.

How do you know when there's a urinary tract infection?

You feel the inflammatory white blood cells as an uncomfortable irritation in the lower abdomen and as burning in the urethra when you urinate. If the kidneys are infected, fever and back pain are also present.

How do you pee if your spinal cord is damaged?

Every muscle in the body is controlled by two nerves. The first nerve travels from the brain down to the spinal cord, and from there a second nerve carries the signal to the muscle. The first nerve is called the upper motor neuron, the second, the lower motor neuron (see figure 85). As the bladder fills with urine, signals from the bladder travel to the spinal cord, signaling the lower motor neuron to contract the bladder. These signals are normally kept in check by the upper motor neuron. Without supervision by the upper motor neuron, as happens with spinal cord damage, the lower motor neuron contracts the bladder with very little provocation from the bladder. This high-strung readiness to contract is called spasticity.

What happens if the lower motor (parasympathetic) nerves to the bladder are damaged?

Instead of a small, irritable bladder, the bladder becomes a big, floppy bag. As urine enters the bladder, the bladder expands until, eventually, it can't expand any more. Finally, the pressure gets so high that urine pushes its way out the urethra and the patient begins to dribble urine. Several hundred years ago, before we had medications to stimulate the bladder, a Dr. Carl Crede described a way to empty a large bladder. You press down on your lower abdomen with a closed fist and lean over. Pushing against the bladder like this forces urine out the bladder. We still use the Crede method today to empty a dilated bladder.

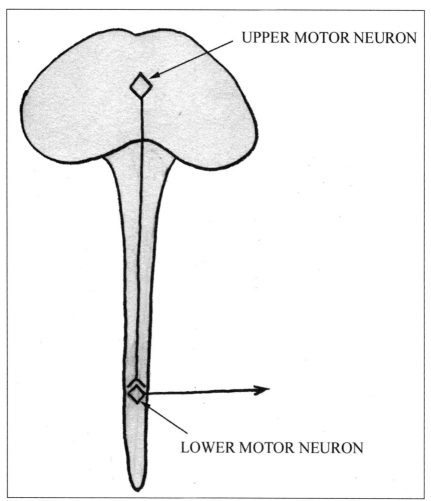

Figure 85

12

~~~~~~~~~~~~~~~~

GENITAL SYSTEM

The reproductive, or genital, system has one job and that's to make sure mankind does not perish from this Earth. In men, the genital system hooks into the urinary system. In women, the two are separate.

What is the prostate gland?

The prostate is a gland the size of a walnut that sits underneath the bladder, encircling the urethra as it leaves the bladder (see figure 86). When sperm pass from the testes into the urethra, the prostate gland and seminal vesicles secrete a nutritious fluid into the urethra for the sperm to swim in.

Once most men hit 50, the prostate tends to enlarge, for unclear reasons. Because the prostate gland completely encircles the urethra, the growing prostate slowly pinches off the urinary stream. Eventually, this problem will need fixing by a urologist, who either slips a tube up the penis and roto-rooters the pinched section or operates and removes the prostate altogether.

Cancer of the prostate is the most common cancer in men, and it is more prevalent than breast cancer in women. Like the breast, the prostate can be examined directly. Unfortunately, it can only be felt through the rectum. With the help of a little KY jelly, a doctor is able to slip his or her finger into the rectum and feel the back of the prostate through the wall of the rectum (see figure 87).

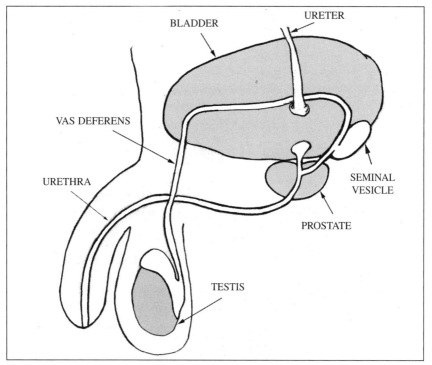

Figure 86

Where are sperm made?

Sperm are made in the testes, or testicles (terms akin to the word "testify" in Latin, as only men were allowed to testify at legal proceedings in ancient Rome). Sperm exit the testes via a tiny tube called the vas deferens and enter the urethra, from which they are ejaculated. During an erection, the urethral connection to the bladder is squeezed off so a man cannot urinate.

Why are the testicles in a scrotum? Wouldn't the body want to keep them well protected in the abdominal cavity?

The testicles actually do start out life in the abdomen—about where a girl's ovaries are found. Sometime before birth, the testicles descend into the scrotum, dragging with them a small cremasteric muscle. If you want

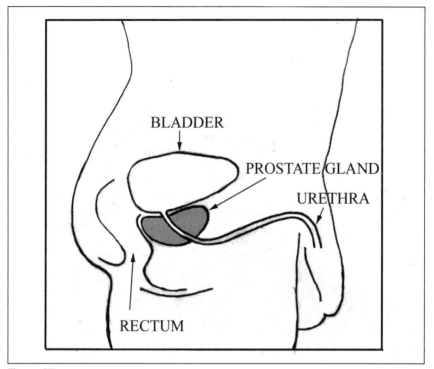

Figure 87

to see the cremasteric in action, gently stroke the inside of the thigh and watch the testicle ascend toward the abdomen ("cremaster" in Greek means suspenders). The reason the testicles descend into the scrotum is that the abdominal cavity is too hot for developing sperm to survive. The testicles need to be a few degrees cooler than body temperature to grow sperm.

Anything that increases a man's estrogen level will make the testicles shrink. Since in men the liver detoxifies estrogen, anything that seriously impairs liver function can raise the estrogen level. Alcohol use is the most common liver toxin leading to elevated estrogen levels, which is why alcoholics with cirrhosis often develop testicular atrophy and stop shaving.

It used to be thought that estrogen-like hormones fed to cows and other estrogen-like chemicals in our diet and environment were lowering male sperm counts, but many studies have failed to confirm this suspicion. One potential source of estrogen in men is obesity, because fat cells contain an enzyme called aromatase that routinely converts testosterone to estrogen. (Because estrogen stimulates some breast cancers to grow, drugs are now being developed to block aromatase to lower a woman's estrogen level.)

What do you do about an undescended testicle?

An undescended testicle cannot be left in the abdomen, because it has a tendency to become malignant later in life. It either has to be pulled into the scrotum or removed from the abdomen.

Why does it hurt so much to be kicked in the balls?

Each testicle is encased in a tough but very pain-sensitive capsule. It's the capsule that hurts, not the testicle. Because the testicles descend from the abdomen, dragging nerves with them, the pain is felt well up into the abdomen.

This same pain-sensitive capsule surrounds each ovary, so when the gynecologist palpates (feels) a woman's ovaries (to check for cancerous enlargement, for example), the doctor has to be careful not to squeeze too hard or the patient will experience the same pain a man feels when kicked in the groin.

What's a circumcision?

At birth, the head of the penis, or glans, is covered by a loose flap of skin called the foreskin. For religious, cosmetic, and health reasons (papilloma virus, which causes cancer of the uterine cervix in women, can grow underneath the foreskin), the foreskin is surgically removed at or near birth.

What's an erection?

The interior of a penis is sponge-like and has lots of channels for blood. There are no muscles in the penis. During sexual arousal, parasympathetic nerves stimulate the release of nitric oxide, which dilates the arteries supplying blood to the interior of the penis. As the spongy interior of the penis fills with blood, the penis becomes erect. It's odd that the parasympathetic nervous system, which is normally activated during times of relaxation, should control such an unrelaxed activity as having an erection. Sympathetic nerves kick in with muscular contractions in the pelvis to ejaculate sperm from the penis, after which they contract the arteries to allow blood to exit the penis.

How does Viagra work?

Nitric oxide dilates arteries by increasing a chemical called cyclic guanosine monophosphate. Viagra works by preventing the breakdown of cyclic guanosine monophosphate.

What are "blue balls"?

During an erection, blood is partially blocked from exiting the penis, which helps to keep the penis erect. Blood is also blocked from exiting the testicles during an erection. If the erection is maintained for 20 minutes or longer, the engorged testicles may swell considerably, distending the pain-sensitive testicular capsules. Ejaculation relaxes the arteries and veins, reestablishing normal blood flow. Allowing the penis to relax without ejaculation still leaves the testicles with a deep ache. The blue refers to blood lingering around, losing its oxygen, and turning blue.

Another cause of sudden severe pain is testicular torsion, or twisting of the testicle, which cuts off the testicle's blood supply. The testicle becomes exquisitely tender and rides a little higher than usual. Emergency surgery is often required to untwist the testicle.

Why do women have periods?

Women are born with a uterus (a womb) to support the development of a fertilized egg into a baby over a period of nine months. Getting ready for a fertilized egg takes some preparation, and each month a woman of childbearing age goes through a 28-day cycle preparing the uterus for such an event. During the first 14 days of the cycle, estrogen is secreted by the ovaries to stimulate the inner uterine wall—the endometrium—to thicken with lots of new blood vessels. Once the egg is released (ovulated) from the ovary at about day 14, the ovary secretes a second hormone, progesterone, to further prepare the uterus for implantation of a fertilized egg. If the fertilized egg never appears, the uterus sheds its endometrium, with all its newly constructed blood vessels, over a period of three to five days. The bleeding process is called menstruation, or period. The cycle then repeats itself over the course of another 28 days.

Monthly periods take their toll on the blood count. Women often have to supplement their diet with extra iron to replace the iron lost in hemoglobin each month.

How does the egg get from the ovary to the uterus?

Thousands of unfertilized eggs are stored in each ovary, each egg containing 46 chromosomes, like every other cell in the body. Every 28 days, under the influence of the follicle-stimulating hormone (FSH), one egg undergoes a process of halving its chromosomes to 23, half the number needed to make a person. At around the 14th day, the ovary ovulates the 23-chromosome egg into the fallopian tube (see figure 88). If, while slowly dribbling down the fallopian tube, the egg encounters a sperm, the sperm penetrates the egg and combines its 23 chromosomes with the egg's 23 chromosomes. It takes five or six days for a fertilized egg to reach the uterus and implant itself on the uterine wall. By the time it reaches the uterus, the fertilized egg has already divided into many cells.

How is a home pregnancy test able to detect an early pregnancy?

Immediately after releasing its egg, the ovary begins producing a third hormone, chorionic gonadotropin, which keeps the ovary producing high levels of estrogen and progesterone to maintain a lush endometrium. As soon as the fertilized egg implants in the uterine wall, it too begins making chorionic gonadotropin, enough to be detected in the urine by a home pregnancy kit. Since it takes at least a week after *implantation* for the level of chorionic gonadotropin to rise to detectable levels, the home pregnancy test should not be performed until 10 days after ovulation. While ovulation should take place on day 14, some months ovulation may occur much later. In other words, a negative home pregnancy test on the heels of a missed period may still turn positive a week or two later.

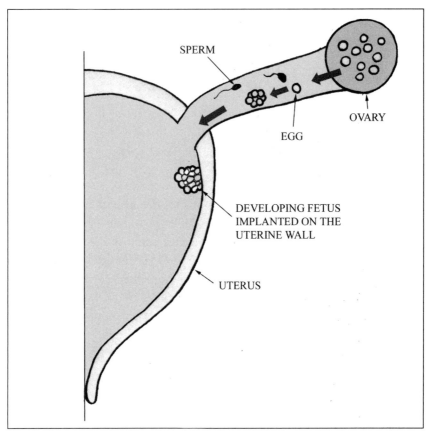

Figure 88

What's the difference between identical twins and fraternal twins?

Normally, only one egg per cycle trims down from 46 to 23 chromosomes, but if for some reason two separate eggs develop and both are released into the fallopian tube (or tubes), both eggs can develop into genetically separate—fraternal—fetuses. Identical twins develop after a single fertilized egg divides into two cells. Sometimes, these two cells separate and develop independently. Since their genetic makeup is identical, the resulting babies are called identical twins.

At what point do the cells of a developing embryo lose their ability to separate and grow into a fetus?

Up until about the stage when there are 8 cells, each cell still has the potential to grow into a complete human being. For a considerable number of cell divisions after the 8-cell stage, each cell retains the ability to become an entire liver, or an entire heart, or even an entire brain. This ability continues in stem cells, which survive all the way into adulthood. Everyone wants to get their hands on stem cells to use them to replace organs that fail. The debate is where to harvest the stem cells. The ideal place would be the patient's bloodstream. Another approach would be to change a fully developed cell into a stem cell and then stimulate it to develop into an entire organ.

Why does a fertilized egg need to attach to the uterine wall?

Since the only way to get nutrients to the developing fetus is via the fetus's bloodstream, the fetus's bloodstream needs to be connected somehow to the mother's blood supply. To do this, the mother supplies her uterine wall and the fetus supplies a placenta. Thousands of tiny blood vessels in the uterine wall invade the placenta and flood it with a lake of mother's blood (containing an anticoagulant to keep the lake of blood from clotting) (see figure 89). From the baby's side, tiny arteries and capillaries from the umbilical cord project into this lake of mother's blood and absorb oxygen, glucose, vitamins, fat, and proteins. Now all the placenta has to do is get those nutrients to the fetus by way of a large vein in the umbilical cord, which enters the fetus through the belly button, or umbilicus.

Does a fetus pee?

Sure. The fetus is suspended in a bag of fluid called amniotic fluid and it just pees into the amniotic fluid. The fetus doesn't make stool yet, because it's not eating.

Why do they tell women to take folate during pregnancy?

Folate, or folic acid, greatly lowers the likelihood of giving birth to a baby with terrible brain and spinal cord deformities, for example, a baby with

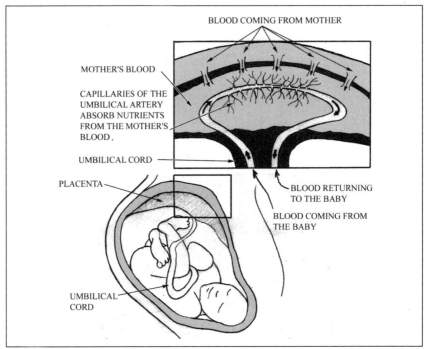

Figure 89

no significant brain tissue at all (anencephaly) or a baby that is paraplegic because the spinal cord is poking out of the back (a condition called spina bifida).

Why is labor so painful?

Labor pains are due to extremely strong contractions of the uterus pushing the baby out. The contractions develop in response to the combined effects of oxytocin released from the posterior pituitary gland and prostaglandins released by the uterus itself. It's unclear exactly what triggers the release of oxytocin.

Oxytocin released from the mother's pituitary at birth is thought to circle back to the mother's brain to foster the warm bonding feelings a mother experiences toward her newborn. The role of oxytocin in men is still unclear.

During labor, prostaglandins thin out the cervix, the opening at the bottom of the uterus through which the baby has to pass. As the cervix thins out, it begins to dilate. Maximal dilation is 10 centimeters. A doctor or nurse monitors labor by manually checking how thin and how dilated the cervix is (see figure 90).

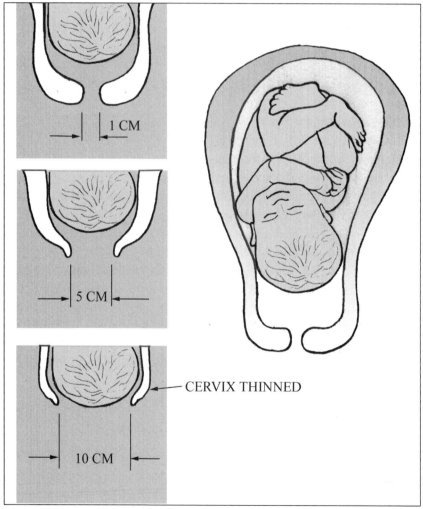

CERVIX THINNED

Figure 90

What is the "afterbirth?"

The afterbirth is the placenta expelled from the uterus after delivery of the baby. Sometimes, the postpartum blood loss with the afterbirth can be dramatic. Since the uterus is made primarily of smooth muscle geared for long, slow contractions, ergot drugs, which stimulate smooth muscle, are used to squeeze the uterus and stop the bleeding.

Ergots were discovered in the Middle Ages, when people ate bread contaminated with a fungus that made the substance. Because smooth muscle is also found in the walls of arteries, the victims who ate the contaminated bread suffered extreme arterial constriction that cut off the blood supply to their arms and legs. Without a blood supply, the arms would slowly die in burning pain, turn black, and fall off as if they were burned off, a process that spawned the nickname St. Anthony's Fire.

What's a Caesarian birth?

If a mother cannot deliver through the cervix and vagina, the baby has to be cut out through the abdominal and uterine walls. Lots of things can forestall a normal delivery. For example, the placenta may have implanted at the bottom of the uterus, plugging up the opening to the cervix. The baby may be lying crosswise instead of head down. The baby may be suffering bouts of inadequate blood flow from the placenta. The baby's head may be too big to fit through the pelvis. Twins may have stretched the uterus so much that the uterus cannot generate sufficient muscular contractions to push out the babies.

Because the uterus is so vascular, Caesarian deliveries (C-sections) are quite bloody, but doctors have been performing them with pretty good success for thousands of years. (It's unclear where the term came from, as Julius Caesar was probably not born by Caesarian section.)

What is preeclampsia?

In about 1 in 20 pregnancies, during the final 3 months, the blood pressure starts to rise, the kidneys start to spill protein into the urine, and the arteries around the body, including those feeding the placenta, go into spasm (constriction). If the spasm is great enough, blood flow to the placenta drops off and the placenta loses its ability to deliver oxygen and nutrients to the developing fetus. To prevent permanent damage to the mother and the fetus, obstetricians will sometimes halt the pregnancy by inducing labor with intravenous oxytocin or by performing a Caesarian section.

What's an ectopic pregnancy?

An ectopic pregnancy is one in which the fertilized egg implants outside the uterus. Almost always, the site is in one of the fallopian tubes, which is called a tubal pregnancy. In a tubal pregnancy, the growing fetus quickly runs out of room. The stretching of the fallopian tube causes tremendous pain, and eventually the growing fetus tears the fallopian tube, often with a great deal of bleeding, which can be fatal. An ectopic pregnancy can also (rarely) occur elsewhere in the abdomen.

What's an abortion?

An abortion is the removal of the fetus from inside the uterus. The fetus can be suctioned off or scraped off with an instrument inserted through the vagina and cervix into the uterus. One of the risks of an abortion is perforation (puncture) of the uterine wall, which becomes quite soft because of new blood vessels growing into the uterine wall, especially around the placenta.

What is menopause?

By the time a woman reaches her late 40s, the ovaries are slowing up their production of estrogen. The reasons for this are unclear. By age 50 or so, the estrogen levels fall so low that the uterine wall cannot undergo its monthly cycle, and menstruation stops.

What is the clitoris?

During fetal development, a nubbin of sexually sensitive tissue goes on to become the head of the penis—the glans (acorn in Latin)—in boys and the clitoris in girls. While this is happening, two flaps of skin are fusing together to become the scrotal sac in boys. In girls, these flaps remain apart to form labia (lips in Latin) at the entrance to the vagina. During sex, the clitoris, much like the penis, becomes engorged.

What is the hymen?

The hymen is a thin membrane covering the entrance to the vagina that is permanently obliterated once sexual activity begins.

What are sexually transmitted diseases?

There are a dozen or so diseases whose primary means of invasion is through some type of sexual contact. Some are more dangerous than others, some are incurable, most are prevented by wearing some protection, such as a condom over the man's penis or a vaginal condom for a woman, and all require treatment of both partners to prevent reinfection.

Syphilis (pronounced SIFF-liss) is a nasty disease because it infects every organ system of the body and can display virtually any symptom. It's also a sneaky disease because it begins as a painless sore on the penis or vagina days or weeks after sexual contact, long after you think to associate the sore with the person who gave it to you. The sore disappears without any treatment, so you're lulled into thinking it's no big deal. However, the syphilis has merely gone underground and will reemerge weeks later as a rash on the palms and soles of the feet, maybe with some achiness and fever. The rash, too, eventually resolves as syphilis submerges again; only this time it reemerges, often years later, in the brain and spinal cord. Syphilis in a pregnant woman is particularly bad news for the fetus. One of the two good things about syphilis is that it cannot live outside the human body, so you can't get it from toilet seats, towels, or rubbing against a syphilitic's clothing. The other good thing about syphilis is that it can be killed by penicillin.

Chlamydia, gonorrhea, and trichomonas are three common but relatively treatable diseases that produce irritation and a cloudy discharge from the vagina or penis. If not treated promptly, each can lead to a chronic infection that spreads up into the fallopian tubes and leaves them scarred. With eggs stranded in the fallopian tubes, the woman becomes sterile (unable to have children). Babies born to mothers with gonorrhea are at high risk of serious eye infections. Since gonorrhea is often difficult to confirm by culture of the vaginal fluids, dilute silver nitrate or an antibiotic is routinely placed in a newborn's eyes to kill any potential gonorrhea bacteria. Doctors have been placing dilute silver nitrate in babies' eyes since the 1880s, when Dr. Carl Crede, a German obstetrician, demonstrated the effectiveness of this treatment in preventing damaging eye infections in newborns.

Herpes, in contrast, is incurable because it's caused by a virus that hunkers down inside nerves, outside the reach of antibiotics, and every so often emerges onto the skin as a crop of painful open sores. You can shorten the period of painful ulcers with acyclovir and similar antibiotics, but you can't stop them. Herpes cannot live outside the body, and thus it requires sexual contact to spread. Unfortunately, you can pass on the virus even if you're feeling fine and have no sores on your skin.

Genital warts (or venereal warts) are also viral in origin and therefore incurable. Sometimes, if the warts get really big, a surgeon can freeze or laser them off, but they often grow back.

Hepatitis B is another sexually transmitted, incurable virus, one that viciously attacks the liver, often leading to cirrhosis. Fortunately, there's a vaccine for hepatitis B.

HIV is another incurable virus you want to avoid at all costs. While it doesn't live outside the body, the stakes are pretty high when engaging in unprotected sex with someone who might harbor the virus.

Lice are tiny insects that itch like crazy. They're visible with the naked eye and so are the tiny white eggs (nits) they lay in the hair. Lice live by grabbing the skin with tiny claws (lice are also called crabs) and sucking the victim's blood. Being insects, they can live on a person's bedding and towels, so the contact with an infected person does not have to be intimate for the lice to be spread.

13

~~~∿∿∿∿∿∿∿∿~~~

HEMATOLOGIC SYSTEM

There are four components to blood: red blood cells, white blood cells, platelets, and proteins.

What is hemoglobin?

Hemoglobin is a protein that carries oxygen in the bloodstream. Each hemoglobin molecule is a conglomerate of four globins—proteins—each of which contains a smaller molecule of heme, which in turn cradles a single iron atom. The iron atom is where a molecule of oxygen binds, so each hemoglobin molecule binds four oxygen molecules. Hemoglobin picks up oxygen in the lungs, where it is plentiful, and releases it in the peripheral tissues, where oxygen is depleted. When you think about it, this is pretty remarkable. Why should a hemoglobin molecule that has grabbed oxygen in the lungs and carried it safely through the heart, aorta, arteries, arterioles, and finally into very thin-walled capillaries suddenly decide to give the oxygen up in the peripheral tissues? The trigger for the release of the first oxygen molecule is the low oxygen level in peripheral tissues. As soon as the first oxygen molecule is released by a globin, the other three globins suddenly change shape, making it more difficult for them to hold on to their oxygen molecules. Conversely, when hemoglobin returns to the lungs to pick up more oxygen, as soon as one oxygen molecule latches onto a globin complex, the other three globins change shape to make it easier for oxygen to attach to them. In other words, hemoglobin is spring-loaded to discharge oxygen in the oxygen-deprived periphery and spring-loaded to bind oxygen in the oxygen-rich lungs.

Is the iron in hemoglobin the reason we need iron in our diet?

Yes. Without iron, we can't make hemoglobin, and our blood count drops—we become anemic. Women are particularly vulnerable to iron deficiency anemia, as they lose iron every month during their period.

Does hemoglobin just float free in the bloodstream?

No. Hemoglobin molecules are carried inside red blood cells because the molecules are small enough by themselves to slip through the kidneys' glomeruli into the urine as hemoglobinuria. Before long, so much hemoglobin would pass into the urine that you'd become anemic. Also, all those hemoglobin proteins would clog up the kidney tubules, and the heme part of hemoglobin would stimulate a kidney-damaging inflammatory reaction.

Why does your skin turn black and blue after you get injured?

A black and blue mark is a bruise, in medical terms, a contusion. Blood released into the skin is broken down into iron, heme, and globin. Heme is broken down to bilirubin, which stains the skin (bilirubin is the same chemical that's mixed with metabolites of cholesterol to make bile).

Why is carbon monoxide so dangerous?

Carbon monoxide results from burning anything containing carbon in the presence of insufficient oxygen, so instead of two oxygen molecules attaching to carbon to form carbon dioxide, only one is attached to form carbon monoxide. Carbon monoxide binds to the iron in hemoglobin much more tightly than oxygen. Once carbon monoxide fills up all the oxygen-binding sites in hemoglobin, forget about breathing, because it won't do you any good. Breathing 100% oxygen will eventually displace carbon monoxide off the hemoglobin, but the fastest way to displace carbon monoxide is to get into a hyperbaric chamber where the atmospheric (and oxygen) pressure can be raised high enough for oxygen to successfully fight carbon monoxide for the hemoglobin-binding sites.

It's easy to be killed by carbon monoxide, because it's odorless. Water-skiers have been killed by carbon monoxide while waiting in the water behind their tow boats with the outboard engine running. What's doubly dangerous about carbon monoxide is that the victims look nice and pink, not dusky and blue, even though they're dying from lack of oxygen. Hemoglobin turns a bright red whether it binds oxygen or carbon monoxide. In fact, the tip-off to carbon monoxide poisoning is that the victim's lips are too red. Be careful around anything that burns, for example, improperly adjusted gas space heaters producing too much carbon monoxide, fireplaces producing carbon monoxide-laden smoke into a leaky chimney, or automobiles with leaky exhaust systems. Always use a carbon monoxide detector around potential sources of carbon monoxide, because you may not recognize your headache and sleepiness as early symptoms of carbon monoxide poisoning.

What's the difference between plasma and serum?

Plasma is blood and its clotting proteins, but without the red cells, white cells, or platelets. Serum is plasma without the clotting proteins. The easiest way to obtain serum is to draw a test tube of blood from a vein and let it sit for awhile to let the blood clot ("serus" is Latin for late, referring to the last part of the blood to remain after clotting). Now spin the test tube in a centrifuge. The mixture of red blood cells, white blood cells, platelets, and blood clot will sink to the bottom of the test tube, leaving in the supernatant a thin, straw-colored serum.

It was only 100 years ago that blood transfusions were finally recognized as the correct treatment of shock. (Prior to that time, shock was thought to be a neurologic problem requiring stimulants such as strychnine.) In their desperate search for a way to keep blood from clotting after being collected in a glass bottle, researchers soon found that citrate, by binding up the calcium in the blood, prevented clotting. The easiest way, then, to obtain plasma is to draw blood and place it in a tube containing citrate, which binds up calcium and prevents blood from clotting. The supernatant left after centrifuging this tube of blood is plasma, containing the clotting factors.

How does the blood know when to clot?

A dozen or more clotting proteins float around the blood, delicately balanced between clotting the blood quickly when an artery, vein, or capillary springs a leak, and not clotting until the leak occurs. In a typical scenario, damaged tissue cells expose a previously hidden surface protein called tissue factor, which triggers a sudden cascade of other proteins to form a complex net of fibrin strands. Meanwhile, the leaking vein is immediately sealed up by platelets, little sticky chemically complex packets floating free in the bloodstream looking for holes in arteries and veins to plug. An adherent clump of platelets releases a signal to the clotting proteins to start clotting around it.

How does aspirin work to thin the blood?

Aspirin prevents platelets from sticking to each other, which delays blood from clotting.

Are there other ways to thin the blood?

Yes, with a drug called heparin or another drug called warfarin. Heparin was discovered in 1916 by medical student Jay McLean, who was actually looking for a substance that accelerated blood clotting. It took another 20 years before Charles Best, the codiscoverer of insulin, devised ways to produce heparin in quantity. Heparin works by wrapping itself around and inactivating a number of the clotting factors.

Warfarin was discovered in the 1940s under the auspices of the Wisconsin Alumni Research Foundation at the University of Wisconsin, after cows started dropping dead from internal hemorrhage after eating clover contaminated with a fungus. When the scientists isolated the chemical being produced by the fungus, they named it Warfarin, after the foundation. Warfarin works by blocking the action of vitamin K, the vitamin necessary for the production of the clotting factors by the liver. Warfarin is the active ingredient in some common rat poisons.

What are clot busters?

In addition to proteins that form blood clots, there are other proteins in the blood that dissolve, or bust up, blood clots as soon as they form. Smoking inhibits the release of these natural clot-busting proteins from the endothelium of arteries. If a doctor can get to a patient in the early stages of stroke or heart attack, she can administer a clot buster and, if God is good, dissolve the clot and reestablish circulation to brain or heart tissue teetering on the brink of dying from lack of blood.

Are there things that make the blood more likely to clot?

Yes, lots of things. Some people are born with defective or insufficient clot-dissolving proteins. Some diseases make proteins that trigger blood clotting. Smoking increases the level of clotting factors in the blood-stream and markedly activates platelets to clot the blood. Estrogen raises the risk of blood clotting. So does anything that slows the circulation of blood, such as sitting on a plane or in a car for a long time.

What does blood type mean?

On the surface of red blood cells are slots for two specific proteins, A and B. What proteins fill those slots determines a person's blood type. Some people fill the slots with only A proteins, some with only B proteins, some with a mixture of A and B, and some with neither, making their blood type O.

Why does your blood need to be typed when donating or receiving blood?

People with type A blood automatically have anti-B antibodies, and people with type B blood automatically have anti-A antibodies. O blood harbors both anti-A and anti-B antibodies, while type AB blood makes neither. If a person with type A blood (containing anti-B antibodies) receives type B blood, the anti-B antibodies will clump the type B red blood cells. The clumped red blood cells clog up small arteries, and as the clumps of red blood cells are destroyed, the hemoglobin inside is released. Free hemoglobin in the bloodstream damages the kidneys, resulting in kidney failure. The clumping of red blood cells from mismatched blood is called a transfusion reaction (it's also called a lawsuit).

On the upside, if your blood is AB, you can receive A or B blood, because you have no antibodies against either. If your blood type is O, you can't receive any blood but O because you have both anti-A and anti-B antibodies. However, if your blood type is A, B, AB, or O, you can always receive type O blood because with neither A nor B on its surface, anti-A and anti-B antibodies have no effect on type O red blood cells. So type O blood is the universal donor, and AB blood is the universal recipient, because it can receive A, B, AB, or O blood.

Why does type A blood automatically have anti-B antibodies if the person has never received type B or AB blood?

It's thought that A and B antigens are contained in the food we eat. People with type A blood only make antibodies against the B antigens they eat, because, to them, only the B antigen is foreign.

What is Rh factor?

Rh is another protein antigen on the surface of red blood cells. It's either there and you're Rh positive or it's not and you're Rh negative. Rh is not as irritating to the immune system as the A and B antigens, so in an emergency an Rh negative person can receive Rh positive blood. The real problem with Rh incompatibility occurs in pregnant women. Suppose a pregnant Rh negative mother gives birth to an Rh positive baby. During delivery, when the placenta pulls away from the uterine wall, the inter-mingled blood vessels of the placenta and uterine wall are torn open, allowing the baby's blood to enter the mother's circulation. Seeing this new Rh antigen, the Rh negative mother now makes antibodies against it. No big deal until she has another pregnancy. If the next fetus is Rh negative, the mother's antibodies won't have anything in the fetus to attack. But if the second fetus is Rh positive, look out. Antibodies against Rh in the mother will cross the placenta and attack the Rh positive red blood cells of the fetus. Not only will the fetus become anemic, but worse than that, the hemoglobin will be released from the red blood cells. Free hemoglobin in a fetus is terrible, because the heme part of the hemoglobin is converted to bilirubin, which enters the fetal brain and causes serious damage. The babies are born retarded, deaf, and seizing.

How do you prevent this tragedy?

Simple. When an Rh negative mother gives birth to an Rh positive baby, give her a shot of antibodies against Rh. Because those antibodies attach to the Rh antigen before the mother's white blood cells can spot them, the mother's white blood cells won't make antibodies against Rh antigen. So, if the mother's second fetus is Rh positive, the mother won't have any antibodies against Rh antigen to cross the placenta and attack the fetus's Rh positive red blood cells.

What is sickle cell anemia?

Sickle cells are red blood cells that curl up into the shape of a sickle when they give up their oxygen molecules in peripheral tissues. Normal red blood cells remain round with a gentle depression in the middle. The reason for the sickle shape is genetic: the hemoglobin has an incorrect amino acid in it that causes the hemoglobin molecule to fold up incorrectly when it releases its oxygen. Sickled red blood cells have a short life span, so the kids become anemic. Also, the sickle shape is ideal for stacking—like a box of Pringle's potato chips—which is exactly what the red cells do. The stacked red blood cells sludge in small arteries and veins, and the sludging triggers the blood to clot, resulting in loss of circulation to the hands and feet, and sometimes the internal organs.

Where is blood made?

In the bone marrow. The next time you eat a chicken leg, look at the dark reddish knob at the tip of the leg bone. That soft chewy interior is bone marrow. Not every bone has marrow, but most do. The bone marrow is a busy place, making red blood cells, white blood cells, and platelets. This rapid production of cells makes the bone marrow particularly vulnerable to anticancer drugs that inhibit the growth of rapidly growing cells. When giving chemotherapy, doctors have to constantly monitor the red cell, white cell, and platelet counts in the blood to ensure the bone marrow is not being suppressed too much.

How do you know if you're anemic?

Being anemic means you don't have enough red blood cells. The easiest way to measure the red cell count is to take a test tube of blood and spin it in a centrifuge. All the red cells settle to the bottom, and by measuring the height of the red blood cells and comparing their height to the height of the entire column of blood (including the supernatant serum), one can easily figure out the percentage of red blood cells in the blood. That's the hematocrit. For a man, a normal hematocrit is 39% to 45%, and for a woman it is 36% to 43%.

How do they measure the platelets in the blood?

Platelets are counted. There should be between 150,000 and 500,000 platelets per cubic millimeter of blood.

What about white blood cells?

Look again at the centrifuged tube of blood. Lying on top of the column of red blood cells is a thin, white layer. The early investigators naturally called the cells in this layer white cells. There should be 5,000 to 10,000 white blood cells per cubic millimeter of blood. More than that suggests an infection or inflammation somewhere in the body.

Are all white blood cells alike?

In general, there are three things white cells have to do, and there's a white cell for each job. The first is to initiate attacks against foreign antigens. This is done by white blood cells called neutrophils, or poly-morphonuclear cells, because of their multishaped nuclei (poly = many, morpho = shape) (see figure 91). The second job is to continue the inflammatory battle after the polys have died in the first wave of attack. This job is handled by white cells called mononuclear cells (or lym-phocytes) because of their simple-shaped nuclei. Some of these mononuclear cells are specialized to make antibodies against the foreign protein, while others are specialized to devour the foreign protein. Both types of lymphocytes remember the antigen to enable a more rapid immunologic response next time. The third job is to clean up the debris from the inflammatory battle. This is done by white blood cells called macrophages.

The orchestration of an immunologic attack involves a lot, I mean a *lot*, of chemicals. Think about what has to be done. Individual white blood cells, which only know how to move and engulf antigens, have to know when and where to leave the bloodstream, crawl to wherever they're needed, find what needs to be eaten, eat it, drag the victim to a lymph node where other white blood cells can analyze it, call up an army of more white blood cells to attack, and remember the culprit for future attack. *I* couldn't do all that, so how is a brainless white cell going to do that? Chemicals at every step—from adhesion molecules along blood vessel walls that nab white blood cells floating in the bloodstream, to cytokines, lymphokines, interleukins, tumor necrosis factors, colony-stimulating factors, interferon, and others—direct white blood cells' movements and production.

A lot of diseases do their damage simply by causing inflammation. In those cases, even without knowing what's precipitating the inflammation, doctors can stop the disease if they can just stop the inflammation. Because there are so many steps involved in mounting an inflammatory attack, there are lots of targets to block an inflammatory response. For example, investigators are trying to reduce the bronchial

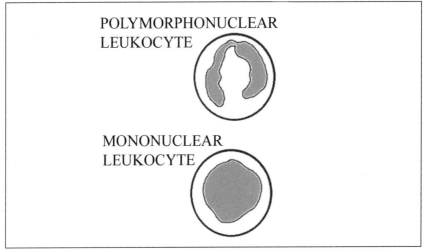

POLYMORPHONUCLEAR
LEUKOCYTE

MONONUCLEAR
LEUKOCYTE

Figure 91

inflammation of asthma by blocking the chemicals that snag circulating white blood cells from the bloodstream.

Do red blood cells live forever?

No. Red cells live only three months, in large part because they have no nucleus and therefore no DNA to make repairs as the cell's equipment deteriorates. After about three months, red cells are destroyed in the spleen and the hemoglobin is removed. After the iron is removed from the heme molecule, the heme is sent to the liver to be metabolized (chemically changed) into greenish-brown bilirubin. Bilirubin is mixed with several metabolites of cholesterol to form bile, which is stored in the gallbladder for the next fatty meal.

Where is the spleen?

Feel the bottom of your rib cage on the left side about in line with your arm pit (axilla). The spleen is right behind those lower ribs (see figure 92). The spleen needs the protection of a bony cage because it has the consistency of a soft sponge. Trauma can easily rupture the spleen, which is loaded with blood, and because of the spleen's spongy architecture, the bleeding will often continue until the patient dies or a surgeon urgently operates to remove the spleen (a procedure called a splenectomy). People without spleens do very well; their livers take over responsibility for removing dead and dying red blood cells from the bloodstream.

What is blood poisoning?

Blood poisoning means that bacteria have gained access to the bloodstream. The scientific name is sepsis. White blood cells go crazy when they detect bacteria in their home territory, and they release lots of potent proteins to alert the rest of the immune system. One of these proteins tells the brain to raise the body temperature. Another potent protein causes blood vessels to leak plasma and white blood cells into the body's tissues to find the invading bacterium. Pretty soon, the leaking blood vessels cause the blood pressure to drop. If it drops so much that the brain and other internal organs do not get enough blood, the patient is in septic shock.

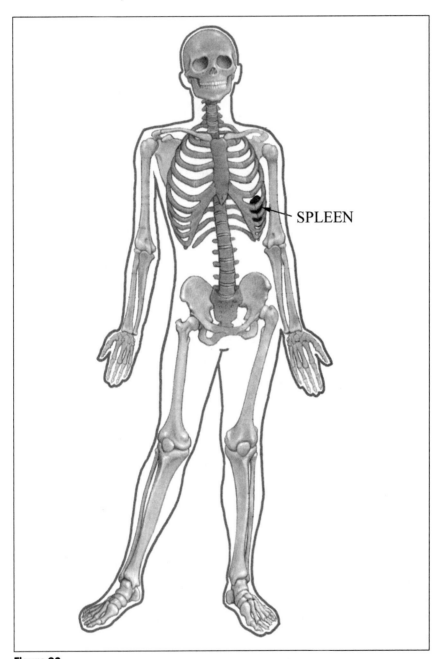

SPLEEN

Figure 92

What's leukemia?

Leukemia is cancer of the white blood cells ("leuko" means white in Greek). The type of leukemia is named after the white blood cell line that is reproducing out of control—for example, myelogenous leukemia for polymorphonuclear cells, and lymphocytic leukemia for lymphocytes. Cancer of the antibody-producing cells is called multiple myeloma.

If you get leukemia, why can't you just kill all the white blood cells?

If you can kill all the white blood cells—and that's a big if—you have the immediate problem of fighting infection. You can put the patient in a sterile environment, but what do you do about all the bacteria in the colon? If they get into the bloodstream, the patient has no white blood cells to defend himself with. Antibiotics don't kill all bacteria and, in fact, the bacteria that do survive antibiotics are, by definition, so powerful that antibiotics can't kill them.

One solution is to kill all the white blood cells with total body radiation, and then to give the patient healthy white blood cells that, hopefully, will take up residence in the bone marrow and begin defending the patient against infections. The problem with this approach is that any white blood cells given to the patient must come from another healthy person whose white blood cells will look at their new host and recognize immediately that the host is foreign and needs to be destroyed. The ensuing attack is called graft versus host reaction. The best way to minimize graft versus host reaction is to take white blood cells from a twin sibling whose genetic makeup is identical to the patient's.

What's hemophilia?

Hemophilia is an X-linked genetic disorder affecting one of the clotting proteins, factor VIII. Without factor VIII, the blood cannot form a firm clot, and with the slightest trauma these kids bleed into their joints or just about anywhere. The treatment is periodic infusions of clotting factors from blood donors.

14

BONES AND JOINTS

Bones provide a giant storehouse of calcium, a manufacturing site for blood, and of course, support against gravity. Fish, in contrast to humans, get away with very thin bones by taking advantage of the buoyancy of water to support their weight.

Why don't toddlers break more bones, with all the falling they do?

Because infants don't yet stand up, their bones don't need a lot of calcium to make them strong. Instead, a baby's bones are primarily cartilage, which is a lot less brittle than calcified bone. Only later, as toddlers develop into youngsters, do the bones fully calcify. With so much pliable cartilage in their bones, toddlers don't suffer as many broken bones as you'd expect, considering all the falling they do.

What's rickets?

Toddlers' bones calcify by laying down calcium on a cartilaginous framework, or matrix, with the help of vitamin D. If calcium is not laid down, as occurs in rickets, the bones remain cartilaginously soft and the children become bowlegged. Also, without adequate calcium, the bones don't grow well and the children tend to be short. Vitamin D assures an adequate supply of calcium by helping the intestines absorb calcium and preventing the kidneys from excreting it. Sources of vitamin D include milk, salmon, sardines, and my favorite, eel. While you're eating breakfast cereal, check the nutrition label for the amount of vitamin D. We need about 400 international units per day. Another very good source of vitamin D is sunlight, because the sun's ultraviolet rays stimulate the synthesis of vitamin D in the skin (as well as melanomas, unfortunately).

What's the difference between rickets and osteoporosis?

In rickets, there's inadequate calcium being laid down on the bones' cartilaginous matrix. In osteoporosis, both the calcium and the underlying matrix are lost. Here's how. Our bones are continually being remodeled in response to demands made on them to support the body's weight. If we don't use our bones, the matrix and the calcium are resorbed. For this reason, heavy plaster casts help broken bones heal faster by forcing the broken arm or leg to lift the heavy cast. Bone resorption is a real problem for astronauts, people confined to bed, people with paralyzed limbs— anyone whose limbs are not used for long periods. The things that keep your bones packed with calcium are plenty of vitamin D, exercise, not smoking, having no more than 2 drinks of alcohol a day, and for women, estrogen, which is why estrogen replacement after menopause is helpful in maintaining a woman's bone density.

Why do young athletic women sometimes develop thinning of the bones (osteopenia)?

Estrogen is necessary to build strong bones densely packed with calcium. In women, estrogen is generally plentiful—unless the hypothalamus fails to tell the pituitary gland to secrete follicle-stimulating hormone, leaving the ovaries without instructions to secrete estrogen. This hypothalamic lapse occurs when the brain becomes aware that not enough food is being eaten to meets the body's energy needs—as if the brain were trying to conserve the body's energy by sacrificing reproduction and stopping the menstrual cycle. Such situations arise when a young woman decides to severely curtail her food intake because she feels she is too fat (anorexia nervosa) or because she is trying to succeed in physically demanding activities that cherish thinness, such as gymnastics, long-distance running, figure skating, ballet, swimming, and cycling. An early sign of falling estrogen production in athletic or anorectic women is the termination of menstrual periods (amenorrhea), while in young girls it is the failure to begin menstrual periods. Without estrogen and without an adequate diet of calcium, phosphorous (bone is calcium phosphate), citric acid, vitamin D, and other nutrients, the bones fail to lay down a dense calcium matrix. If bones don't form a dense calcium matrix by the time they stop growing (somewhere around 20 to 25 years of age), they cannot make up the deficiency later in life. The bones remain thin for the rest of the person's life. The situation is worsened by smoking, which impairs the function of estrogen, and by alcohol, which interferes with the laying down of new bone. The only real solution is to increase nutrition and lighten up on exercise. Even though the problem is low estrogen levels, estrogen pills alone are ineffective in restoring bone density to normal, because other, as yet unknown, factors contribute to the osteopenia. For example, there is some evidence that leptin, the chemical indicator of fat stores, participates in bone growth. In women aggressively trying to shed all fat, the falling leptin levels may interfere with proper bone growth. Young girls must drink plenty of milk, get plenty of sunshine to make vitamin D, and engage in sports and athletics to make their bones densely calcified, but overdoing the exercise or dieting excessively may cause fragile bones later in life.

What is a stress fracture?

A stress fracture is a tiny crack in the surface of a bone occurring with vigorous physical activity as shock-absorbing muscles fatigue. Any bone can suffer a stress fracture with a repetitive activity such as marching, but osteoporotic bones are particularly susceptible. The treatment of a stress fracture is to rest the bone and let it heal by itself.

Where do you find cartilage in the body?

Cartilage forms the flexible part of the nose and the ears. Cartilage also lines the surfaces of bones in joints. Covered with a little mucus, two cartilages in a joint can rub against each other very smoothly. As we age, however, joint cartilage thins out and pain develops as bones rub against bones. Another place cartilage is found is between the vertebral bodies, the bony cubes that stack up to make our spinal column. In between the vertebral bodies is a slab of cartilage, called an intervertebral disc ("inter" means between), that gives the spine flexibility and cushions it when we jump up and down.

What's a slipped disc?

Intervertebral discs don't actually slip, but they do crack, allowing the center of the disc to ooze out. A disc is constructed like a toilet seat, with a firm outer rim and a soft mushy center. As we age and suffer repeated back trauma over the years, cracks develop in the outer rim, allowing the squishy center to squeeze out through the cracks like toothpaste. This leakage of disc material is called disc herniation. Disc herniation is generally not painful unless the herniated disc material presses against a nerve root coming out of the spinal cord, called a pinched nerve (see figure 93). Injury to a nerve root is called a radiculopathy. A disc herniation in the neck causes a cervical radiculopathy, and a disc herniation in the low back causes a lumbar radiculopathy, while a disc herniation lower would cause a sacral radiculopathy. Cervical nerve roots leave the spinal cord to supply the muscles of the arm, while lumbosacral nerve roots are headed to the muscles of the leg. This is why the pain of a cervical radiculopathy radiates from the neck into the arm and the pain of a lumbosacral radiculopathy radiates down the leg.

What's the difference between a ligament and a tendon?

A ligament is a tough band of tissue that holds bones together. People with lax ligaments can move their joints through a wide range of motion, meaning they are double-jointed. During pregnancy, a hormone called relaxin is released by the placenta to loosen the ligaments holding the bones of the pelvis together, which accommodates the growing baby and allows its head to slip through the pelvis during birth.

The discovery of relaxin is a perfect example of an observant person asking why. Frederick Hisaw, a zoologist in the 1920s and 1930s, was investigating the pocket gopher, which had become a pest in the area.

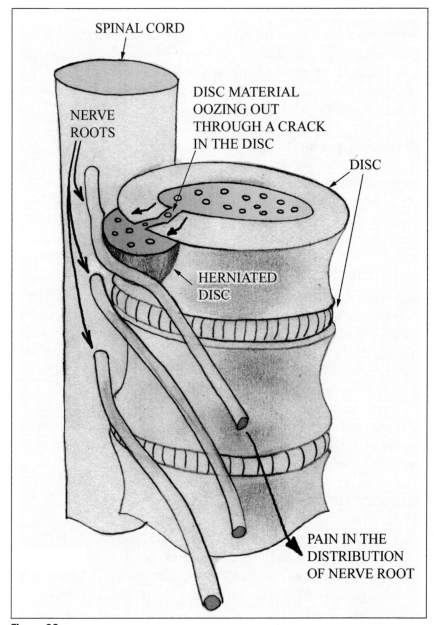

Figure 93

Hisaw noticed something odd: some of the gophers had a gap between two of their pelvic bones. Why was this, he asked? Further observation led Hisaw to discover that the gap widened at the time of delivery. It was not long before he and his colleagues tracked down relaxin.

The most commonly injured ligaments are in the knee, where four ligaments hold the femur against the tibia—two on the outside of the knee joint and two within the knee joint. The two ligaments on the outside of the knee joint are the medial collateral ligament, along the inner side of the knee joint, and the lateral collateral ligament, along the outside of the knee joint (see figure 94). The two ligaments deep within the knee joint are the anterior and posterior cruciate ligaments ("cruciate" means crossed because the anterior and posterior cruciate ligaments form an X).

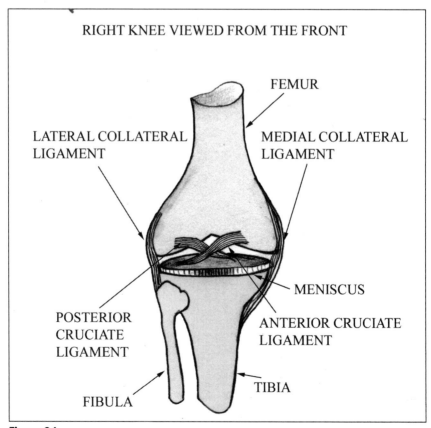

Figure 94

The purpose of muscles is to move bones. Muscles attach to the bones by narrowing into rope-like tendons that you can easily feel and see. For example, as you make a fist and wiggle your fingers, look at and feel the tendons crossing the front and back of your wrist en route to the fingers. Other easily felt tendons are behind the knee as you bend the knee against resistance (the hamstring muscle tendons), the quadriceps tendon above and below the knee cap (patella), and of course the Achilles tendon, connecting the gastrocnemius muscle in the calf to the calcaneus (heel) bone in the foot. So ligaments attach bone to bone and tendons attach muscle to bone.

What's the medial meniscus in the knee joint?

When bones come together at a joint, the surfaces of the bones are covered with a layer of cartilage that is lubricated with synovial fluid. In the knee, the weight placed on the tibia is so great that a thick slab of cartilage, called the meniscus, covers the top of the tibia (see figure 94). The inside section of the meniscus is the medial meniscus and the outside section is the lateral meniscus.

What's a bursa?

A bursa is a tiny pillow of fluid around joints, positioned to allow tendons to slide over them.

What's a ganglion?

A ganglion is a cyst (bubble) of fluid on a tendon, usually a tendon on the back of the hand. On occasion, ganglions form over a joint. Ganglions are treated by sucking out the fluid with a needle, or, when that fails, surgery.

How many bones are there in the human body?

An orthopedic surgeon was once asked this question on the witness stand by an attorney hoping to discredit his testimony. The orthopedist responded that he didn't know, but he was happy to name them all while the attorney kept count.

Beginning in the skull, note that the back of the skull curves in quite high, at about the level of the nose. Below the little bump on the back of the skull (the occipital notch) are other bumps, called spinous processes, fins of bone running down the spine attached to each vertebral body. The first cervical (neck) vertebra is the atlas because it, like the mythical Atlas holding the world on his shoulders, holds up the globe of the skull. The skull and the atlas rotate as a unit around the second vertebra—the axis. The most prominent spinous process is the 7th cervical vertebrae, at the base of the neck. The shoulder blade, or scapula, rests on the back of the chest wall. The clavicle, or collar bone, stretches between the sternum (breastbone) and a small part of the scapula peeking over the shoulder called the acromion. The purpose of the clavicle is to stabilize the shoulder joint when the arm is pushing, pulling, and lifting heavy objects. (The shape of the clavicle resembles an old-fashioned clavis, or key in Latin.) The upper ribs also insert on the sternum, while the lower ribs insert on a piece of cartilage attached to the sternum. The lowest ribs—the floating ribs—don't reach all the way to the sternum. The upper arm bone is the humerus, which connects to two bones in the forearm: the ulna and the radius. Having two bones in the forearm allows us to flip-flop our hands and twist a screwdriver: the ulna bone remains stationary while the radius rotates at its base near the elbow, flip-flopping the distal part of the radius over the ulna. (Distal means far away from the center of the body; proximal means close to the center of the body.)

At your waist, you should be able to feel the brim of the pelvis, the ilium, and be able to trace it back to the flat sacral bone at the bottom of the spine. Where the ilium and sacrum join is the sacroiliac joint, which you can't feel but which often hurts when arthritis sets in. At the bottom of the sacrum you can feel your tailbone, or coccyx, named after the beak of the cuckoo (cuckoo in Greek is "coccyx").

In the leg, the head of the femur rotates in a basin called the acetabulum (which apparently resembled an old vinegar cup, as "acetum" is Latin for vinegar and "abulum" is Latin for a small cup.) The bone protruding from your hip is not the hip joint but a bony projection of the femur called the greater trochanter ("trochanter" means runner in Greek). The bottom of the femur forms the upper part of the knee joint.

The main bone in the lower leg is the tibia. The thin fibula bone lateral (away from the midline) to the tibia functions more as a place for muscles to attach than as a supporting structure. Together, the tibia and fibula look like a brooch, which is what fibula means in Latin. The bottom of the fibula forms the outside ankle, or lateral malleolus, and the bottom of the tibia forms the inside ankle, or medial malleolus ("malleolus" means little hammer in Latin; recall the malleus bone, or hammer, in the middle ear).

What's the soft spot on a baby's scalp?

The soft spot is a large gap between plates of skull bones resting atop the brain. A baby's brain needs elbow room inside the skull to finish growing. To accommodate this, the baby's skull is not a single bone but seven separate bones floating free. The large triangular gap between the four largest plates (two frontal and two parietal) is called the soft spot, or fontanelle (see figure 95). By gently resting your finger on the fontanelle, you can feel pulsations of the brain as blood is pumped through it ("fontanelle" means small fountain in Latin). Once the brain stops increasing in size at about age 12, the skull plates fuse together, forming sutures between them. Two of the sutures, one down the middle from front to back and the other from ear to ear, can readily be seen on a closely shaven head. If, for some reason, one of the sutures closes before the brain has fully grown, the growing brain will bulge out whatever part of the skull is still unfused, causing quite a cosmetic problem. To correct the distortion, a neurosurgeon will operate and remove the fused suture. The new edges of the skull bone eventually grow together after the skull has had time to establish its normal shape.

How does our jaw open and close?

Right in front of your ear, feel the joint where the jaw is hinged. Now feel it better by sticking your index finger into your ear canal while you open and close your jaw. This joint is called the temporomandibular joint, because is connects the mandible (jaw) to the temple part of the skull.

What is lordosis?

Lordosis is the normal incurving of the spine in the neck (cervical spine) and the low back (lumbar spine).

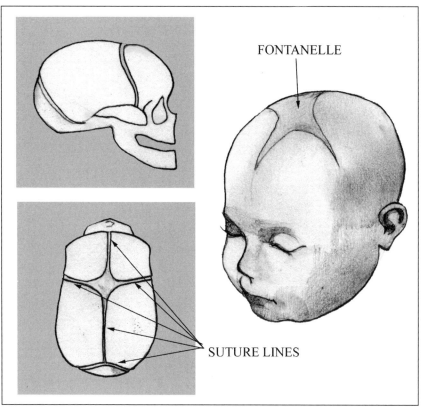

FONTANELLE

SUTURE LINES

Figure 95

What is kyphosis?

Kyphosis is an excessive front-to-back outcurving of the thoracic (chest) spine causing people to walk bent over (see figure 96). Lots of elderly people develop kyphosis as they develop osteoporosis.

What is scoliosis?

Scoliosis is a side-to-side curvature of the spine (see figure 97). There are many causes for scoliosis, including weakness of the muscles holding up the spine and abnormalities of the vertebral bones themselves.

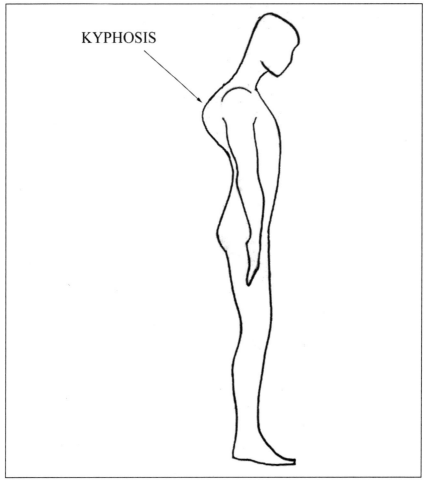

KYPHOSIS

Figure 96

What is a dislocated shoulder?

The shoulder is an inherently unstable joint because it has to allow for such a wide range of arm movement. Unlike the knee, which moves only front to back, the shoulder joint has to accommodate movement in every direction. To do this, the shoulder joint, a ball-and-socket joint, uses a very shallow socket known as the glenoid cavity, which does not grab the head of the humerus like the acetabulum does the head of the femur. To

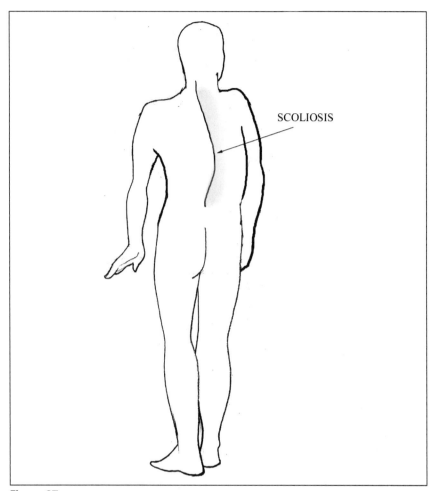

SCOLIOSIS

Figure 97

keep the head of the humerus tight against the socket, the shoulder joint relies on lots of ligaments, muscles, and tendons to hold the shoulder together. It performs wonderfully 99% of the time, but once in a while a sudden force can pop the head of the humerus out of joint. Usually, the humerus pops forward in front of the glenoid cavity, occasionally behind or below it. By manipulating the humerus just right, a doctor can slip the head of the humerus back into place.

What's the difference between a shoulder dislocation and a shoulder separation?

A shoulder separation refers to a different joint. In a shoulder separation, the collar bone, or clavicle, separates from the acromion in the shoulder.

What is a torn rotator cuff?

The intricate apparatus of ligaments, muscles, and tendons holding the head of the humerus against the glenoid cavity is called the rotator cuff. Wear and tear, or acute trauma, can inflame the rotator cuff. As part of the inflammatory response, small bits of scar tissue—adhesions—develop. If the pain is severe enough to prevent a person from using his shoulder, the adhesions can build up and restrict shoulder movement, called a frozen shoulder.

What's gout?

Gout is an extremely painful, acute inflammation of a joint due to deposition of uric acid crystals in the joint. The most common site for gout is the big toe. Uric acid, a chemical containing waste nitrogen derived from the breakdown product of DNA, normally stays in solution in the bloodstream. When the uric acid level rises too high, it crystallizes in joints.

What's a bunion?

A bunion is a bulbous protuberance around a deformed joint, usually at the base of the big toe. When a person wears high-heeled pointy shoes, the weight of the body is focused onto the base of the big toe, shoving it into the shoe and distorting the joint (see figure 98). Surgery is sometimes needed to correct the deformity and relieve the pain.

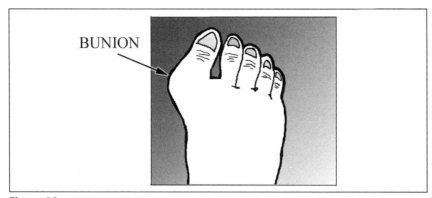

BUNION

Figure 98

15

~~~~~~~~~~~~~~

NEUROLOGIC SYSTEM

There are only two real mysteries in this world. One is the nature of the origin of the universe and the other is how the brain works.

From a distance, the brain is like an ice cream cone. The ice cream part is the cerebral hemispheres, where we do all our intellectual work, while the cone part, or brainstem—the oldest part of the brain—controls ancient functions shared by all animals: consciousness, sleep, eye movements, pupillary reaction, eye closure, facial sensation, facial movement, hearing, swallowing, articulating sounds, blood pressure, rotating the head, tongue movements, blood pressure, pulse rate, and respirations.

Each cerebral hemisphere is divided into four large sections called lobes: the frontal lobe in front, the occipital lobe in back, the parietal lobe situated between them, and the temporal lobe on the side.

Nerves that start and end in the brain or spinal cord are part of the central nervous system, while nerves that extend from the brain or spinal cord to locations out in the body are part of the peripheral nervous system.

How do nerves work?

There are something like 200 billion nerve cells in the brain, and all of them work pretty much the same way. Each has a bushy tail of dendrites, a cell body, and a single axon. Electrical signals enter a nerve cell through its dendrites ("branches of a tree" in Greek). Thousands of different nerve cells may be signaling the dendrites of a single nerve cell at any one time. If enough dendritic signals occur at the same time, the cell body fires off an electrical signal that shoots down a single axon to stimulate the dendrites of another nerve cell. The actual signal between nerve cells is chemical, not electrical. The axonal tip is loaded with tiny cannon balls of a single neurotransmitter, such as dopamine, acetylcholine, epinephrine, norepinephrine, serotonin, or GABA (see figure 99). When the axonal signal reaches the axonal tip, the cannonballs discharge their neurotransmitter onto the next nerve cell's dendrites (or directly onto its cell body). The connection between an axon and the dendrites or cell body of another neuron (nerve cell) is called a synapse. There are 50 to 100 trillion synapses in the human brain! In the peripheral nervous system, an axon stimulates a muscle to contract, almost always by releasing the neurotransmitter acetylcholine.

It took until 1921 before anyone proved that neurons release neurotransmitters. In that year, Dr. Otto Loewi dreamt the definitive experiment: bathe a spontaneously beating heart—with its nerves still attached—in a salt solution, and then stimulate the vagus nerve, the nerve that slows the heart. Then take that solution and dip another spontaneously beating heart into it—this time without any attached nerves. If the heart slows, as it did for Loewi, then the vagus must have released a neurotransmitter into the bathing solution. The neurotransmitter was later identified as acetylcholine.

Why does it take a year for a baby to start walking and two years before he or she starts talking?

Just looking at the size of a baby's head plainly indicates that a baby's brain is not fully developed. In fact, it will take another 20 years, maybe longer, to become fully developed. Much of brain development from fetus to childhood and extending through the teenage years entails migration of nerve cells to critical locations in the brain, elaborating the connections between nerve cells and upgrading the speed of communication.

Nerve cells talk to one another via axons. Like wires carrying electrical impulses, axons, too, have to be insulated from one another to prevent

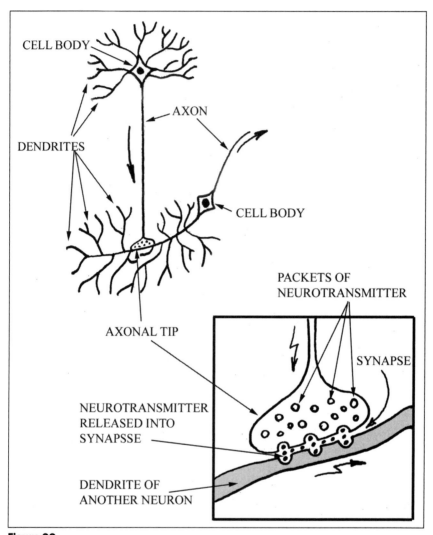

CELL BODY

DENDRITES

AXON

CELL BODY

AXONAL TIP

PACKETS OF
NEUROTRANSMITTER

SYNAPSE

NEUROTRANSMITTER
RELEASED INTO
SYNAPSSE

DENDRITE OF
ANOTHER NEURON

Figure 99

the electrical impulse from jumping—short-circuiting—to an adjacent axon. Unlike electrical insulation, however, the jacket of insulation, called myelin, around each axon also speeds electrical impulses down the axon (see figure 100). Babies don't have much myelin, but as myelin is laid down during the first few years of life, the neurologic abilities gradually improve.

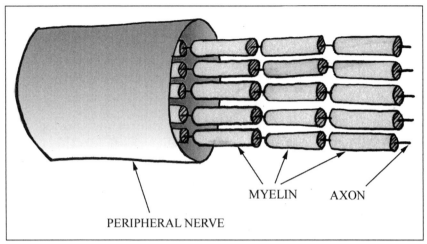

MYELIN   AXON

PERIPHERAL NERVE

Figure 100

Myelin development begins in the brain and heads south into the spinal cord. You can track the growth of myelin down the nervous system by tracing the progression of an infant's milestones down the body. By one month, an infant is tracking his parents with his eyes. By two months, he's smiling at them. By three months, his neck can fully support his head. By four months, his shoulder control is good enough that he can reach out and swipe at things. By five months, he is grasping. And by six months, his abdominal and back muscles have enough neurologic control to enable him to sit alone. Further myelination from six months until about one year can be seen as improved balance and improved finger dexterity, refining his grasp from thumb and all four fingers to, by one year of age, picking up raisins with pincer movements of his thumb and index finger.

What about the dendrites during the first few years of life?

Dendrites grow a great deal during the first four or five years of life, in fact, more than they need to. Dendrites are a nerve cell's antennae, so the more elaborate its dendrites, the more signals a nerve cell can pick up from other nerve cells. The peak of dendritic growth occurs between age 3 and age 5. After that, the dendrites begin to drop out if they're not used.

Conversely, enriched environments with plenty of stimulation keep the dendritic tree lush.

Lead is particularly harmful to toddlers and preschool children because it prunes the dendritic tree. For this reason, lead was banned from paint and gasoline, but there are still plenty of old apartment houses with chipping and flaking lead paint on walls and windowsills. Toddlers are particularly at risk of lead poisoning, as they will put anything into their mouths, including paint chips and, especially, their fingers after playing in flaking paint on the floor and windowsills.

What is "gray matter"?

Gray matter is where cell bodies line up and congregate. Clusters of cell bodies are called gray matter because they turned gray when brains were preserved by the early pathologists. The axons and myelin remained white, so white matter refers to the axons and myelin. Because cell bodies decide whether to fire an axon, collectively, the cell bodies in the gray matter analyze incoming information and decide what to do about it, hence the expression "use your gray matter." Another common term for a cluster of cell bodies is ganglia.

Where is the gray matter in the brain?

Cell bodies are distributed in three general locations, one toward the base of the brain, called the basal ganglia, another encircling the brainstem, called the limbic system, and a third at the surface of the brain, called the cerebral cortex ("cortex" means bark) (see figure 101). Here's why there are three locations. For millions of years, reptiles did very well using their small collections of gray matter situated atop the brainstem—what we would now call the basal ganglia. When mammals first developed, a new layer of gray matter—the limbic system—had to be grafted onto the existing reptilian brain. Later mammals needed even more gray matter, so a third layer was stacked over both the limbic system and the reptilian-basal ganglia. This third layer became the cerebral cortex, located high up near the surface of the brain. In between the cerebral cortex and the two layers of deeper gray matter is a layer of white matter representing the axons of the cerebral cortex.

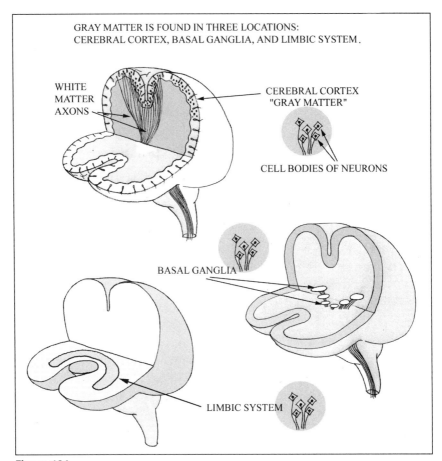

GRAY MATTER IS FOUND IN THREE LOCATIONS:
CEREBRAL CORTEX, BASAL GANGLIA, AND LIMBIC SYSTEM.

WHITE
MATTER
AXONS

CEREBRAL CORTEX
"GRAY MATTER"

CELL BODIES OF NEURONS

BASAL GANGLIA

LIMBIC SYSTEM

Figure 101

Why did another layer of gray matter need to be grafted onto the reptilian brain?

In other words, what do mammals do that reptiles don't? The answer is not so obvious. Velociraptors were certainly as good at hunting as lions; they were surely as strong and as fast, and based on what we know from snakes and crocodiles today, they experienced anger (assuming fighting was associated with anger), fear (assuming escape entailed fear), and pleasure (assuming sex was pleasurable for them). What mammals do that reptiles don't do is feel emotions beyond anger, fear, and pleasure. Pet alligators and snakes don't respond to cuddling. Mammals, in contrast, nurture and care for their young. They have a sense of family and community. They play and bond with one another. They live and hunt in packs, and they guard and protect members of the pack. For this, you need more than the reptilian brain had to offer.

What eventually developed was a small collection of gray matter, called the limbic system, located immediately above and encircling the brainstem. The limbic system developed with two things in mind. First, emotions had to be connected to memory, because emotionally charged events needed to be remembered. You don't want a child touching a hot stove more than once. (The converse is also true: emotionally insignificant events, such as boring school classes that don't evoke an emotional response, will not be remembered.)

Attaching an emotional handle to an event not only makes it easier to remember, but it also makes us *want* to remember it. Present a novel toy to an infant and watch the caution, anxiety, curiosity, excitement, fascination, and even fear on his face as he inspects it, emotions only to be supplanted by joy as he plays with it. The emotions generated by the child's limbic system enable him to solidify his memory of the toy. In order to facilitate the job of attaching emotions to memories, the limbic system developed adjacent to the hippocampus—the new-memory center in the temporal lobe (see figure 102).

The second task for the developing limbic system was to express emotions, with changes in heart rate, blood pressure, breathing, blushing, sweating, bowel control, and all the other features of the fight or flight response. To do this, the limbic system was attached to the hypothalamus, the part of the brain that sends out signals to express our emotions physically through the sympathetic and parasympathetic nervous system (see figure 103).

Later, as mammals began to use their brains for more challenging activities such as hunting in packs and living in groups, the cerebral cortex expanded to provide the necessary intellect. The arrival of primates (man, monkeys, and apes) brought an even broader range of emotions, such as humor, regret, disappointment, pride, shame, jealousy, and compassion, requiring the limbic system to expand upward into the cingulate gyrus, a very old section of cerebral cortex deep in the brain. To experience and respond to this broadening range of emotions in primates,

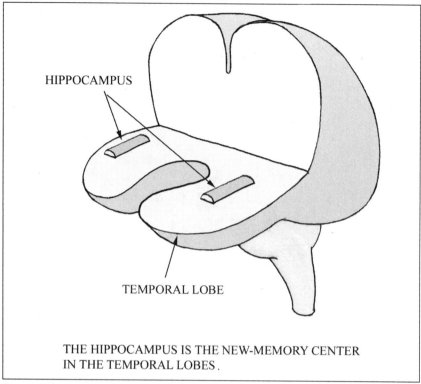

THE HIPPOCAMPUS IS THE NEW-MEMORY CENTER
IN THE TEMPORAL LOBES.

Figure 102

the cerebral cortex, particularly in the frontal lobes, established extensive connections with the limbic system.

How do we establish new memories?

New memories are logged into the brain through the temporal lobes, via the hippocampus and neighboring temporal lobe cortex. Everything we see or feel or hear or taste or smell must pass through the hippocampus and adjacent temporal lobe cortex to be remembered. We know this based on an unfortunate surgical mishap in the 1950s, when a patient underwent surgery to remove one of his temporal lobes in an attempt to control his seizures, which were emanating from that temporal lobe. Unbeknownst to the surgeon, the hippocampus in the other temporal

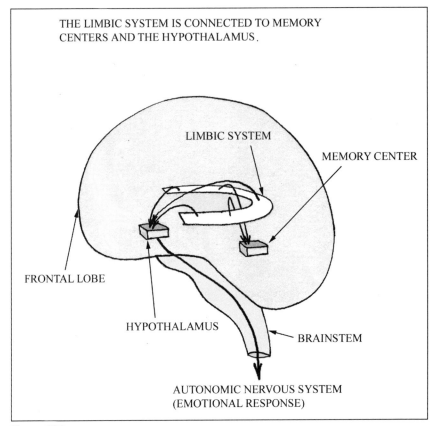

THE LIMBIC SYSTEM IS CONNECTED TO MEMORY CENTERS AND THE HYPOTHALAMUS.

LIMBIC SYSTEM

MEMORY CENTER

FRONTAL LOBE

HYPOTHALAMUS

BRAINSTEM

AUTONOMIC NERVOUS SYSTEM (EMOTIONAL RESPONSE)

Figure 103

lobe had never developed and the patient had been going through life with only one functioning hippocampus, which the neurosurgeon cut out. From that day forward, the patient could not lay down a single new memory, but he could still recall everything that happened to him up to the day of surgery. The fact that he could recall old memories indicated that old memories are stored outside the temporal lobes and are accessible without the help of the temporal lobes. Also, because people with damage to the temporal lobes can still remember for about an hour, working memory—the scratch pad of the brain from which immediate memories are taken for long-term storage—is also thought to lie outside the temporal lobes in the frontal lobes. The actual chemistry of a memory trace is still unknown.

Why do smells evoke immediate memories?

All sensory information entering the brain—vision, touch, pain, hearing, temperature—except smell, must first stop in the thalamus to be analyzed. The thalamus is an egg-shaped structure resting atop the brainstem and functioning as a triage agent for the cerebral cortex, deciding—based on what the cortex has told it—which new information is important enough to interrupt the concentration of the cerebral cortex.

Smell is the only sensation that bypasses the thalamus and connects directly into the temporal lobe, as it directly stimulates memory and emotional centers in the temporal lobe to allow animals to smell their way through the world (see figure 104). By bypassing the thalamus, the mere whiff of something can elicit in us an immediate memory of some distant experience and simultaneously evoke an immediate feeling of reverie, beauty, love, disgust, and so on. Though sounds do stop in the thalamus, they are analyzed by the temporal lobes, where they are able to take advantage of the lobes' memory and emotional centers. It takes only two or three notes of a song to recall the rest of the song, as you experience intense feelings of patriotism, fear, desire, hope, sadness, excitement, rebellion, reverie, passion, beauty, love, happiness, and many more, often associated with a memory of a particularly emotional moment or period in your life. Music's grip on our temporal lobe emotions is far stronger than that of either vision or touch.

Why do soldiers feel no pain from bullet wounds until they reach safety and only then realize they've been shot?

Since pain must first stop in the thalamus before reaching (and disturbing) the cerebral cortex, it is likely that in times of extreme stress, such as on the battlefield, the cerebral cortex either ignores thalamic pain signals or prevents them from leaving the thalamus altogether.

Why does your hand jerk away from a burning hot surface before you even realize it's hot?

Because the pain signal in the hand bolts to the spinal cord and back out to the arm muscle before heading north to alert the brain. When this fast

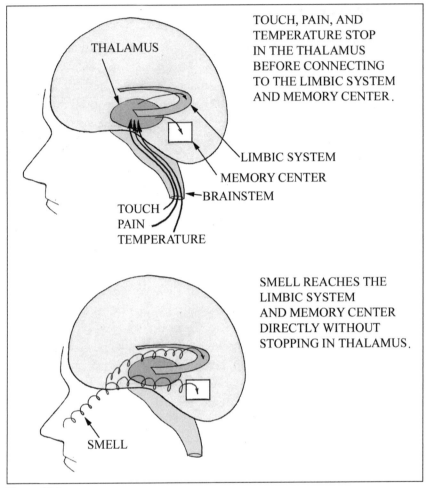

Figure 104

pain signal does reach the thalamus, it is immediately sent to the parietal cortex to determine exactly where in the body the pain is coming from and what type of pain it is (extreme heat, pin, cut, crush, bite, etc.).

How come there are times when you can't tell where the pain is coming from?

Those pain signals are ascending to the brain along a second pain system, one that slowly wends its way up the spinal cord, sending offshoots to the vomiting center in the brainstem and the sympathetic nervous system in the hypothalamus, and finally reaches the thalamus before being sent to the frontal lobes and cingulate gyrus, where the agony and suffering of pain arise.

Two different kinds of pain have evolved in man: fast pain and a phylogenetically older slow pain. Fast pain, the sharp pain felt when you first hammer your finger nail ("ouch!") is immediately felt, is well localized, and elicits a quick withdrawal flinch. Slow pain, the terrible throbbing pain that follows ("owwwww"), is slower in onset, is poorly localized (the whole finger hurts, not just the nail), and elicits prolonged muscular spasm, immobilizing the painful area. Fast pain has a low threshold, but then mercifully stops when the painful stimulus stops. Slow pain has a higher threshold, but once that threshold is crossed, there follows a crescendo of deeply aching, emotionally charged agony accompanied by nausea, sweating, hyperventilation, and heart pounding, all of which far outlast the stimulus. The type of stimulus causing fast pain is accurately discerned, while slow pain all feels about the same—severe, deep, aching, tearing, throbbing, and burning—regardless of the stimulus. By connecting slow pain to the frontal lobe instead of the hippocampus in the temporal lobe, painful suffering may be remembered but not the pain itself, thank God, or else there'd be only one childbirth per family.

How is a tiny brain, such as a bird's, able to perform such complex activities as building a nest or migrating thousands of miles?

It is quite amazing that a tiny bird brain can accomplish such complex activities as building a nest, raising young birds, and flying to distant locations without getting lost. The limitation of a small brain is that the behavior cannot be changed. Given a particular situation, a bird will respond the same way every time. The ability of the human brain to change its response is one of its greatest feats. For example, male mammals, ranging from mice to bulls to men, eventually suffer a declining interest in mating with the same female. When presented with a new mate, however, the male responds immediately with renewed sexual interest. Even his sperm count rises. Your average stud bull is so governed by this instinct that he won't even mate twice with the same cow until he has first mated with all the other cows in the herd. The phenomenon is called the Coolidge effect. Only the huge endowment of gray matter in man could permit a change in this kind of animal behavior.

How do we feel emotions such as sadness, joy, jealousy, guilt, lust, boredom, rage, anxiety, fear, remorse, and hope?

Emotions are produced by the release of neurotransmitters such as acetylcholine, serotonin, dopamine, epinephrine, and others. How a chemical dripping onto a nerve cell is translated into a complicated emotion such as hope is another of the brain's quiet mysteries.

What's the hypothalamus?

The hypothalamus is an ancient area of the brain located right above the brainstem that helps the brainstem regulate the more primitive functions of the body, such as appetite, thirst, temperature regulation, and sleep, and also controls the endocrine system and the autonomic nervous system. As its name implies, the hypothalamus is situated under the thalamus.

Appetite, thirst, and temperature regulation are governed by extremely sensitive hypothalamic cells that can detect the temperature of the body, the concentration of salt in the blood, and whether it's time to eat. Based on the saltiness of the blood, the hypothalamus can adjust the amount of water in the body by either instructing us to drink water or instructing the kidney (through antidiuretic hormone in the posterior pituitary) to retain water. Two major hypothalamic hormones control our eating: NPY, which tells our brains we're hungry, and melanocortin, which says we're full (see figure 105). Each of these hormones is in turn controlled by hormones released from various organs. Just before we eat, ghrelin secreted by the stomach signals the hypothalamus to release NPY. Once food passes from the stomach into the intestines, the intestines release cholecystokinin, which shuts off NPY release and stimulates melanocortin release to make us stop eating. Cholecystokinin only works for a short time. To keep us from eating between meals, the intestines and colon release PYY, which sustains the release of melanocortin. PYY and cholecystokinin also work by inhibiting the stomach from emptying, which contributes to our sense of fullness. How much food it takes to shut off NPY and turn on melanocortin is governed by leptin, a hormone secreted by fat cells to alert the brain to our fat stores, and by insulin, which reflects our carbohydrate stores. The more leptin and insulin, the less we eat; the less leptin and insulin, the more we eat.

The hypothalamus controls the endocrine system by instructing the anterior pituitary gland to release FAT PIG: **F**ollicle-stimulating hormone, **A**drenocorticotropic hormone, **T**hyroid hormone, **P**rolactin, **I**nterstitial cell-stimulating hormone (or luteinizing hormone in women), and **G**rowth hormone. Special releasing hormones made in the hypothalamus are sent to the anterior pituitary via a private blood supply connecting the hypothalamus to the anterior pituitary. For example, during periods of stress, the hypothalamus releases corticotropin-releasing hormone to stimulate the anterior pituitary to release its hormone, adrenocorticotropin, which kicks

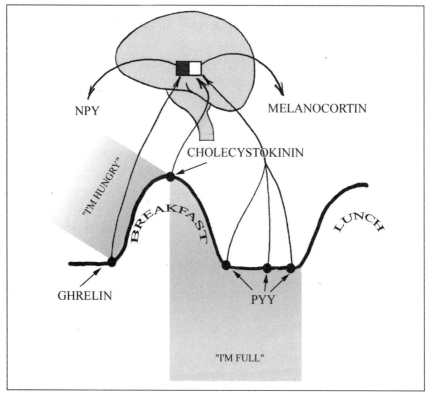

Figure 105

the adrenal glands into action for a fight or flight response. The same corticotropin-releasing hormone descending from the hypothalamus is either detoured into the brain or, more likely, synthesized elsewhere in the brain to heighten the state of anxiety during periods of stress.

The hypothalamus also instructs the posterior pituitary to release its two hormones—antidiuretic hormone and oxytocin—but in a slightly different way from the anterior pituitary gland. Nerve cells in the hypothalamus extend down into the posterior pituitary gland to release antidiuretic hormone and oxytocin directly into the general circulation.

The hypothalamus controls the autonomic nervous system by sending nerves down to the brainstem and spinal cord, and from there out to the blood vessels, glands, heart, intestines, and skin to perform their autonomic functions.

What is anorexia nervosa and is the hypothalamus involved?

Anorexia nervosa is an eating disorder that usually affects young women, occasionally young men. Anorexia nervosa patients develop an intense fear of gaining weight because they see themselves as too fat, no matter how thin they actually are. They eat small portions of vegetables or they may prepare a meal for others but not eat any of it. Running out of nutrients, the internal organs begin to fail, bones become brittle, and starving to death becomes a real risk.

Anorexia nervosa differs from bulimia in that anorexics don't eat. Bulimics eat a lot—in binges—and then vomit it back up and then either diet (like anorexics) or use water pills, laxatives, and enemas to control what they perceive as excessive weight.

Hypothalamic hormones may go out of whack in anorexia nervosa, but whether they cause the starvation or result from the starvation is unclear. So far, attempts to replenish or stimulate or even block hypothalamic hormones have not had success in treating this life-threatening disease.

What is depression?

Depression is sadness. All of us become sad from time to time, but when periods of sadness extend for weeks and months, when nothing becomes enjoyable, and when a person starts losing weight from loss of appetite, can't sleep, can't concentrate, and even considers suicide, it's time for outside help. One particular form of depression involves repeated bouts of depression interspersed with periods of feeling upbeat—maybe too upbeat. Being such a person, or living with such a person, makes it difficult to step back and see the cyclical nature of the depression. Cyclical depression, with or without interspersed bouts of upbeat behavior, is characteristic of bipolar disorder, formerly known as manic-depressive disorder. The importance of recognizing this disorder is that it's treatable with medications.

Depression is our most common emotional disorder. The cause of depression is still unclear, but some depression is situational. Everyone has an internal sensor comparing where we think we are in life with where we think we could have been or should have been. Depression may occur when that gap becomes too wide. What people have trouble seeing is that they are more accomplished and more worthy than they think, and that where they think they could have been, or should have been, is unrealistic. In other words, the gap is not as wide as they think and there are ways to shrink it.

Why do drugs such as Prozac, Effexor, Paxil, and Zoloft help depression?

While it's generally believed that the limbic system and frontal lobes are where depression occurs, it's less clear why depression occurs. Drugs such as Prozac, Effexor, Paxil, and Zoloft, and regular exercise, all of which raise the brain's serotonin levels, seem to help depression, suggesting that low serotonin is involved in sadness.

Why does sunshine help depression?

During the long Alaskan winters, when the sun barely rises, it's common for people to become depressed, but the suicide rate doesn't increase until the spring, when the sun begins to shine again and people emerge from their depression. Those who don't emerge and see their acquaintances improve become doubly depressed and even suicidal.

While sunshine is always uplifting, the emotional appeal of sunshine may have a chemical basis. Sunshine, you recall, stimulates the skin to make vitamin D. Scientists are beginning to suspect that vitamin D may be acting on the brain to improve mood.

Do any vitamins help depression?

Folate deficiency is common in depression, more so in older depressed people. Antidepressants appear to work better when supplemented with folate, and in older people high-dose folate alone improves depression.

Because folate is destroyed by cooking, the best sources of folate are fresh fruits and vegetables. If you supplement your diet with folate pills, keep in mind that folate taken alone can worsen an already existing vitamin B12 deficiency, and that simply adding vitamin B12 may be ineffective if your intestines have trouble absorbing it. In that case, vitamin B12 must be given by injection.

What is mania?

Mania is an unproductive, hyperactive, euphoric skipping from task to task or idea to idea. A person suffering mania is a maniac, from the Greek "mene" for moon, akin to "luna" in Latin (lunar and lunatic).

What happens when someone lapses into a coma?

Consciousness is analogous to having your lights on. For this, you need an electrical generator located in the brainstem and a lightbulb screwed into each cerebral hemisphere. The generator in the upper brainstem is known as the reticular activating system. When a person is conscious, the reticular activating system is generating electricity and both lightbulbs are intact. The upper brainstem is therefore the most important square inch of the human body; without it, a person is unconscious. The most serious threat to the upper brainstem, other than a bullet, is increased intracranial pressure. Anything inside the skull that doesn't belong there—a brain tumor, a blood clot, brain swelling, hydrocephalus—may raise intracranial pressure. As intracranial pressure builds, brain structures under pressure shove their way through gaps and around membranes to escape the high pressure. Eventually, the rising intracranial pressure presses these structures downward against the brainstem with enough force to cut off the brainstem's blood supply and permanently eliminate any chance that the patient will ever regain consciousness. Overwhelming pressure against the brainstem such as this is called herniation.

Doctors can actually see rising intracranial pressure with an ophthalmoscope. Normally, fluid inside optic nerve axons and blood within optic nerve veins are flowing inward toward the brain. Raised intracranial pressure dams up the flow of axonal fluid and venous blood, causing the tip of the optic nerve (the optic disc) to swell. A swollen optic disc is called a "choked disc" or papilledema. Seeing papilledema through an ophthalmoscope, a doctor or optometrist immediately suspects raised intracranial pressure as the cause.

What is hydrocephalus (water on the brain)?

The brain is a hollow organ. In the center of the brain is a lake of spinal fluid called ventricles. Cerebrospinal fluid (or spinal fluid, for short) is continually being synthesized by clusters of cells hanging from the walls of the ventricles. One of the functions of spinal fluid is to wash away metabolic waste products accumulating from the brain's daily activity. The drain sites for spinal fluid lie over the surface of the brain, embedded in major veins returning blood to the heart. To get spinal fluid from the ventricles inside the brain to its drain sites over the surface of the brain, spinal fluid has to exit the ventricles through several small holes at the base of the brain and then circulate up over the surface of the brain in a water jacket of spinal fluid surrounding the brain. Any process that obstructs this circulation of spinal fluid will cause the fluid to dam up into the ventricles, ballooning them up. The condition of having dilated ventricles is called hydrocephalus, a Latin term meaning water on the brain. As back pressure in the ventricles rises, the ventricles press upward against the cerebral hemispheres and downward against the reticular activating system in the upper brainstem. The patient slowly loses consciousness as his lightbulbs dim. If the pressure rises too high, the damage can be permanent and even fatal. The patient may become brain dead, with no chance of ever waking up or even breathing on his own.

Why do some comatose patients suddenly wake up after 2 years in a coma?

If a patient is unconscious, either the reticular activating system is malfunctioning or both lightbulbs are broken. You're better off having a malfunctioning reticular activating system, because if it ever does get restored, electricity will be sent to structurally normal cerebral hemispheres. If both lightbulbs are broken, meaning the hemispheres are damaged, that person's lights will always be a little dim.

The miraculous emergence from coma after 2 years occurs only in patients with brainstem injuries. Sometimes it takes that long for the reticular activating system to reorganize its electrical wiring to start generating electricity again, but when it does, the patient wakes up and is himself again. Patients who are unconscious because of damage to both hemispheres have to repair both cerebral hemispheres, a daunting task given the complexity of the cerebral hemispheres.

Can the brainstem be damaged without affecting the reticular activating system?

Yes. Because the reticular activating system is only in the upper part of the brainstem, it is not affected by damage occurring lower in the brainstem. Injury to the middle section of the brainstem interrupts all the brain's signals funneling down through the brainstem to control the face, arms, and legs. In other words, damage midway down the brainstem paralyzes all the muscles in the body from the nose down, except for the respiratory muscles, which are controlled by the respiratory center in the *lower* brainstem. Because the reticular activating system is spared, these patients are awake, aware of what's going on, even though they're totally paralyzed (except for their eye movements). This condition is called being locked in. One of the first persons to be described with the locked-in syndrome, long before it was ever understood, was a character in *The Count of Monte Cristo*. Locked-in patients can communicate by moving their eyes. In fact, one locked-in victim was able to write a book by signaling each letter using his eye movements alone.

Do anesthetics work by shutting down the reticular activating system?

It is still unknown whether general anesthetics work by shutting down a specific region of the brain or the whole brain.

How long can someone go without blood flow to the brain before suffering brain damage?

If you cut off all blood flow to the brain, it takes only a few seconds before the brain loses consciousness, and other 4 to 5 minutes before permanent brain damage occurs. The few-second rule was established during the French Revolution, when mobs killed royalty and nobles by guillotine. After their heads fell into the basket, doctors standing over the baskets were able to get the victims to move theirs eyes left and right to command for a only a few seconds. Today, we know how long it takes to lose consciousness by monitoring patients' heart rhythms with wires attached to the chest wall. If the heart suddenly stops beating, it takes only a few seconds to faint. Similarly, if you are lying in bed with a very low blood pressure and suddenly stand up, fainting is almost immediate. The reason it takes only a few seconds for a brain suddenly deprived of oxygen and glucose to lose consciousness is that, unlike muscle, the brain does not store glycogen or any other source of energy. The brain is continuously dependent on the energy it receives from the blood to stay conscious. Cut off the blood supply and the brain immediately shuts down.

Low oxygen, however, with no disturbance in blood flow—for example, suffocating during a severe asthma attack or epiglottitis—is nowhere near as dangerous to the brain as cutting off its oxygen supply by interrupting blood flow to the brain. While permanent brain damage may occur within 4 to 5 minutes of the ceasing of blood flow to the brain, patients suffering low oxygen with no disturbance of blood flow may endure far longer periods with no permanent neurologic deficits. For this reason, patients who suffer a cardiac arrest outside the hospital and are resuscitated by chest compression alone do surprisingly well compared to those resuscitated by chest compression and mouth-to-mouth ventilation.

What happens after 4 to 5 minutes of no oxygen?

People who survive more than 4 or 5 minutes without oxygen end up with widespread damage to the cerebral cortex, leaving their brainstem and perhaps even parts of the basal ganglia and limbic system still functioning. With an intact brainstem, these patients are able to look about, swallow, breathe, and grimace, all without meaningful contact with the outside world. The doctor's term for such patients is vegetative.

What are breath-holding spells?

Young children in a hissy fit or a crying jag sometimes forget to breathe until they're blue in the face and pass out. While it's scary to parents, the low supply of oxygen to the brain does no permanent harm, because the child starts breathing again soon after he faints.

Why do we sleep?

For something we spend a third of our life doing, we know surprisingly little about sleep. Some authorities think we sleep in order to review the day's experiences and place the important ones into long-term memory. Maybe we sleep to clean the brain of toxic metabolites, or maybe we sleep to regenerate more adenosine triphosphate (ATP) and more neurotransmitters. Creative thinking can certainly occur during sleep, best exemplified by the famous dream of Friedrich Kekule. In the 1860s, while struggling to figure out the chemical structure of benzene, the German chemist dreamt of a snake seizing its own tail and immediately awoke with the answer: benzene was a six-carbon ring, not a six-carbon chain. This discovery of the hexagonal structure of benzene went on to form the basis for most of organic chemistry.

We are awake because of continual stimulation by a dense network of cells in the upper part of the brainstem called the reticular activating system. For a person to sleep, the reticular activating system must be turned off. How this happens is unclear, but adenosine is thought to play an important role. As you recall, the body's energy molecule is ATP, adenosine triphosphate. As the day wears on and the brain uses ATP for thinking, feeling, and movement, ATP is broken down to adenosine diphosphate, adenosine monophosphate, and just plain adenosine. When enough adenosine attaches to adenosine receptors in the hypothalamus and the base of the frontal lobes, the hypothalamus and basal frontal lobe shut down the reticular activating system and the brain goes to sleep.

Another chemical that helps us drift off to sleep is the neurotransmitter serotonin, the deficiency of which seems to lead to depression. In fact, one of the symptoms of depression is difficulty falling asleep and staying asleep. Serotonin may be the reason mothers give their kids a warm glass of milk before going to bed: milk contains L-tryptophan, an amino acid converted by the brain to serotonin.

How does caffeine keep us awake?

The effects of caffeine have been known ever since shepherds discovered that their sheep would not go to sleep after eating the beans of coffee plants. Caffeine works by blocking adenosine receptors, which prevents the brain from seeing the rising level of adenosine, so we don't get tired.

Caffeine uses a second mechanism to keep us awake by taking advantage of messenger molecules. When brain cells are stimulated by adrenalin, a messenger molecule inside the nerve cell relays that message to various parts of the cell. Caffeine inhibits the breakdown of that messenger molecule.

Caffeine also keeps us awake by gently stimulating pleasure centers in the limbic system, just as cocaine, heroin, amphetamine, alcohol, marijuana, and smoking do, only less. The mild stimulation of the limbic system makes us feel pleasantly invigorated. It also helps explains why coffee is so addictive. A Coke or Pepsi contains about a half a cup of coffee's worth of caffeine.

Why do we yawn when we're tired?

No one knows for sure why we yawn. Yawning does not get more oxygen to the brain.

What happens during sleep?

Soon after pounding the pillow, we descend over a period of 30 to 40 minutes from drowsiness (stage 1 sleep) into deep sleep (stage 4), and then over the next half hour we ascend back into light drowsiness (stage 1 again) (see figure 106). At this point, during the second episode of stage 1 sleep, begins the first dream of the night. All our voluntary muscles become limp except in the eyes, which dance about, presumably viewing the dream. Inexplicably, the penis, which contains no muscles, develops an erection. After 5 to 10 minutes of these rapid eye movements (REM sleep), we descend again into stage 4 sleep and then back up to stage 1 for another dream. With each succeeding cycle—perhaps 8 to 10 during the night—the descent becomes shallower and the dreams longer until we finally awaken, often stepping right out of a dream.

What is sleep paralysis?

Sleep paralysis is the inability to move or speak on awakening in the morning or on descending into sleep, which generally lasts seconds to minutes. The spell can be broken if the person is touched by someone else, like in the case of Snow White. The spells can be accompanied by terrifying awake nightmares or feelings of impending death. The patho-physiology (mechanism) is thought to involve remnants of REM sleep when our limbs normally become limp.

What is narcolepsy?

The same intense urge to fall asleep that strikes us late at night strikes nar-coleptic patients during the day, usually when their mind drifts, sometimes during embarrassing situations, but rarely in dangerous ones. A friend of mine had to quit his surgical residency program after it was discovered that the reason he would fall asleep holding retractors (instruments to keep the wound open during surgery) was because he was narcoleptic. At night, nar-coleptic patients differ from normal people by beginning REM sleep dreaming as soon as they drift off into stage 1 sleep, instead of waiting for the second episode of stage 1 sleep. Narcoleptics recall these initial dreams, called hypnagogic hallucinations, as being particularly vivid. Similarly graphic dreams on awakening are called hypnopompic hallucinations. Nar-coleptics may also suffer sleep paralysis on awakening in the morning. Other narcoleptics suffer from a condition called cataplexy. When suddenly startled, or suddenly struck by something particularly funny, they instantly collapse to the floor for seconds or minutes of total body limpness, as with REM sleep, but without losing consciousness or dreaming. Being weak with laughter is a fragment of cataplexy in everyone.

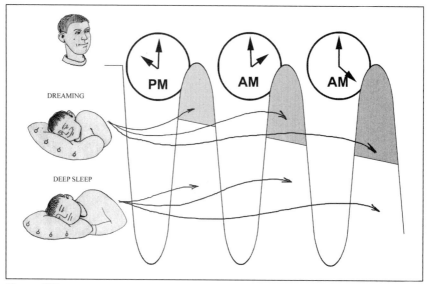

Figure 106

Why does your body suddenly jerk as you're descending into sleep?

The jerk center is located in the brainstem and is normally kept in check by an awake cerebral cortex. As the cerebral cortex drifts off to sleep, the jerk center is unleashed to send bolts of electrical discharges to the limbs. Sudden bodily jerks are part of a larger startle response, typically occurring in response to a loud noise. Some families around the world startle with such intensity that when surprised by a sudden command, they react by repeating the command and then doing it! This could include ripping off their shirts, striking the person next to them, or stirring their tea with their finger. In North America, these people are known as the Jumping Frenchmen of Maine.

What is sleep apnea?

Not everyone who nods off during the day has narcolepsy. Some people just don't sleep well at night because they periodically stop breathing (apnea) and are awakened by the resulting lack of oxygen. The lousy night's sleep makes them sleepy the next day. The usual cause is a fat neck obstructing the airway as the patient's pharyngeal muscles relax during sleep.

What is SIDS?

SIDS, or Sudden Infant Death Syndrome, is the unexplained death of a sleeping infant. Infants who sleep on their stomach are more vulnerable to SIDS than those who sleep on their backs. One thought is that by nuzzling their face into the bedding, these infants rebreathe their own expired air. Why only a few infants are unable to tolerate the prone (face down) position is unclear, but parents are now instructed to place their infants on their backs when putting them to sleep.

What are night terrors?

Night terrors, which occur in young children about an hour or so after going to sleep, are blood-curdling shrieks from which the child cannot be aroused, only to be forgotten by the morning. After descending into deep sleep, these children become temporarily stuck in stage 4 sleep, but why that should cause hysterical crying is unclear.

What is jet lag?

Jet lag is that worn-out, tired but wired feeling lasting a few days after flying across several time zones. Going east is worse than going west. Travelers going from New York to Los Angeles find it easy to go to bed at 8 P.M. (11 P.M. in New York) and sleep a little longer. Travelers going from Los Angeles to New York, however, find 11 P.M. in New York (8 P.M. in L.A.) too early to retire. The same kind of fatigue and feeling out of sorts is often suffered by people working the night shift and sleeping during the day.

Sleep is one of the daily rhythms of the body. Other things that tend to wax and wane on a regular basis throughout the day are blood pressure, body temperature, sexual desire, hunger, bowel movements, alertness, and fatigue. The waxing and waning are controlled by hormones released from the endocrine glands—particularly cortisol—and neurotransmitters such as melatonin and serotonin, all of which seem to be coordinated by a small cluster of nerve cells in the hypothalamus called the suprachiasmatic nucleus. As part of the hypothalamus, the suprachiasmatic nucleus is perfectly situated to regulate the release of hypothalamic hormones and neurotransmitters. While the suprachiasmatic nucleus has its own daily rhythm, that rhythm can be modified by the amount of daylight a person sees. Nerves from the retina connect directly to the suprachiasmatic nucleus in order to fine-tune the body's daily rhythms.

What happened to the reptilian parts of our brains? Do we still use those parts of the brain to move our muscles?

Yes indeed. We still use the basal ganglia, but not as reptiles do. Reptiles use their gray matter for strength, speed, and coordination, while we use our basal ganglia only to control how much we move and how fast. So if our basal ganglia don't work, as happens in Parkinson's disease, movements become sparse and slow. In other basal ganglia diseases, we move too much, a condition called movement disorders. The four movement disorders are tics and chorea, or little flickers or brief movements of one or more parts of the body, akin to being fidgety; a tremor of a hand or arm when sitting quietly; ballism, or wild flinging movements of an arm or leg (from the word "ballistic"); and athetosis, or slow writhing movements of the hands, arms, trunk, and neck, which are held, even at rest, in strange postures.

Until primates came along, reptiles and mammals had no need for fine control of their paws and claws. Primates, though, had to develop an entirely new system to permit fine-hand coordination. The system that developed involves two separate nerves. The first nerve, called the "upper motor neuron," begins in the brain, where the decision is made to move a muscle. The upper motor neuron travels downward into the spinal cord, where it stops and fires its neurotransmitters at the second nerve. The second nerve, called the "lower motor neuron," begins in the spinal cord, exits the spinal cord as a nerve root, and snakes its way under and around bones to the muscle it's going to move. When a lower motor neuron signal reaches its axonal tip, the neurotransmitter (usually acetylcholine) is released onto a special receptor in the muscle called the neuromuscular junction, which sends an electrical signal throughout the muscle, stimulating it to contract.

Where are the upper motor neurons in the brain?

The cell bodies for upper motor neurons are located in a single strip of the cerebral cortex at the rear of the frontal lobe. The motor strip was mapped in the 1930s by Dr. Wilder Penfield and Dr. Herbert Jasper in Montreal. In the operating room, Penfield removed a portion of the skull bone from an anesthetized patient, let the patient awaken from anesthesia, and then with a small electrical wire touched the surface of the brain. (Since the brain itself has no nerves that sense pain, the stimulations were painless.) When the wires touched the motor strip, the patient's limbs moved. What Jasper and Penfield found as they marched the electrical probe around the motor strip was that the upper motor neurons controlling the legs lay between the two hemispheres of the brain, and the upper motor neurons controlling the arm, hand, face, lips, and tongue extended down the motor strip (see figure 107). More important, they found that those muscles needing delicate control, such as the lips, tongue, shoulder, and fingers, had a lot more representation in the motor strip than the hip or back muscles. For example, try swinging your leg in a clockwise rotation. Now draw a circle counterclockwise in the air. Suddenly your leg is rotating in a counterclockwise direction, as the massive number of shoulder fibers in the motor strip dominate the relatively few hip rotator fibers.

All axons descending from the motor strip funnel through a narrow area deep in the brain. In cross section, the bundle of upper motor neurons forms the outline of a pyramid, so another term for upper motor neuron is pyramidal tract fiber. The fibers coming from the basal ganglia are called extrapyramidal fibers. The pyramidal tract fibers from one side of the brain cross in the lower brainstem to supply the muscles on the opposite side of the body.

What happens if you damage the pyramidal tract?

Originally, the pyramidal tract evolved to fill a need for fine motor control of the hand and fingers, not strength, as reptiles and mammals were already quite strong without the benefit of a pyramidal tract. Eventually, though, as the pyramidal tract became more developed in apes and man, it took over control of strength, too. Consequently, injury to a

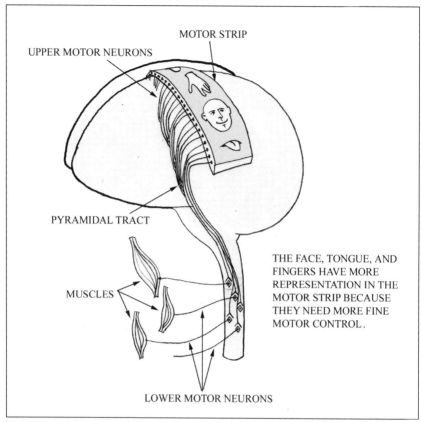

UPPER MOTOR NEURONS

MOTOR STRIP

PYRAMIDAL TRACT

MUSCLES

THE FACE, TONGUE, AND FINGERS HAVE MORE REPRESENTATION IN THE MOTOR STRIP BECAUSE THEY NEED MORE FINE MOTOR CONTROL.

LOWER MOTOR NEURONS

Figure 107

pyramidal tract on one side of the brain paralyzes the opposite side of the body and impairs fine coordination of the opposite hand. Thus, when grandma suffered a stroke affecting her right side, she suffered a lack of blood flow to the pyramidal tract in the left side of her brain. Even if she recovers strength, her fine dexterity will likely be impaired, reflecting residual pyramidal tract damage.

The third thing that happens with pyramidal tract damage is spasticity—stiffness. Together, the stiffness, weakness, and loss of fine coordination of pyramidal tract damage make a person's movements clumsy and awkward. From this comes the endearing term spastic, or spaz, to refer to any awkward, clumsy person.

Basal ganglia dysfunction can also cause movements to become slow and stiff, but not weak. It usually takes a doctor to distinguish the slowness and stiffness of basal ganglia dysfunction from the slowness and stiffness of pyramidal tract dysfunction.

Why do your knees jerk when the doctor taps them?

The doctor is tapping the tendon connecting the quadriceps muscle to the tibial bone below the kneecap (patella). Buried in all tendons is a tiny specialized muscle called the Golgi tendon organ, which monitors how much the muscle is being stretched. When the tendon is tapped, the Golgi tendon organ thinks the quadriceps muscle has suddenly been stretched and sends a signal to the spinal cord to contract the muscle back to its proper length, which you see as a knee jerk.

Slow stretching of the Golgi tendon organ resets the tension in a muscle, which may explain why you feel looser and more relaxed after stretching. It may also explain why a yawn is so satisfying.

Why do the police make you walk a straight line when they suspect you of drinking while driving?

The police are testing your cerebellum, the brain's major balance center, which happens to be particularly sensitive to alcohol. The cerebellum is a very old structure, having evolved in the earliest fishes and reptiles. It is situated behind the brainstem, close to the semicircular canals in the inner ear (see figure 108). In fact, once signals from the semicircular canals enter the brainstem, they head straight for the cerebellum. So the cerebellum, brainstem, and semicircular canals work together to control balance.

To understand what the cerebellum does, just hang around a bar, because alcohol loves the cerebellum. When you think of a drunk, what do you think of (besides panhandling)? The way they walk: they look like they're on board a reeling ship during a sea storm trying to walk to the bow of the ship when there's no handrails or ropes to keep them from falling overboard. They place their feet wide apart to steady themselves and even then they're swaying from side to side. Each step, which requires lifting one leg and balancing briefly on the other, makes their imbalance,

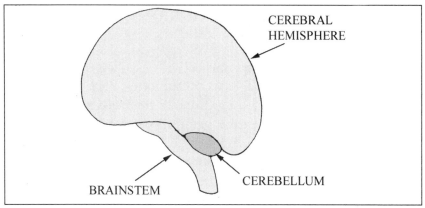

Figure 108

or ataxia, that much more obvious. The police test cerebellar balance by having the suspect walk a straight line: an intoxicated person can't do it without falling to one side. The cerebellum also controls coordination of the hands, so that when asked to touch his nose, the suspect's finger wobbles back and forth as it nears his nose.

Why do some people's hands shake when they're holding a knife and fork or a glass of water?

A tremor like this usually runs in families and is appropriately called familial tremor. Generally, such tremors remain a cosmetic problem until, after decades of slowly worsening, they begin to interfere with handwriting, eating, and other fine motor activities. In some patients, the tremor causes the head to bobble and the voice to tremble, à la Katharine Hepburn. The problem is thought to stem from a poorly understood chemical abnormality of the cerebellum.

Are sights, sounds, and touch sensations analyzed in different parts of the brain?

Yes. Vision is received in the occipital lobes, sounds are received in the temporal lobes, and skin sensations are analyzed in the parietal lobes.

After stopping in the thalamus, why are skin sensations sent to the cerebral cortex?

Without a cerebral cortex, you can still feel the sharp edges and flat surfaces of, say, a cube, but without a cerebral cortex, that's all you'll feel. To mentally assemble what you touch into a three-dimensional image, you need a cerebral cortex. Like the motor strip, sensations are organized into a sensory strip in the parietal lobe with lots of attention devoted to the lips, face, and hands, and less to areas like the thighs or chest.

You have two eyes and two occipital lobes. Which eye goes to which occipital lobe?

You'd think the left eye would go the left occipital lobe and the right eye to the right occipital lobe, but that's not how it works. In each eye, the left half of the retina sees the right half of the visual world because the left half of the retina is looking at the world through a tiny pupil. Similarly, the right half of each retina sees the left half of the visual world. So far so good.

Ganglion cell axons from each half of the retina skirt along the surface of the retina to the optic nerve. Inside each optic nerve, axons from the left side of the retina stay on the left side of the optic nerve and axons from the right side of the retina stay on the right side of the optic nerve.

The reason for this strict separation of retinal axons is that the inside axons of each optic nerve are going to cross to the opposite side of the brain. The site of crossing is called the optic chiasm. Once the inside axons cross, all the nerve fibers from the left half of both retinas are on the left side of the brain and all of the nerve fibers from the right half of both retinas are on the right side of the brain (see figure 109).

What this means is that when the retinal axons reach the occipital lobes, the left occipital lobe sees the right half of the visual world and the right occipital lobe sees the left half of the visual world. This allows the occipital lobes to display images in full panorama, something that couldn't happen if each eye funneled all its fibers to its own hemisphere. It also means that damage to one occipital lobe prevents someone from seeing his right or left visual world. This can be a real problem for people who want to drive, or even pedestrians stepping off a curb.

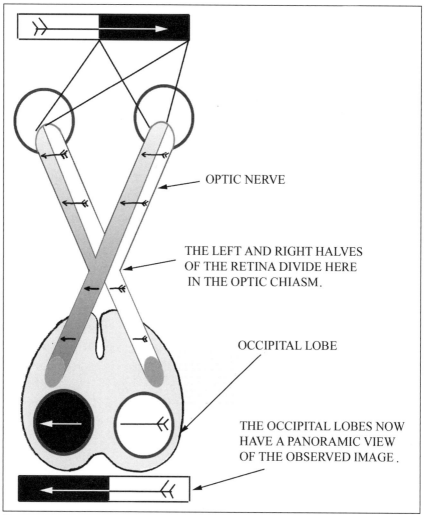

OPTIC NERVE

THE LEFT AND RIGHT HALVES
OF THE RETINA DIVIDE HERE
IN THE OPTIC CHIASM.

OCCIPITAL LOBE

THE OCCIPITAL LOBES NOW
HAVE A PANORAMIC VIEW
OF THE OBSERVED IMAGE.

Figure 109

Why does the left side of the brain control the right side of the body and the right side of the brain control the left side of the body?

Once the brain decided to split an image between the two hemispheres, with the left occipital lobe seeing the right half of the visual world and right occipital lobe seeing the left half of the visual world, all the motor and sensory systems followed suit, so that the left hemisphere controls movement and sensation on the right side of the body and vice versa.

Why are some people right-handed and others left-handed?

No one really knows, but it may have something to do with the speech center. Speech is controlled by a small but vital area called Broca's area, after Dr. Paul Broca, who first described it in 1862. (Paul Broca was a French neurologist who, in describing Broca's area, pioneered the radical concept of cerebral localization. Prior to this time, the brain was thought to be a homogenous network of neurons, each area equally capable of carrying out all cerebral functions.) Where would you put Broca's area if you were in charge? Right next to the lips and tongue in the motor strip, since the lips and the tongue do the talking. But do you put the speech center in the right hemisphere or the left hemisphere? The hemisphere you choose is going to get some favored treatment, because the speech center needs the latest in motor development to articulate accurately what you want to say. If you favor one part of the motor strip, you might as well favor the whole motor strip, making the opposite side of the body dominant. In the large majority of people, Broca's area is in the left hemisphere, so most people are right-handed. Why the left hemisphere is favored over the right hemisphere, and why Broca's area remains in the left hemisphere in the majority of left-handed people, is anybody's guess.

What happens when Broca's area is damaged?

The person's speech becomes marred by spelling and grammatical mistakes, or aphasic—more than simply slurred, which would be analogous to sloppy handwriting. Speech in people with Broca's aphasia is slow, halting, hesitant, made with great effort, and devoid of the little helper words necessary to make sentences flow. A typical sentence would still convey the gist of what the aphasic patient wanted to say—such as "dog . . . backyard"—but without the prepositions, conjunctions, adjectives, and adverbs that make for full speech. Oddly enough, some patients with Broca's aphasia can still communicate by singing what they want to say, thus using the "Yankee Doodle center," located somewhere outside Broca's area.

How does the brain understand speech?

For that, the brain needs another specialized area to decipher written, spoken, and (in the case of Braille) felt symbols. Ideally, such a deciphering center would be located midway between the temporal lobe (where spoken words are received), the parietal lobe (where Braille is received), and the occipital lobe (where written words are received). In 1874, Dr. Carl Wernicke discovered such a center in the posterior left temporal lobe, now called Wernicke's area (see figure 110). Wernicke's area also participates in the expression of speech by helping to choose the right phonemic sound bits to make real words.

Except for the upper brainstem, Wernicke's area is the single most important spot in the human body. Here's why. Without Wernicke's area, we could not understand spoken words, printed words, sign language, or Braille. Without Wernicke's area, we would also choose the wrong sound bits when speaking and writing. We all do this from time to time, but we immediately hear the error and correct it. Without Wernicke's area, however, we would never recognize our own nonsense words because without Wernicke's area we cannot decipher and monitor our own speech to ensure we are saying what we want to say. Patients with Wernicke's aphasia speak words never before heard, blithely speaking with all the intonations of normal speech (intonations are the singsong quality of speech, such as the rise of disbelief or the fall of a solemn pronouncement). The patient thinks he's speaking just fine, because he can't monitor his own speech for errors. Meanwhile, you're sitting there like the RCA Victor dog listening to "There's a strabble in my kreedisfran," trying to make sense of gibberish that sounds like English because it has the proper intonations of speech.

Wernicke's aphasia is much more devastating than Broca's aphasia. At least in Broca's aphasia, where the speech is slow and halting and sometimes even absent, the patient can still use his intact Wernicke's area to understand what's being said to him. In Wernicke's aphasia, the person can neither understand language nor make his wants known through language. The patient is trapped in a virtually subhuman existence, unable to communicate with those around him.

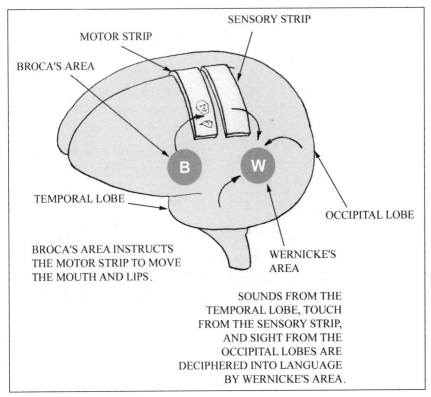

SENSORY STRIP

MOTOR STRIP

BROCA'S AREA

B   W

TEMPORAL LOBE

OCCIPITAL LOBE

BROCA'S AREA INSTRUCTS
THE MOTOR STRIP TO MOVE
THE MOUTH AND LIPS.

WERNICKE'S
AREA

SOUNDS FROM THE
TEMPORAL LOBE, TOUCH
FROM THE SENSORY STRIP,
AND SIGHT FROM THE
OCCIPITAL LOBES ARE
DECIPHERED INTO LANGUAGE
BY WERNICKE'S AREA.

Figure 110

Is aphasia the same as autism?

No. Aphasia is an isolated disturbance of language filled with spelling and grammatical mistakes. The emphasis is on *isolated disturbance*. An aphasic patient's emotional and intellectual reactions are normal. In autism, the language disturbance involves more than just the ability to speak. It involves the motivation to speak, paying attention to what's being said, and understanding the speaker's tone of voice. Autistic children—autism always starts in early childhood—are withdrawn, focused on and even obsessed with some internal thought, emotionally uninvolved with those around them, unable to read body language and speech intonations, impulsive, and hypersensitive to sensory stimulation, including sounds, touch, and odors. Many if not most are mildly mentally retarded, but some have superior skills in art, math, or music. Clearly, autism involves a more widespread disturbance of brain function than an aphasic's isolated disturbance of expressing or understanding language. The pathologic physiology (or pathophysiology) of autism is unfortunately still very unclear.

Why is the right hemisphere called the "artistic" hemisphere?

While the left hemisphere is adept at assembling and juggling bits of information, such as numbers and speech sounds, the right hemisphere is more attuned to the intonations and emotional overtones of speech, the reading of facial expressions, and the appreciation of shapes and forms, shadows and space. Left hemispheric people like written directions; right hemispheric people like maps.

What is cerebral palsy?

Cerebral palsy is any kind of acquired brain damage suffered before, during, or just after birth (acquired means that, at the time of conception, when the sperm united with the egg, the brain was genetically normal and that it would still be normal if not for the cerebral injury). In cerebral palsy, the injury can affect upper motor neurons, the basal ganglia, or the cerebral cortex—individually or in any combination. In other words, if the brain injury spares the cerebral cortex, intelligence is normal. Speech may be slow and thick, the hands may be uncoordinated, and the gait may be stiff and clumsy, but if you can get past all that, you'll find their memory, reasoning, judgment, and emotions to be normal.

What's the difference between cerebral palsy and mental retardation?

Mental retardation is any kind of brain damage, including genetic damage, that hinders the childhood development of intellect. The damage almost always involves the cerebral cortex or, rarely, the white matter alone. Since cerebral palsy may or may not involve the cerebral cortex, it may or may not cause mental retardation.

What's a learning disability?

A learning disability is a problem with one of the skills of learning, such as reading, writing, spelling, or math, amid otherwise normal intelligence.

What's dyslexia?

Dyslexia is one of the learning disabilities. Dyslexic children have a problem reading because, apparently, they have a problem matching letters or letter combinations to their sounds, which is the basis for reading. It's unclear where the problem is in the brain.

What's a stroke?

A stroke is the sudden destruction of brain tissue because of a sudden disruption of the blood supply to that part of the brain. The blood supply can be disrupted because an artery or vein has occluded or hemorrhaged, or because the blood pressure has suddenly dropped. The term "stroke" refers to the suddenness with which the brain no longer functions—the victim is struck down. Depending on what part of the brain is affected, the patient may suddenly become ataxic (cerebellum), paralyzed on one side of the body (pyramidal tract), unable to speak (Broca's or Wernicke's area), or blind in one direction (occipital lobe).

Sometimes, the neurologic deficit is short-lived, lasting perhaps a few hours. In those cases, the disruption of the blood supply is only temporary. Any disruption of blood supply that causes an organ to malfunction without actually killing the tissue is known as ischemia. A short-lived episode of cerebral ischemia is called a transient ischemic attack, or TIA. The neurologic improvement, however, is misleading because the next episode may be right around the corner, and it might be permanent this time. It's not uncommon for people to ignore a spell of trouble speaking or weakness on one side of the body, only to suffer a full-blown stroke within hours or days. Fortunately, the stroke may be preventable if the patient can get to the doctor in time, which is a lot better than waiting for a stroke to occur and then having to rely on clot busters.

What's the risk of using clot busters in strokes?

The risk of clot busters is bleeding, particularly when they are used to break up clots in the brain. Here's why. When brain tissue loses its blood supply, two things happen to raise the risk of hemorrhage into the brain. First, dead tissue softens as the cells decompose. Second, along with brain tissue, blood vessels in infarcted tissue disintegrate, too. So, if the clot busters are given after brain tissue has already died, or if the clot busters fail to bust open the clot and the tissue goes on to die, the disintegrating blood vessels may begin to leak blood into the already softened brain tissue. With clot busters on board, the leaking blood vessels won't clot off. The result can be a major hemorrhage.

Which stroke is more likely to be associated with right-sided weakness—one involving Broca's area or one involving Wernicke's area?

Broca's area, because it lies right next to the motor strip, while Wernicke's area is distant from the motor strip.

If you have a stroke, does it wipe out your memory?

Not unless you suffer numerous strokes damaging lots of areas of the brain, because memories seem to be stored in multiple places in the brain. How and where memories are stored and later retrieved is another of the brain's mysteries. One thought is that duplicate copies of memory traces are stored at different sites within the cerebral cortex, depending on the sensation that detected the event or the emotion associated with the event. Thus, a visual memory trace would be stored in the occipital region of the brain, an auditory trace in the temporal lobes, and a touch trace in the parietal lobes, corresponding to where vision, hearing, and touch are received in the brain.

Is there anything you can do to improve your memory?

The hippocampus is one of the few places in the brain where new brain cells continually replace old brain cells. Why there is a turnover of hippocampal neurons is unclear. Using the hippocampus appears to enhance hippocampal function. For example, London taxi drivers spend an average of two years learning the locations of streets in London before taking an exam to be a licensed London taxi driver. Magnetic resonance imaging (MRI) scans of their brains reveal a larger than normal posterior hippocampus where maps of our environment are thought to be laid down, and the longer the taxicab drivers drive, the larger their hippocampus. For mice, physical exercise has been shown to shorten the time it takes to solve mazes. Other animal studies have provided good evidence that physical exercise increases the number of new hippocampal neurons, raises the level of chemicals used in memory, and improves the physiology of memory.

Why are some people able to give speeches with no notes?

Perhaps they are following the example of the ancient Greeks by mentally walking through their house and placing the items to be remembered in each room. Others associate what needs to be remembered with visual images and then assemble the visual images into a story.

What's a seizure?

Neurons communicate with each other in a nice, orderly fashion. A seizure begins when one neuron becomes irritable and starts firing off signals uncontrollably. In some mysterious way, that neuron is able to convince its neighbors to do the same, and pretty soon the whole neighborhood is firing away. If those firing nerve cells happen to be in the motor strip, the opposite hand or leg or face will start twitching. If they happen to be in the temporal lobe, the temporal lobe does its thing. For example, the patient may smell something, or remember something, or experience some emotion as part of the seizure—all functions of the temporal lobes. Obviously, every time you have an episode of déjà vu or smell something out of the blue, you don't have a seizure. The key feature of a temporal lobe seizure is that the memory or the smell is always the same, because the seizure always starts from the same cluster of renegade nerve cells. If the seizure activity in one temporal lobe spreads to the other temporal lobe, the patient loses awareness and enters into a twilight state, engaging in automatic, purposeless activity such as picking at his clothes or walking around in a daze.

How is a seizure different from epilepsy?

A person who suffers recurrent seizures has a seizure disorder, or epilepsy.

Lots of people have spells of one type or another. How do you tell if those spells are seizures?

Sudden jerking of an arm, or arm and face, is pretty good evidence of a seizure, but some seizures are difficult to recognize as seizures. The best way to tell if a spell is a seizure is to hook the patient up to an EEG (an electroencephalogram) and hope that he has a spell while being monitored. If the spell is a seizure, the EEG will detect the sudden change in the brain's electrical activity.

What's an EEG (an electroencephalogram)?

An EEG is nothing more than an antenna in the form of wires pasted to the scalp to detect the brain's electrical activity. Wires from the pads are connected to a machine that amplifies and records the brain's electrical activity on paper or on disc. It seems simple enough, but when Dr. Hans Berger, the first person to record the electrical activity of a human brain (in 1924), decided to try it out on his son, the community went nuts and accused Berger of trying to maim his own son. At least they cared.

What happens if seizure activity in one area of the brain suddenly spreads to all areas of the brain?

When electrical chaos spreads throughout the brain, the person loses consciousness, falls down, and convulses. If all his muscles contract simultaneously, he becomes stiff. If the muscles contract in a coordinated fashion, the limbs jerk back and forth.

Eventually, for as yet unknown reasons, a seizure does stop. For the next few hours, however, the patient feels groggy and dull, until the accompanying chemical chaos is corrected. Sometimes, seizures don't stop and the patient enters into a perpetual state of epilepsy, or status epilepticus.

What do you do if someone has a convulsion in front of you?

Not much, because the seizure should stop in a few minutes. During those few minutes, however, every muscle in the body is contracting, so there's no coordinated movement of the diaphragm or the chest wall. In other words, a convulsing patient is not breathing. In a minute or so, he'll turn blue, but the brain is protected from lack of oxygen during the seizure by a large increase in blood flow to the brain. This means there is no need to stick something in the patient's mouth to help him breathe. Anyway, you won't be able to insert anything into his mouth, as the jaw is usually clenched shut. If you keep trying, the only thing you'll do is chip a tooth for him to aspirate. The most important thing to do during a seizure is cradle the head so it doesn't smack against the concrete or other hard surface. When the seizure stops, everything relaxes, including the epiglottis. If he vomits after the seizure, the epiglottis won't close and the stomach contents will be aspirated into the trachea. All that acid in the stomach will wreak havoc on delicate lung tissue, so to prevent aspiration, turn the patient on his side after the seizure to direct vomitus out of the mouth. And don't be surprised if he soils himself as his urethral or anal sphincter muscles relax.

What is your alpha rhythm?

During calm rest with your eyes closed, the brain's electrical activity oscillates back and forth at anywhere from 8 to 13 times a second, a state called alpha activity. So, if an EEG records alpha activity, your mind is in neutral. Why the brain's electrical activity oscillates rhythmically at all may have to do with reverberating circuits between the thalamus and cerebral cortex.

Why do you need to wear a baseball helmet at bat?

Getting hit in the head with a baseball traveling 60 to 90 miles per hour will knock a person out and might even damage the brain, although that shouldn't kill you. But an epidural hematoma will, and that's why you need to wear a helmet. To understand what happens, take a saw and saw off the skull bone. What do you see? Not much, because a thick membrane covers the brain. This membrane, called the dura, which is from the same root as durable, is tough. The space outside the dura, between the dura and the skull, is called the epidural space. Right underneath your temple is a very thin temporal bone, and along the inside surface of the temporal bone, facing the epidural space, runs a small artery (the middle meningeal artery) (see figure 111). A baseball striking the temporal bone may crack this thin bone, sending the ragged edges of the bone into the wall of the artery. Blood leaking from the arterial tear accumulates rapidly in the epidural space at arterial pressure—enough to raise a column of mercury 100 millimeters or more. Normally, the pressure inside the skull is about 13 millimeters of mercury or less. The massive rise in epidural pressure presses the dura against the brain with such force and speed that patients can be rendered comatose within a half hour or less and dead within a hour. And yet the treatment is so simple. Cut the skin overlying the temporal bone and drill a hole through the thin temporal bone. As soon as the epidural space is entered, blood will squirt out through the hole and relieve the pressure on the brain. All that's left to do is to suck out the hematoma, find the bleeding middle meningeal artery, and coagulate the bleeding point with special electrical tweezers.

Can you also bleed beneath the dura?

Yes. That's a subdural hematoma, which has its own good and bad points (see figure 112). A subdural hematoma is under much less pressure than an epidural hematoma because the source of the subdural blood is a bleeding vein, not an artery. That's the good news. The bad news is that in order to tear a subdural vein, at least in young people, the brain has to be struck so hard that the underlying brain is usually damaged. The reason young people need much more force than old people to tear their subdural veins has to do with shrinkage of the brain as we age. Subdural veins carrying blood from the brain jut across the subdural space to feed large veins along the inside of the skull bone. As we age, the brain shrinks a little and pulls away from the skull, stretching the subdural veins and making them vulnerable to tearing from what would otherwise be mild

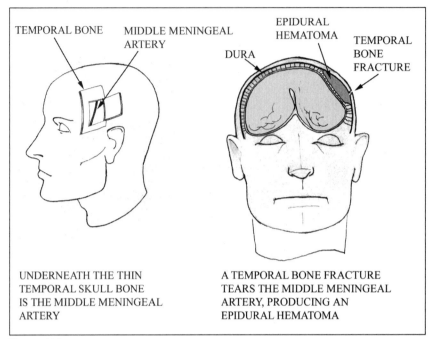

TEMPORAL BONE   MIDDLE MENINGEAL   EPIDURAL
                  ARTERY   HEMATOMA   TEMPORAL
                              DURA   BONE
                                                     FRACTURE

UNDERNEATH THE THIN   A TEMPORAL BONE FRACTURE
TEMPORAL SKULL BONE   TEARS THE MIDDLE MENINGEAL
IS THE MIDDLE MENINGEAL   ARTERY, PRODUCING AN
ARTERY   EPIDURAL HEMATOMA

Figure 111

head trauma. In young people, the brain is still pressed up against the skull, making it much more difficult to tear these bridging subdural veins. In young people, the force has to be quite substantial, and it ends up damaging the brain as the subdural veins are torn.

What's a subarachnoid hemorrhage?

While aneurysms can occur on any artery in the body, the arteries lying under and between the lobes of the brain are particularly prone to aneurysms. Resting gently atop the whole surface of the brain is a delicate membrane called the arachnoid (so named because delicate fibers in the arachnoid resemble spider legs—"arachne" is spider in Greek). Underneath the arachnoid—in the subarachnoid space—is a water jacket of cerebrospinal fluid encasing and cushioning the brain and spinal cord. Cerebral aneurysms form on arteries passing through the sub-

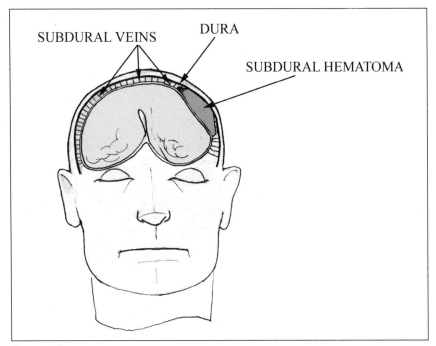

Figure 112

arachnoid space on their way to the brain, and bleeding from them results in a subarachnoid hemorrhage.

Because these arteries have not yet entered the brain, hemorrhage from a subarachnoid aneurysm usually spreads over the surface of the brain. If, however, the hole in the aneurysm happens to be pointing right at the brain, the hemorrhage may penetrate into the substance of the brain, which is much more destructive to the brain than bleeding over its surface. Bleeding over the surface of the brain can still be lethal if pressure inside the skull rises too high and the neurosurgeon is unable to relieve it.

One of the more common complications of a subarachnoid hemorrhage is hydrocephalus. Blood in the spinal fluid clogs up the cerebrospinal fluid drain sites over the surface of the brain, causing spinal fluid to back up into, and balloon out, the ventricles. A neurosurgeon can relieve the rising intraventricular pressure by drilling a small hole in the skull bone and slipping a catheter through the substance of the brain into the dilated ventricles. The other end of the catheter, or shunt, is threaded under the skin into the abdomen, where the high-pressure spinal fluid can now drain and be reabsorbed.

The good thing about aneurysms is that they often give a warning that they are about to blow by leaking a day or two prior to hemorrhage. That warning leak causes a bad headache radiating into the neck or down the back, often with nausea and vomiting.

Why does the warning leak cause pain in the neck and back?

Because the water jacket of spinal fluid encasing the brain extends down the spinal canal to encase the spinal cord. When an aneurysm bleeds into the spinal fluid, the blood spreads throughout the spinal fluid, over the surface of the brain, and around the spinal cord in the neck and back. The blood is very irritating and causes a chemical meningitis, with pain and stiffness of the neck extending down the back.

What can you do if you recognize the warning leak from an aneurysm?

First, don't do anything to raise the blood pressure, because that might make the aneurysm bleed again. Next, get to a hospital, where a neurosurgeon will operate to pinch off the neck of the aneurysm with a tiny clip. Instead of clipping the aneurysm, wires can sometimes be delicately threaded up the aorta and directly into the aneurysm to stimulate formation of a blood clot within the aneurysm.

What is meningitis?

Meningitis is inflammation of the meninges, a two-part membrane overlying the brain. The emphasis here is overlying the brain, not in the brain, because if the inflammation gets into the brain, the disease process is no longer meningitis, but encephalitis. The inner part of the meninges is the pia mater, which carries blood vessels bound for the brain, and the outer part is the arachnoid. Between them, in the subarachnoid space, circulates cerebrospinal fluid.

The cause of meningeal inflammation is almost always either blood from a subarachnoid hemorrhage or a viral, bacterial, or fungal infection. Bacterial meningitis is a life-threatening medical emergency because it can kill a patient, often within a day or two if antibiotic treatment is not administered immediately. Fungal meningitis is less imminently life threatening.

How do you know when you have bacterial meningitis?

Fever and a headache should always raise a suspicion, especially if the headache radiates into the back of the neck and down the back. Add onto that a stiff neck, nausea, vomiting, and lethargy, and meningitis becomes pretty likely.

How is the diagnosis of meningitis made?

The only way to confirm the diagnosis of meningitis is to find white blood cells in the spinal fluid that have been shed there from the inflamed meninges and to culture some of the spinal fluid in the microbiology lab. All of this, of course, requires a sample of spinal fluid, and the only way to get it is by sticking a needle into the spinal fluid and drawing off a sample. That's what a spinal tap, or lumbar puncture, does (see figure 113). The patient lies on his side, while the doctor numbs up a patch of skin over the low back, inserts a long needle through the numb patch into the epidural space, and advances the needle through the dura, across the subdural space, and across the arachnoid, into the spinal fluid. After a lumbar puncture, the holes in the dura and arachnoid seal up. The same basic process is used by anesthesiologists to block the pain of childbirth, except that instead of puncturing the dura, the needle is only inserted into the epidural space before injecting the anesthetic.

Isn't there a risk of hitting the spinal cord when you do a spinal tap?

No, because the spinal cord does not extend down the entire length of the spinal column, leaving a large subarachnoid space for cerebrospinal fluid to be tapped into. The spinal cord terminates a little more than halfway down the back, opposite the first lumbar vertebra. Nerve fibers headed for the legs, bladder, penis, and vagina leave the lower spinal cord in the thoracic (chest) region and continue down the spinal canal as nerve roots to exit at the appropriate lumbar and sacral levels.

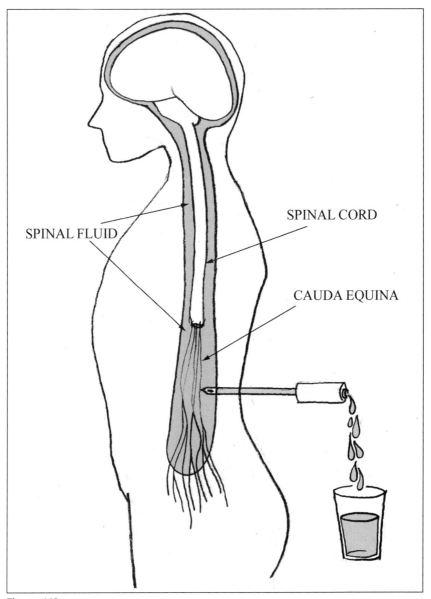

SPINAL FLUID

SPINAL CORD

CAUDA EQUINA

Figure 113

In a fetus, the spinal cord does line up with its corresponding vertebral body, but as the child grows, the spinal cord does not lengthen as fast as the spinal canal, leaving the spinal cord only about 60% as long as the spinal canal.

The bushy tail of nerve roots in the lower spinal canal reminded the early anatomists of a horse's tail, hence the name cauda equina (tail of a horse). In a lumbar puncture, the spinal tap needle is inserted into the lower end of the spinal canal, slipping between the nerve roots of the cauda equina and thus avoiding any possibility of damage to the spinal cord.

What is multiple sclerosis?

Sclerosis is an old-fashioned term for scarring. In multiple sclerosis, the scarring occurs in multiple sites in the spinal cord and brain (including the optic nerves). Each bit of scarring is due to inflammatory stripping off of myelin from axons anywhere in the brain or spinal cord. No one knows what triggers the inflammatory reaction. After the inflammation settles down, the myelin is repaired, but repair jobs are never as good as stock myelin, so the person is always left with a little residual injury at the site of the injury plaque. Over the years, as the number of plaques accumulates, the neurologic impairment becomes more obvious.

Many of the inflammatory plaques in multiple sclerosis occur around tiny blood vessels in the brain, suggesting that something harmful is leaking into the brain from the bloodstream. Based on this and other evidence, some investigators have focused on the brain's tiny blood vessels. The vasculature of the brain has long been known to be special, ever since it was observed that injecting india ink or other dyes into an animal's bloodstream would stain every internal organ but the brain. What makes the brain's endothelial cells so impervious to chemical dyes is a special reinforcement between endothelial cells, forming a blood-brain barrier. Medications to tighten the blood-brain barrier may someday be an effective treatment for multiple sclerosis.

What is mad cow disease?

In mad cow disease, certain proteins, called prions, inside neurons begin to unfold (no one knows why). Once one protein unfolds, it induces other proteins to do so, and before long the insides of neurons become choked with clumps of unfolded proteins. Because prions can be transmitted to another person or animal, they are considered infectious agents. Why the stomach does not digest them when they are eaten is unclear, but an uninfected cow can contract the disease if it is allowed to eat the remains of another infected cow.

In the 1950s, a similar problem was found in Papua New Guinea, where people traditionally ate the brains of their recently dead tribal members. Yuk. Their neurologic illness was called kuru. Jakob Creutzfeldt disease is still another transmissible prion disease resulting in rapid loss of intellect, muscular jerking, paralysis, and death. For a while, kids were getting this terrible disease after receiving growth hormone that had been harvested from people who had died of Jakob Creutzfeldt disease. Corneas taken from people who had died of Jakob Creutzfeldt disease also killed a fair number of corneal transplant recipients. We're a little more careful now to ask why organ donors died before harvesting their organs for transplantation.

What is Tourette's syndrome?

Tourette's syndrome is an inherited movement disorder consisting of uncontrollable twitches and utterances often associated with obsessive-compulsive behavior and aspects of attention-deficit disorder. The twitches can include eye blinks, facial grimacing, head jerks, foot twitches, and even more complex movements such as straightening a tie. The utterances can range from clearing the throat, sniffing, grunting, and barking to frank cursing. The pathophysiology is thought to originate in the basal ganglia, so intelligence is unaffected.

What is Alzheimer's disease?

Alzheimer's disease is another disease due to the accumulation of protein clumping in brain cells, but these abnormal proteins are not transmissible. The disease typically begins in the gray matter of the temporal lobes and hippocampus, so an early symptom is inability to remember from one day to the next. Eventually, all the gray matter is involved and the patient begins to forget remote memories and lose his reasoning, judgment, and insight. (Reasoning is the ability to solve a problem that has only one correct answer. Judgment is the ability to solve a problem that has more than one solution and requires you to judge the best solution. "Why" questions require judgment. Math problems require reasoning.) The key to diagnosing Alzheimer's disease is that, despite severe memory loss, problems with reasoning and judgment, and loss of insight into their cognitive problems, the victims retain their social graces. Social graces are controlled by the frontal lobes, which in Alzheimer's disease maintain some normal function.

Misplacing your keys, forgetting conversations, forgetting people's names, forgetting why you walked into a room, and forgetting telephone numbers probably do not signal the beginning of Alzheimer's disease. Forgetting these kinds of things is far more likely due to preoccupation, boredom, distraction, and depression than to true Alzheimer's disease. The time to get concerned about memory loss is when it's accompanied by loss of judgment and reasoning and lack of acknowledgment or insight into the memory loss.

How do you prevent Alzheimer's disease?

Face it, genetics is the number 1, 2, and 3 causes of Alzheimer's disease. The best you can do is try to stay mentally active. Recently, 800 older Catholic nuns, priests, and brothers without Alzheimer's disease were followed for four and a half years. Those who read books, magazines, and newspapers, went to museums, did crossword puzzles, and played cards and checkers were less likely to be part of the 12% who developed Alzheimer's disease.

There is mounting, but still inconclusive, evidence that the statins, drugs that lower cholesterol, protect against Alzheimer's disease. Likewise, hypertension and elevated homocysteine levels are being viewed with strong suspicion as contributors to Alzheimer's disease. Folate deficiency may very well be important, too, perhaps because folate helps metabolize homocysteine.

Does boxing damage the brain?

Under the microscope, the brains of Alzheimer's patients contain nerve cells loaded with abnormal protein. Something quite similar to this is present in the brains of boxers who become punch drunk—slow moving, slow thinking, and poor memory, poor judgment, and impaired insight, in other words, demented. A professional boxer's fist is capable of delivering 52 g's of force—equivalent to being hit by a 13-pound bowling ball at 20 miles per hour. Repeated blows to the head such as this are thought to jar proteins loose from intact brain cells. These proteins are then picked up by nerve cells and eventually stifle nerve function.

You don't have to strike your head against something rigid to get brain damage. Severe whiplash, where the head is snapped back and forth with violent force, can injure delicate axons coursing through the brain. Babies and toddlers are particularly vulnerable to this because they don't have strong neck muscles to prevent the head from being snapped back and forth. So no matter how angry you get at a young child, never pick him up and shake him violently. Many people have inadvertently caused brain damage in infants and toddlers doing just that, and have gone to jail.

Is Muhammad Ali punch drunk?

He may have some elements of being punch drunk, but what he really has is Parkinson's disease with slowed and sparse movements. All that repeated head trauma damaged his basal ganglia.

What is the evidence that the frontal lobes control social behavior?

Suspicion that the frontal lobes were involved in proper social behavior was given a big boost by Phineas Gage. In 1848, Gage was an upright, God-fearing man who had the unfortunate job of tamping down dynamite for the railroad. One day, Gage's tamping rod caused some of the dynamite to explode, which propelled the rod into his frontal lobes. Coworkers took him to the doctor, who without anesthesia and without the help of a neurosurgeon simply pulled the steel bar out of his brain. Phineas miraculously survived this ordeal, but could not return to work because of a dramatic change in his personality. He lost his restrained demeanor and became ornery, impulsive, irresponsible, uncaring, and a bit of a ladies man, even though his intellect, speech, and motor function remained pretty much intact.

Even more profound personality changes were suffered by patients who underwent prefrontal lobotomies in the 1930s, 1940s, and 1950s. In one version of the procedure, a psychotic or otherwise difficult-to-handle patient, or even a violent criminal, would be made to sit still under local anesthesia while the doctor inserted a thin ice pick through the thin bone over each eye, deep into each frontal lobe. He would then work the knife from side to side in order to cut the frontal lobe white matter. Looking back, it's hard to believe doctors performed this procedure, because the patients were rendered apathetic and passive, devoid of any emotional contact with those around them. Today, the most common trauma to the frontal lobes is auto accidents, when unrestrained front-seat drivers and passengers are slammed against the windshield.

What does it mean to be psychotic?

A person is psychotic when he has delusions. The easiest definition of a delusion is any idea believed by only one person in the world and judged by experts to be impossible. Until that person can convince others that it's not impossible, the person is considered to be psychotic. As history has taught us, being labeled psychotic is in part determined by prevailing societal beliefs. If Mr. Psychotic is able to convince another person to believe his delusion, and they're the only two people in the world who believe it, the two are called folie a deux.

When conversing, psychotic patients have trouble logically connecting their thoughts, a condition called loosening of associations; worse still is the flight of ideas, in which there is no connection whatsoever between one thought and the next. In tangential speech, each thought carries the speaker in a new direction, but at least each thought is connected to the previous thought. Circumstantial speech is characterized by excessively detailed inclusion of irrelevant details that obscure the main point the speaker is trying to make.

What's a hallucination and how does it differ from an illusion?

An illusion is a distorted image of something real, as with a mirage. A hallucination is an image that has no origin in reality. Thus a ghost is an illusion if there's smoke in the air, a hallucination if the air is clear.

Some of the most vivid hallucinations occur after taking LSD-25. In the 1930s, chemists discovered that the ergots isolated from fungi to prevent postpartum bleeding were actually a family of ergot chemicals whose backbone was lysergic acid (LSD). When Albert Hofmann, a Swiss chemist hoping to find new, useful medications, tried synthesizing derivatives of lysergic acid in the 1940s, he accidentally inhaled the 25th derivative (LSD-25) and experienced vivid hallucinations and euphoria.

What's the difference between an organic psychosis and a functional psychosis?

If the cause of the psychosis is identifiable, such as amphetamine abuse, brain tumor, or encephalitis, then it is an organic psychosis. If the cause of the psychosis cannot be identified, it is a functional psychosis. The lay term for functional psychosis is "crazy."

What is the chemical reason for organic and functional psychoses?

It's not clear why functionally psychotic people hear voices, or why they believe the television talks to them, or why they think their thoughts are being controlled by someone directing radio waves into their head, but delusions such as these often clear up with medications that block the neurotransmitter dopamine.

Dopamine is an interesting neurotransmitter. Insufficient dopamine in the basal ganglia diminishes our movements, as in Parkinson's disease. If you give too much dopamine to Parkinsonian patients, not only do they develop too many movements, but as the dopamine floods the limbic system, the patients begin to suffer hallucinations. So in one area of the brain dopamine increases motor activity, while in another part of the brain dopamine produces hallucinations. In still another part of the brain, namely, nucleus accumbens, situated between the brainstem and the frontal lobes, dopamine release creates a sense of pleasure and euphoria. When rats with electrodes in their brains are allowed to control the stimulation of their own nucleus accumbens, they will stimulate themselves to the point of exhaustion, even death.

Nucleus accumbens is where you experience that warm "ahhhhh!" when smelling freshly baked bread or sinking your teeth into a delicious sandwich. Nucleus accumbens (along with brain centers connected to it) is also where drugs such as nicotine, alcohol, cocaine, heroin, methamphetamine, and marijuana, and inhalants such as toluene, evoke their euphoria.

Even the anticipation of experiencing something emotionally or physically pleasurable activates nucleus accumbens. This may be why gambling is so addictive, or why people get better when given placebos—because they expect to improve, not because the medicine or therapy have any direct effect. A good example of placebo effect occurred in the 1950s, when patients with angina were undergoing surgery to increase blood flow to the heart. In the surgery, an artery along the inside of the chest wall was stripped from the chest wall and attached to the heart. Patients were doing great until one day a patient developed a complication on the operating table after the chest incision had been made but before the surgeon was able to do the procedure. When the patient awoke from anesthesia, he, too, felt great, and his angina was gone. This prompted scientific studies in which patients with angina were subjected to sham (fake) operations, and you guessed it, those who received the sham operations did as well as those who received the real operation.

If dopamine really increases in the brain in response to an expected reward, you might expect Parkinson's disease, a disease of dopamine deficiency, to improve as part of the placebo effect. Today, surgery is being done on Parkinsonian patients suffering severe tremors. Dopamine-secreting cells are being implanted into their brains to increase the chemical dopamine, and sure enough the tremors improve. Sham operations—the same operation without implantation of dopamine secreting cells—also improve involuntary tremors in more than one-third of patients, indicating a release of dopamine from the placebo operation.

The placebo effect is used extensively by all health care providers: medical doctors, alternative medicine doctors, acupuncturists, and chiropractors. What they say to the patient is something like this: First, I believe you (so if you're angry that no one believes you, you can stop being angry). Second, I know what's wrong with you (so you can stop being anxious about your illness and relax), and here is the explanation for what's going wrong in your body. Third, I'm going to give you something that will make you better. (That something can be almost anything. If it's medicine, the dose is kept low so that more pills can be administered to create the illusion of being given a lot of medicine.) Last, feel free to call me at any time before your next visit to discuss your symptoms or your treatment.

Using this simple, upbeat, reassuring approach, a health care provider could prescribe peanut butter and improve many patients' complaints.

Why are drugs so addictive?

When first used, addictive drugs evoke a pleasurable sensation from dopamine that is released in nucleus accumbens (and perhaps from other neurotransmitters elsewhere in the brain). After a while, repeated use of the drug reduces the number of dopamine receptors in nucleus accumbens, so the drug fails to evoke the same intense, pleasurable feeling. When the drug is stopped, though, the addict experiences a painful craving characterized by anxiety, depression, irritability, rest-lessness, and fatigue—true psychic pain—and will do anything to feel good again. Drug addiction changes the way you take care of yourself and those you love. Forget about food, forget about sex, forget about friends. The obsession for a fix focuses all your attention. You become selfish with your time, spending it all on planning how to get that next fix. You withdraw, protecting your money and your drug supply, suspicious that someone will deprive you of what you absolutely need to stay alive. It's worth it to lie, to cheat, or steal—even from your friends and loved ones—in order to stop the craving.

Drugs don't have to make you high to become addictive. Smoking, for example, controls your appetite, helps you concentrate, calms your nerves, and improves your mood, all without making you goofy or causing you to stare off into middle space. Yet smokers will walk a mile for a Camel.

Cigarette addiction doesn't hold a candle to intravenous drug addiction. Intravenous drug addicts will use dirty needles and contam-inated drugs that are likely to carry the infectious agents for AIDS, hep-atitis, heart-valve infections, brain abscess, you name it. Intravenous drug addicts couldn't care less that cocaine permanently damages heart muscle, or that cocaine wreaks havoc on cerebral arteries, making strokes and heart attacks a fairly common problem, even among occasional users.

Whatever ill effects drugs have on the body, marketing them with finger-popping names such as ecstasy has made drugs hip and slick, and as familiar and harmless as an old friend. How could lover's speed, clarity, ecstasy, boomers, yellow sunshine, Georgia home boy, grievous bodily harm, special K, roofies, ice, crank, crystal, and speed be anything but cool?

If a person never suffered a stroke, heart attack, or dangerous infection, would cocaine and methamphetamine be so bad? More specifically, does repeated use of cocaine and methamphetamine permanently damage the brain?

Probably. In one study of cocaine-dependent and methamphetamine-dependent young men, MRI scans demonstrated actual shrinkage of their temporal lobes. In another study, crack cocaine users who had abstained from the drug for six weeks still had atrophy of their frontal lobes. In other studies of abstinent cocaine and amphetamine users, the levels of N-acetyl-aspartate, a chemical found only in brain cells, remained below normal in the frontal lobes, indicating a permanent loss of brain cells. In still other studies using sophisticated magnetic proton spectroscopy, methamphetamine users abstinent for three years still had reduced brain levels of dopamine and serotonin. Neuropsychological tests of abstinent cocaine and methamphetamine users reveal persistent cognitive deficits. Cocaine fed to animals in doses equivalent to that used on the street causes brain cell damage readily visible under the microscope.

Does marijuana cause brain damage?

The evidence for brain damage from long-term marijuana use is less clear. Like cocaine, amphetamines, nicotine, and alcohol, marijuana stimulates the release of dopamine in nucleus accumbens, but not as much as cocaine or amphetamines do. This may explain why withdrawal from marijuana is a lot easier than withdrawal from cocaine and amphetamines. That's the good news. The bad news is that marijuana has a special liking for the hippocampus and interferes with the synaptic connections between hippocampal nerve cells, which explains why marijuana users have such trouble laying down new memories when stoned. As for permanent damage, there are no autopsy studies proving hippocampal damage from marijuana, but synthetic marijuana given to rats causes dendrites in the hippocampus to twist and break. Also, hippocampal cells grown in a petri dish die when exposed to levels of marijuana found in a marijuana smoker's bloodstream. Evidence such as this explains why long-term heavy users of marijuana have such trouble laying down new memories long after stopping their marijuana use. Moderate marijuana smokers (6 joints or less a day), on the other hand, do seem to make a good recovery of their memory function.

Rather troubling is a recent PET scan study of gray matter in marijuana users. PET scans use radioactive chemicals to provide extremely sensitive measurements of the brain's chemical activity. The study revealed that those people who began using marijuana at age 16 or younger had less gray matter than those who began after age 16, with the greatest effect occurring in the frontal lobes. Whether this was due to a direct effect of marijuana on neuronal development during the teenage years or a secondary effect due to marijuana's effect on pituitary, ovarian, and testicular hormones is unclear (hormones affect brain development).

One nagging problem with long-term heavy use of marijuana (more than 20 days a month) is loss of motivation, which of course makes it difficult to become motivated to quit. The brain centers causing loss of motivation are not yet known. Nevertheless, if a long-term marijuana smoker can somehow convince himself to give up marijuana, the loss of motivation generally improves, at least for mild and moderate users.

What does the drug ecstasy do in the long run?

Ecstasy appears to damage the neurons containing serotonin. Some, but not all, studies have demonstrated abnormally low levels of serotonin in the brains of ecstasy users long after the drug has been stopped, suggesting permanent brain damage. Recent studies have also reported persistent memory problems long after ecstasy has been stopped.

What about alcohol—does it cause brain damage?

For any one person, it is not entirely clear how much total alcohol must be drunk over a lifetime before intellectual decline, imbalance, and incoordination set in. In most people, evidence of permanent brain damage should be apparent by the time a person has drunk 300,000 grams of alcohol. Since each drink of beer, wine, or liquor contains approximately 13 grams of alcohol, that's about 23,000 drinks, or about 5 drinks a day for 13 years. For some, of course, drinking as few as 3 or 4 drinks a day may lead to serious brain damage. Not all the damage may be due to alcohol per se, because heavy alcohol users don't always mind their diet and end up vitamin deficient, especially thiamine deficient, which by itself will cause brain damage.

Moderate social drinking (1 to 6 drinks a week), however, may actually offer some modest protection from dementia (and coronary artery disease). Unfortunately, the rate of car accidents and liver damage rises with social drinking, and 1 to 6 drinks a week can quickly turn into 7 to 12 drinks or more. Binge drinking, particularly, is rough on the brain, at least in rats. In rats, 2 to 4 days of binge drinking has been shown to cause significant nerve cell death in the olfactory bulbs and their connections to memory centers in the temporal lobes. Whether this translates into similar damage in humans is unclear, but it is known that the younger a person is when he starts drinking, the smaller the hippocampus is, as demonstrated by magnetic resonance imaging (MRI).

How dangerous is alcohol, cocaine, marijuana, and smoking to a developing fetus?

Billions of nerve cells in a developing fetal brain are undergoing cell division, cell growth, migration, and specialization. For a brain to end up normal, everything has to be done at just the right time in just the right place. Chemistry-altering drugs such as alcohol, cocaine, marijuana, and tobacco slow down and pervert the delicate formation of a fetal brain. With enough stimulation from parents, however, most of these infants do catch up for the most part. Unfortunately, mothers who care so little about their babies that they smoke and do drugs during pregnancy are less likely to provide that extra stimulation necessary for the baby to catch up.

How many brain cells do we lose as we age?

Beginning around age 55, our brains begin to shrink, as much as 10 to 15% in some brain regions. The primary reason for the shrinkage is not loss of nerve cells, but shrinkage of nerve cells. The shrinkage may translate into mild forgetfulness, but true intellectual decline is usually due to something more serious, such as Alzheimer's disease.

What are migraine headaches?

A migraine is a headache caused by the release of chemicals from nerves in the scalp. These chemicals dilate and irritate arteries in the scalp, resulting in a headache. Because all arteries dilate a little with each heartbeat (which is why arteries pulsate), many migraine patients suffer a throbbing or pounding headache in cadence with the heartbeat, especially in the temples, where the large, superficial temporal artery travels just under the skin (feel it in your own temples, or in front of the temporomandibular joint). A migraine is often unilateral (affecting only one side of the head) and associated with visual scintillations (sparkles and jagged lines), nausea, vomiting, and photophobia (glare from lights, forcing patients to retreat to a dark room). Many doctors refuse to diagnose migraine unless the patient has these other associated features, when in fact the majority of recurrent headaches without these associated features also respond to migraine medication, even those that occur during times of tension and stress, following head trauma, or around a woman's period.

What is Bell's palsy?

Bell's palsy causes sudden paralysis of one side of the face, including the forehead. People freak because they think they're having a stroke, but the reason for the paralysis is the pinching of the facial nerve on its way from the brainstem to the muscles of the face. In order to get onto the face, the facial nerve has to pass through a tiny tunnel in the skull bone behind the ear lobe. If, for any reason, the facial nerve swells, the short section squeezing through the tunnel pinches itself and stops functioning. The vast majority of people recover just fine, but once in a while the pinching is so severe that the nerve fibers actually die and have to regrow. If nerve fibers that used to supply the salivary glands end up going to the tear glands, whenever a person sees and smells tasty food, his eyes shed crocodile tears. Other patients with misdirection involuntarily close their eye when they smile because the nerve fibers that should go to the lips and cheek mistakenly have grown back to the eye-closure muscles.

Why do some football players suffer spinal cord injuries?

In general, spinal cord injuries occur because some players are born with narrow spinal canals. The spinal cord begins at the bottom of the brainstem and descends through an elevator shaft of bone called the spinal canal. A normal spinal canal provides plenty of elbow room for the spinal cord to move about when the neck is suddenly flexed or extended. If the spinal canal is congenitally narrow, however, what would normally be mild trauma to the neck can deliver a judo chop to the spinal cord (see figure 114). The spinal cord is pretty delicate. Its cross-sectional diameter is no bigger than a dime, and packed into that narrow cable are all the signals connecting the brain to the body. A direct blow to the cervical spinal cord by sudden flexion or extension of the neck can render an athlete quadriplegic.

Why do they immediately put a collar on you after an accident?

Because if you fractured one of the cervical vertebrae, that vertebra might slip backward and strike the spinal cord. Even if you didn't fracture a cervical vertebra, you might have torn a ligament holding adjacent vertebrae together. Without that stabilizing ligament, the vertebra are no longer fixed to one another. If one vertebra slides over the one below, the sudden sharp angulation of the spinal canal can injure the spinal cord (see figure 115). Since X rays don't detect a torn ligament, two X rays are taken: one with the neck flexed and the other with the neck extended. If one of these views shows the vertebra to be out of alignment or overly separated from its neighbor, suggesting a torn ligament, the patient may have to wear a rigid frame for a while, until the ligament heals and the vertebral bodies are stable again. If a rigid frame does not work, a neurosurgeon or orthopedic surgeon can operate and wire the two vertebra together to prevent further separation or slippage.

Where are lower motor neurons located?

The cell bodies for lower motor neurons are in the center of the spinal cord. The axons of lower motor neurons exit the spinal cord in bundles called nerve roots. Nerve roots exit the right and left side of the spinal

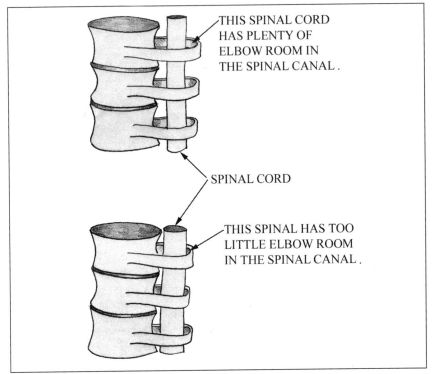

THIS SPINAL CORD HAS PLENTY OF ELBOW ROOM IN THE SPINAL CANAL.

SPINAL CORD

THIS SPINAL HAS TOO LITTLE ELBOW ROOM IN THE SPINAL CANAL.

Figure 114

cord in a nice, orderly fashion, one for each vertebral body—kind of like railroad tracks leaving a railroad station. Soon after leaving the spinal cord, behind the clavicle and under the shoulder, the lowest four cervical roots and the highest thoracic root—C5, 6, 7, and 8 and T1—enter the brachial plexus, an area analogous to a railroad switching yard where fibers from these nerve roots redistribute themselves and exit as peripheral nerves headed for the arm and hand (see figure 116).

In the lumbosacral region, nerve roots from L1 to L5 and S1 to S5 redistribute themselves in the lumbosacral plexus, deep in the abdomen. The biggest nerve exiting the lumbosacral plexus is the sciatic nerve, which courses underneath the buttock (gluteus maximus) and down the back of the leg through the hamstrings and gastrocnemius muscles to reach the foot. The sciatic nerve supplies the hamstring muscles (which flex the knee) and all the muscles below the knee, thereby controlling all movement of the foot.

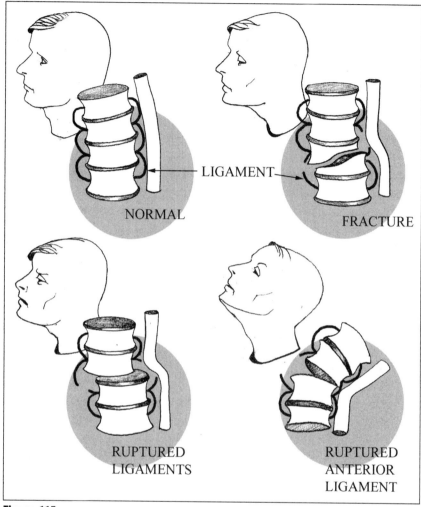

LIGAMENT

NORMAL

FRACTURE

RUPTURED LIGAMENTS

RUPTURED ANTERIOR LIGAMENT

Figure 115

What is polio?

Polio is a terrifying, highly contagious viral disease affecting the lower motor neuron cell bodies in the spinal cord. Now under control, polio once would strike a child with fever, headache, and neck stiffness and virtually overnight render the child paralyzed in an arm, a leg, both arms,

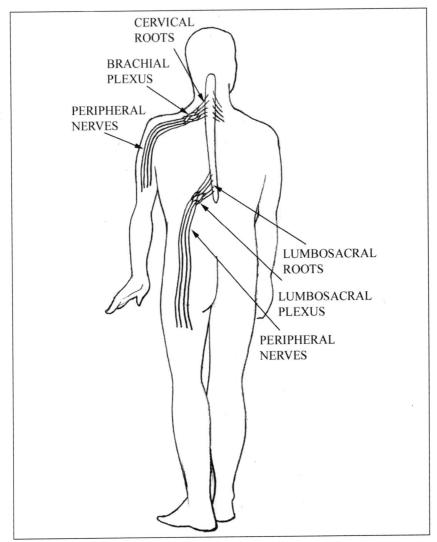

Figure 116

both legs, or the entire body. During World War II, American soldiers fighting in North Africa suffered a fair number of cases of polio, yet it was rare in the local population. It turns out that if a baby became infected with polio virus, the virus never got beyond the intestines and simply settled in for a long, peaceful coexistence with its host. In other words, polio had become a menace because of the development of sanitation. The demise of polio came with the Salk vaccine and, after that, Sabin's weakened polio virus, which after being taken orally lives in the intestines and induces its host to make antipolio antibodies.

What is Lou Gehrig's disease?

In 1938, the great New York Yankees baseball player Lou Gehrig contracted what looked like a slow form of polio, and he slowly became weaker and weaker, until he died in 1941. In his touching farewell speech at Yankee Stadium in 1939, Gehrig made the famous statement saying he still considered himself the luckiest man on the face of the earth. To this day, the cause of his disease, amyotrophic lateral sclerosis, remains unknown.

What is a dermatome?

A dermatome is the strip of skin supplied by one nerve root. Dermatomes are sequentially stacked atop one another over the skin (see figure 117). Dermatomes to remember are the 5th cervical (C5) for the shoulder, the 4th thoracic (T4) for the nipple, and T10 for the umbilicus (belly button).

Why do people suffering a heart attack have pain radiating down the left arm?

Referred pain is pain produced in an internal organ but felt far away in the chest wall, neck, arm, or leg. Pain fibers from both the heart and the inside of the arm enter the spinal cord at the T1 level. When the heart is in pain, the brain is tricked into believing the pain is coming from the left arm.

Other examples of referred pain are right shoulder pain during a gallbladder attack, pain in the middle of the abdomen from appendicitis occurring in the right lower abdomen, and pain in the left side during heavy exercise from intestinal ischemia (because of blood being diverted from intestines to muscles).

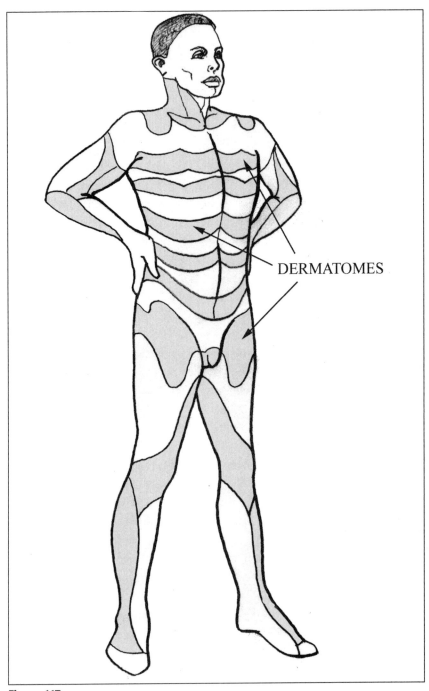

DERMATOMES

Figure 117

What are pressure points?

Pressure points are highly tender spots scattered around the body—where a tendon attaches to a bone, where a nerve crosses a bone, or where a nerve connects to a muscle. Pressure points are important to know about because they enable a parent—with little effort and without leaving any bruises—to make a child follow any instruction. The handiest one is the radial nerve, which wraps around the back of the humerus in the radial groove (see figure 118). The radial nerve extends to the muscles on the back of the forearm that elevate the wrist and extend the fingers. To find the radial nerve, locate the bottom tip of the deltoid muscle where it narrows to insert on the humerus bone. Now slip your fingers backward between the deltoid and triceps muscles and feel for the humerus bone. Your child should be on his toes by now asking what he can do for you.

Why is your hand sometimes numb when you wake up in the morning?

Because you've slept in a position that compressed a nerve going to the hand. There are three nerves supplying the hand: the ulnar nerve supplying the little and ring fingers; the median nerve supplying the thumb, index, and long fingers; and the radial nerve supplying the skin over the back of the thumb and index finger.

The same thing happens in the leg when it goes to sleep after sitting too long in one position. You're resting your leg on a nerve.

If you rest on a nerve too long, eventually the motor fibers will be affected, too. This can happen on a honeymoon when the wife sleeps with her head sweetly cradled on her husband's arm. The weight of her head compresses the radial nerve in the spiral groove en route to muscles along the back of the forearm, the muscles that lift up the wrist. You can imagine the bride's consternation over her choice of a life partner when she awakens in the morning to find her new husband hysterically prancing around with a wrist drop.

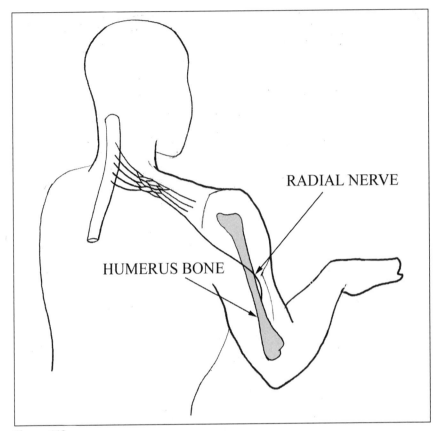

RADIAL NERVE

HUMERUS BONE

Figure 118

What's the funny bone?

When you bang the back of your elbow and get that stinging electric sensation shooting down your arm into the little finger, you've struck the
funny bone—the ulnar nerve en route to the hand. Bend your elbow
about halfway and feel a little groove on the inside back of your elbow
where the ulnar nerve passes through (see figure 119). People who lean
on their elbows a lot can slowly damage the ulnar nerve and cause the
muscles in their hands to waste away (atrophy). To stop any further
damage, surgeons will sometimes operate and move the ulnar nerve from
the ulnar groove to a position in front of the elbow.

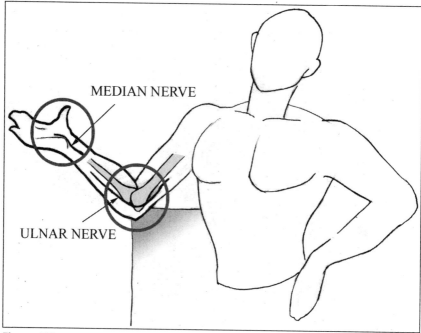

MEDIAN NERVE

ULNAR NERVE

Figure 119

What is carpal tunnel syndrome?

"Carpal" means wrist, and "tunnel" refers to a tunnel in the wrist bones through which the median nerve passes to reach the thumb muscles and overlying skin. For various reasons, the median nerve may become compressed in the carpal tunnel. Symptoms are often worse at night, causing the patient to wake up in pain and shake his hand. To relieve pressure off the median nerve, a surgeon simply unroofs the carpal tunnel.

Why does rubbing a tender spot ease the pain?

Every nerve in the body is made up of thousands of axons. Some of the axons carry motor signals to muscles and others carry sensory information from the skin to the spinal cord, including sensations such as vibration, joint position sense, pain, and temperature. The nerve fibers carrying vibration enter the spinal cord and immediately form a physiologic gate. This gate limits the number of pain signals allowed into the spinal cord. By rubbing the skin, you stimulate those vibratory fibers and tighten up the gate so fewer pain signals get through. TENS units, or transcutaneous electrical nerve stimulators, work in a similar fashion by electrically stimulating peripheral nerves with low-level current to tighten up the gate. Conversely, if you have a disease such as diabetes that selectively damages vibratory nerve fibers in peripheral nerves, more pain signals get through and the limbs can be in constant pain.

What's a polyneuropathy?

"Poly" means many, so a polyneuropathy is a disturbance of many peripheral nerves in the body. The symptoms usually begin in the axonal tips, where the nerves are most vulnerable to anything that impairs the delivery of nutrients from the cell body. Hence, the numbness and tingling of a polyneuropathy usually begins in the feet, because those nerves have the longest axons in the body.

Polyneuropathies are commonly caused by diabetes and alcohol. Guillain Barre syndrome is an abrupt immunologic polyneuropathy in which antibodies attack the myelin of peripheral nerves, often completely paralyzing the patient within days and forcing him onto a ventilator to breathe. Eventually, the myelin is repaired and the patient recovers.

What happens if the sensory nerves are totally damaged?

Sensation is vital to maintaining our exposed tissues. For example, if sensory nerves to the eye are cut or otherwise severely damaged, the patient will lose his eye because the eye is no longer protected from various types of trauma. If sensory nerves in the nose, hands, and feet are lost or severely damaged—as happens in leprosy—the nose, fingers, and toes will be lost. In leprosy, the nerve damage is caused by a slow-growing bacterium, a cousin of tuberculosis, and is thus somewhat contagious. Because of the use of multiple antibiotics, the disfigurement of leprosy is far less common nowadays, but leprosy is still one of the most feared infectious diseases worldwide.

What are muscle cramps, and why do we get them?

A muscle cramp, or charley horse, is a sustained painful muscle contraction. Cramps usually occur in the calf, but any muscle can suffer a cramp. Why a muscle should persist in contracting probably has to do with dehydration and changes in the serum sodium, potassium, calcium, and magnesium after exercise.

Why does a body become stiff after death?

The stiffness that sets in after death is known as rigor mortis. Normally, muscles contract when an electrical impulse enters the muscle and stimulates the release of calcium within muscle fibers. When the contraction is finished, the calcium is taken back up, a process that requires energy from ATP. Dead people don't make ATP, so when a person dies there's no ATP to retrieve calcium accumulating in muscle fibers. As a result, postmortem muscles remain in a contracted state, hence the slang term "stiff" for a dead body.

When trying to show how strong you are, why do you "make a muscle?"

The short answer is that the biceps muscle—in fact, any muscle—is strongest when fully contracted. Have a friend make a muscle while you place your left palm under your friend's elbow and grab his wrist with your right hand. Trying to straighten out your friend's arm (by overcoming his fully contracted biceps muscle) is a lot harder than allowing him to fully extend his arm and keeping him from flexing it. The same principle applies to the triceps. With the arm bent (triceps fully lengthened), try to prevent your friend from extending his arm. This is considerably easier than trying to bend a fully extended arm with the triceps fully contracted.

Here's why. On a microscopic level, muscles are composed of millions of interdigitating strips of tiny muscle fibers, each fiber loaded with little protein "oars" extending to the sides. To contract, the protein oars scull the individual muscle fibers past one another like, to mix metaphors, the bristles of two hairbrushes being pushed against each other. A contracted muscle is stronger than an extended muscle because more of the individual muscle fibers are overlapping and binding to one another.

What are some important muscles of the body?

Certain muscles are easy to see or feel. For example, when the jaw is biting down or clenched in anger, you can see and feel the bulging temporalis muscle in the temple and the masseter muscle along the angle of the jaw. Extending from the mastoid bone to the sternum is the prominent sternocleidomastoid muscle. Because the mastoid bone lies behind the axis of rotation of the skull, the left sternocleidomastoid turns the head to the right, and the right sternocleidomastoid turns the head to the left. To feel your left sternocleidomastoid muscle contracting, push your right hand against the right side of the jaw while you try to keep your chin in the midline. You can feel both sternocleidomastoids contracting by forcefully pushing your forehead forward against your hand.

Try feeling the following muscles as they contract (see figure 120). The deltoid muscle forms the contour of the shoulder and raises the arm; the biceps—the "make a muscle" muscle—flexes the forearm; brachioradialis flexes the forearm when the thumb is pointed up; the triceps on the back of the upper arm extends the forearm; and the pectoralis muscles on the front of the chest pull the arms together.

The muscles that allow you to make a fist are not in the hand; they're in the forearm. A grip is formed when tendons traveling across the inside of the wrist curl the fingers inward. The muscles for those tendons are up in the forearm near the elbow. As you make a tight fist, feel those muscles contract while their tendons pop out at the wrist. Now watch what happens to your wrist as you make a grip: the wrist rises. Try making a fist with the wrist hanging limp: no grip. Needed to first lift the wrist, the muscles on the back of the forearm are essential to forming a firm grip.

The muscles in the hand serve to spread and close the fingers and lift the thumb up out of the plane of the palm. Hold your hand out, palm up. If you're a monkey, your thumb will be lying flat in the plane of the palm. Human thumbs are lifted up, away from the palm, by the thenar eminence, that ball of muscle at the base of the thumb. Feel the thenar eminence contract as you slowly press the thumb against the little finger.

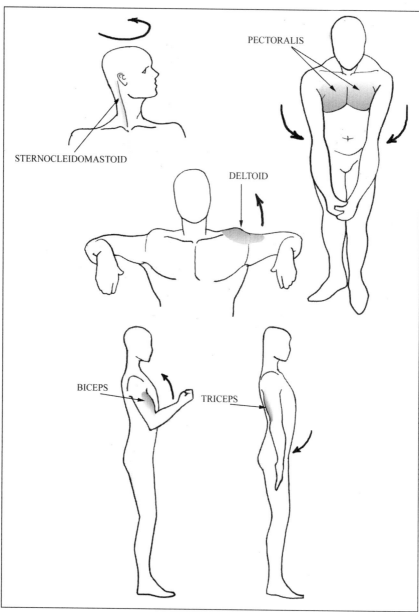

Figure 120

In the legs, the gluteus maximus extends the hip (see figure 121). You can't see the muscle that flexes the hip, the psoas muscle, because it lies along the back wall of the abdomen. (The psoas muscle of a castrated bull, or steer, cooks up into a tender filet mignon because a steer has never used his psoas muscle for mounting.) The quadriceps on the front of the thigh extends the knee, while the hamstrings on the back of the thigh flexes the knee. Gastrocnemius points the foot downward to step on the gas. Tibialis anterior, the broad muscle in the front of the lower leg, pulls the foot upward.

What is muscular dystrophy?

Muscular dystrophy is a slow deterioration of muscles. The cause is genetic malfunction of a key muscle protein, and because there are many key muscle proteins, there are many forms of muscular dystrophy. The most common muscular dystrophy is Duchenne muscular dystrophy, which affects boys (it's X-linked) beginning around the age of 4 or 5. By their teenage years, kids with Duchenne muscular dystrophy can barely walk. Eventually, the disease affects even the respiratory muscles.

What is rabies?

Rabies is a virus passed through the saliva, in other words, through the bite of infected animals, especially dogs, cats, foxes, bats, raccoons, skunks, coyotes, wolves, and jackals. Squirrels, rats, mice, hamsters, guinea pigs, gerbils, and chipmunks rarely, if ever, get rabies.

Rabies virus enters a nerve at the wound site and slowly travels up the nerve to the spinal cord and then into the brain. All this can take weeks to months, long after the bite has been forgotten. If the victim is to survive, antirabies antibodies must be administered before the virus reaches the brain. Otherwise, the death is slow and torturous, beginning with painful muscle spasms and quickly advancing to paralysis of the swallowing muscles, extreme agitation, and finally, delirium mercifully ended when the patient lapses into a terminal coma.

Rabid animals are usually pretty obvious: previously nocturnal animals start showing up on your doorstep during daylight hours. They look sick

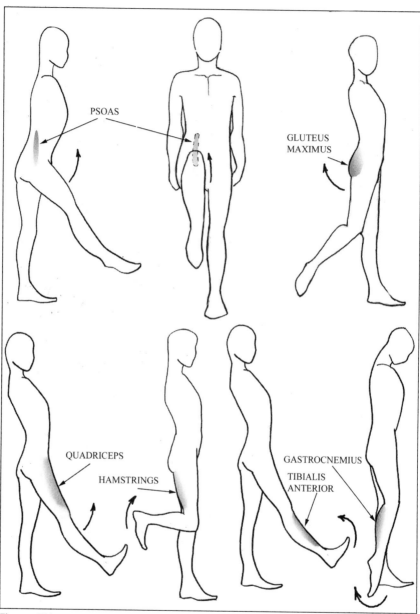

Figure 121

and approach humans without fear. Bats, though, God bless 'em, can look fine and still be infected.

If you are bitten by an animal, wash out the wound with lots of soap and water. It's important to get Animal Control to capture the animal, because the doctor wants to know whether the animal is rabid before beginning a series of antirabies antibody injections.

The horrible death from rabies only heightens our respect for Louis Pasteur, who courageously began working with rabies-infected tissue in the 1880s. By grinding up the spinal cord of an infected animal and injecting it into another animal, Pasteur and his colleagues quickly established that the disease could be transmitted from one animal to another. One colleague, Emile Roux, discovered that when left exposed to the air the infected spinal cord would slowly lose its infectivity, or virulence. He then showed that by injecting the less virulent spinal cords, he could protect animals from the more virulent spinal cords. Suddenly, a child appeared on Pasteur's doorstep having been bitten repeatedly by a rabid dog a few days previously. Left with no choice, Pasteur injected the child with his least virulent spinal cord, and he followed over the next ten days by injecting from more and more virulent spinal cords. The child survived without harm and Pasteur became even more renowned than he already was, though much of the credit belonged to Emile Roux.

How does snake venom kill you?

It depends on the snake. There are generally two kinds of venomous snakes: the cobra/coral snakes and the vipers (rattlesnake, cottonmouth, copperhead). Cobra and coral snake venom paralyzes nerves. Viper venom causes hemorrhaging by destroying blood vessel walls and preventing the blood from clotting.

What does black widow spider venom do?

Black widow venom prevents motor nerves from shutting off. As the venom spreads through the body, muscles develop intensely painful contractions, especially in the abdomen. (Tetanus toxin also triggers painful muscle spasms by preventing motor nerves from shutting off, but its mechanism of action is slightly different.)

16

—~~~~~~~~~~~~—

HOW DOCTORS MAKE A DIAGNOSIS

Doctoring looks pretty easy. A patient offers his complaints, then the doctor orders some tests, figures out what the problem is, and recommends medicines, surgery, or physical therapy to cure the problem. In fact, however, after that first visit, the doctor rarely knows the true cause, or etiology, of the patient's illness. The doctor will simply have a list of possible etiologies. That list is called an etiologic differential diagnosis. How, then, does a doctor take a patient's complaints and formulate an etiologic differential diagnosis?

ESTABLISHING A DIFFERENTIAL DIAGNOSIS

The first step is to determine which organ system the patient's signs and symptoms are coming from. Like any machine, the body works by coordinating its 14 organ systems: skin, immunologic, eyes, ears, respiratory, cardiac, gastrointestinal, endocrine, vascular, urologic, genital, hematologic, bones and joints, and neuromuscular. When organ systems malfunction, the body reacts in two broad ways—with symptoms and signs. Symptoms are things a person complains about, such as fatigue, shortness of breath, dizziness, pain, double vision, and trouble thinking. Signs are abnormal physical findings a doctor discovers on physical examination, such as swollen glands, a rapid heart rate, an enlarged liver, or a breast lump. By taking a history and performing a physical exam, the doctor tries to determine which organ system the patient's complaints are coming from.

Unfortunately, every organ of the body contains other organ systems within it. The liver, for example, contains blood vessels, blood, and lymph. Likewise, cough and shortness of breath could be due to pathology in the respiratory system or in its blood vessels, blood, or lymphatics within the lungs. The list of organ systems that could be harboring the pathology causing the patient's signs and symptoms constitutes the anatomic differential diagnosis.

The second step in the diagnostic process is to take each anatomic site and list all the possible categories of disease that could be affecting each site. There are eight categories of disease: drugs, infections, genetic, immunologic, tumor, trauma, mechanical, and organ dysfunction. *Drugs* refers to any external inanimate agent. Besides drugs, this category includes medications, intravenous agents, vitamin deficiency, radiation, and hypo- and hyperthermia. *Infections* includes any infectious agent. Genetic disease processes include genetic, degenerative (deterioration of an organ system for no known reason), and congenital illnesses with no known cause. An immunologic disease process is one in which antibodies and white blood cells do the damage in the absence of infection. *Tumors* are tumors. *Trauma* is any sudden crush, tear, perforation, rupture, dislocation, or dissection of an organ. The force can come from outside the body or as a spontaneous event inside the body. *Mechanical* insults cause their damage by exerting pressure, compression, obstruction, constriction, distension, torsion, intussusception, herniation, prolapse, aneurysmal swelling, or diverticular swelling. *Organ Dysfunction* is what happens to the presenting organ system when another distant organ system malfunctions, for example, the slowing of mentation with hypothyroidism.

Since each site in the anatomic differential diagnosis could be causing the patient's signs and symptoms, each of the eight etiologic categories must be considered for each site in the anatomic differential diagnosis. By listing the anatomic differential diagnosis across the top of a grid and the eight etiologic categories down the side, a doctor can establish a complete etiologic differential diagnosis (see figure 122).

	ANATOMIC SITES			
	Site 1	Site 2	Site 3	Site 4
DISEASE PROCESS				
Drugs				
Infection				
Genetic				
Immunologic				
Tumor				
Trauma				
Mechanical				
Internal Organ Dysfunction				

Figure 122 Differential Diagnosis Chart

PATHOPHYSIOLOGY

The *mechanism* by which the etiologic agent causes a disease process is its pathophysiology, short for pathologic physiology. Thus an etiologic agent, through a pathophysiologic process, causes an organ system to malfunction, resulting in the patient's signs and symptoms. Cocaine, for example, causes strokes via different pathophysiologies: by raising the blood pressure; by causing intense arterial constriction and thereby preventing blood from passing through the artery; by causing blood to clot more readily; by hastening atherosclerosis; and by settling in the walls of arteries and precipitating an inflammatory reaction called arteritis.

PRIORITIZATION OF THE ETIOLOGIC DIFFERENTIAL DIAGNOSIS

Having established the etiologic differential diagnosis, the doctor prioritizes the list of etiologies, placing at the top of the list those life-threatening diseases that pose the most serious and imminent risk to the patient, and that hence need to be ruled out immediately before they have a chance to do serious damage.

TESTS

Tests are ordered at each step in the process—to confirm malfunction of an organ system, to confirm the etiologic agent, and to understand the pathophysiology. A CAT scan, for example, is an X-ray test that, with the help of a sophisticated computer program, allows us to look inside the body. The images come out as slabs, as if the CAT scan machine had sliced up the body like a baloney slicer. An MRI also slices images of the body, but it doesn't use X-rays, so it's somewhat safer. An MRI also provides more detailed images than a CAT scan does. The risk of X-rays is that they can damage the chromosomes in a girl's ovaries or a boy's testes. If those chromosomes happen to be the ones that make a future baby, the baby may be malformed in some way. To minimize that risk, a heavy lead apron is spread over the lower abdomen and groin, because X-rays cannot penetrate lead.

A SPECT scan is a test in which a radioactive chemical is injected intravenously. The patient is then slid under a Geiger counter. Since the radioactive chemical remains in the bloodstream, the images generated reflect primarily blood flow. In the brain, damaged brain tissue shuts off its own blood supply, so an area of low SPECT scan activity is presumed to represent an area of brain damage. A PET scan differs from a SPECT scan in that the radioactive chemical does not remain in the bloodstream, but is taken up by cells and utilized. The PET scan, therefore, is a direct measurement of cellular activity.

An arteriogram is an X-ray of the body after dye is injected into an artery. Typically, a person is positioned supine (flat on his back) on an X-ray table. Numbing medicine is injected into the skin over the pulsating femoral artery near the groin (which you can feel on yourself). The femoral artery is then punctured with a needle, and through that needle a thin catheter (tube) is threaded. The catheter is advanced up the aorta against the flow of blood or down the femoral artery, depending on the clinical problem. Using considerable skill, the radiologist maneuvers the catheter into the correct artery. Then a syringe of dye is injected through the catheter and as the dye flows into the artery, an X-ray is taken to provide a detailed image of the arterial lumen and the anatomic distribution of the artery.

An ultrasound is a test that forms images of the internal organs by bouncing high-frequency sound waves off them. The image of the internal organs isn't a lifelike photograph, but with a little training you can make out surprising detail of the organs.

A biopsy is a sampling of an organ. This is usually done by sticking a large bore needle through a numbed patch of skin into, say, the kidney and then pulling the needle out. In the lumen of the needle is a core of the kidney.

Blood tests come in three varieties. One type of blood test checks for damage to an internal organ, another checks the performance of the internal organs, and the third checks for foreign substances in the blood. Blood tests for internal organ damage are based on the principle that when an internal organ is damaged, it releases its contents into the bloodstream. Such tests detect damage to the liver, heart, and pancreas.

Tests of function measure how well an organ is functioning. For example, a blood test of the lungs would measure the level of oxygen and carbon dioxide in the blood. Blood tests for kidney function measure the levels of creatinine and urea-nitrogen, two chemicals normally cleared by kidneys. Tests of foreign substances measure the level of, say, antibiotics or anticonvulsants in the bloodstream.

DOCTORING

It should be clear now why medical training takes so long. Prospective doctors have to learn the signs and symptoms of each organ system, how to elicit those signs and symptoms from a patient, the disease processes that affect each organ system (inflammation, ischemia, metabolic disturbance, cancerous invasion, etc.), specific etiologic diseases, how they trigger their disease process, and their proper surgical and nonsurgical treatments. This requires a fundamental understanding of biochemistry, anatomy, physiology, pathology (disease processes under the microscope), pharmacology, radiology (X-rays, CAT scans, MRI scans, arteriography, and ultrasound), and laboratory testing.

17

FINAL THOUGHTS FOR TEENAGERS

As you grow out of your teens and experience more of the world, you'll encounter a dizzying array of new ideas, facts, and assertions about one thing or another. One of the things you will soon realize is that people will tell you anything to get your love and money. Fortunately, each of us was born with a sensitive neurologic structure deep within the brain called a bullshit detector to alert us to things that don't make sense. Here are some tips on how to look at things more critically.

The conclusions and assertions you hear and read are the product of a three-part syllogism. The first part is the general principle, or "law." The second part is the facts. And the third part is the conclusion—the "therefore," where the general principle is applied to the facts at hand. Sometimes the general principle is wrong, sometimes the facts are wrong, and sometimes the general principle is misapplied to the facts (and sometimes all three of these problems apply). Suppose somebody tells you you shouldn't smoke. That's a conclusion based on a syllogism. The general principle is that smoking is bad for you, the assumed facts are that you don't want to do something bad to your body, and the conclusion naturally follows that you should stop smoking. Are the general principle and the facts correct? Take the general principle that smoking is bad for you. That's true, but smoking is not all bad. There are some good qualities to smoking, such as calming your nerves, helping focus your attention, reducing your appetite, and aiding social interaction. There are plenty of 80- and 90-year-old people who smoke. So when you say smoking is "bad," how bad is it? Specifically, what risk do I face by smoking?

To answer that, you need to understand how to assess risk. Half of growing up is learning how to assess risks. The other half is deciding whether to accept the risk. (The "third half" is learning how to relinquish control and let those around you assess and accept risks as they see fit.) Risk assessment is very simple if you follow Judge Learned Hand's straightforward formula: take the likelihood that the bad consequence will happen and multiply that by the damage done if it does occur. For example, the risk of stained teeth from smoking is high, but the damage done is minor, so that risk is relatively small. The risk of cancer from smoking is lowish, but the damage done is usually fatal, making that risk higher—call it a moderate risk. A relatively small risk of smoking also applies to chronic bronchitis, wrinkling of facial skin, and dulling of the senses of smell and taste, while the same moderate risk that applies to cancer also applies to atherosclerosis and emphysema. When the risks of cancer, atherosclerosis, and emphysema are combined, smoking poses a moderate to moderately high risk overall.

As for the "fact" that you don't want to do something bad to your body, that needs to be challenged. Not everyone believes that a life of working out, eating like a monk, meditating, no smoking, no binge drinking, no drugs, and no unprotected sex with multiple partners is the way to go. Lots of people would gladly shave a few years off their lives to live it up.

Step three—applying the general principle to the facts—can also be slippery, because all you see is the conclusion, and you have to figure out whether the conclusion truly follows from a proper application of the general principle to the facts. Just because A came before B does not mean that A caused B unless all the other causes of B have been ruled out. For example, John wants to kill Jane. Jane is murdered. Therefore, John killed Jane. The certainty of that conclusion is obviously wrong, because the proper general principle was that John was the only one who wanted to kill Jane. In fact, there may have been many people who wanted to kill Jane. The same problem applies to the following medical syllogism. XYZ medicine is known to improve depression. This patient's spirits improved after taking XYZ medication. Therefore, XYZ medicine improved the depression. Maybe, but you can't say for sure until you know that XYZ medicine is the only thing that could have improved the depression. In this case, there may be many other reasons the depression could have improved.

How about a case where a person falls and strikes his head and three months later develops multiple sclerosis? He now asserts that the head trauma caused his multiple sclerosis. You could know that conclusion to be true only if head trauma were the only cause of multiple sclerosis. Maybe the cart is before the horse. Maybe he fell because he had undiagnosed multiple sclerosis. Take the assertion that people who exercise retain their intellect longer than sedentary people. All you have is regular exercise and retained intellect in old age. While one would like to believe that regular exercise results in an intact intellect in old age, maybe those who make it to old age with an intact intellect are the only ones left to exercise. Or maybe a third factor, such as a positive attitude, makes a person want to go out and exercise and at the same time keeps minds sharp in old age.

Even harder than scrutinizing claims asserting how to live a long and healthy life is deciding for yourself what makes a full and satisfying life. Then you can decide how much risk you need to take to reach those goals against how much risk you're willing to take, a very personal decision. Whatever you decide now will undoubtedly change as you test out how much satisfaction you get from trying different things in life. One of the great things about America, perhaps the greatest thing, is that everyone is free to screw up their lives in their own unique way. While there will always be some self-righteous crusader monitoring your every behavior, feeling compelled and justified to announce your every mistake in life, ultimately, the decision about how you treat your body is your own. I hope reading this book will help you make the best decisions for you. God's speed.

GLOSSARY

Abortion. Artificial termination of a pregnancy.

Abscess. A walled-off collection of pus.

Accommodation reflex. The rounding up of the lens and constriction of the pupil when viewing something up close.

Accutane. An anti-acne drug that works by slowing the production of sebum and inhibiting the bacteria that infect clogged pores.

ACE inhibitors. Drugs that block angiotensin-converting enzyme, thereby protecting arteries from the harmful effects of angiotensin II.

Acetabulum. The socket into which the head of the femur inserts to form the hip joint.

Acetylcholine. A neurotransmitter.

Acne. Collections of oily whiteheads and blackheads on the skin surface, formed when sebum and dead hair cells clog pores. Infected whiteheads and blackheads become pimples.

Acromegaly. Excessive growth of soft tissues and bone due to overproduction of growth hormone secretion.

Acyclovir. A drug active against herpes virus.

Adenoids. Lymphoid tissue at the back of the nasal chambers.

Adenosine triphospate (ATP). By packing lots of energy into its phosphate bonds, adenosine triphosphate is able to release that energy at will for thousands of chemical reactions.

Adhesions. Scar tissue binding together two tissues, for example, two sections of intestines, pleura and the chest wall, joints and adjacent soft tissue.

Adiponectin. A protein released from fat cells that makes cells more sensitive to insulin. The release of adiponectin is inhibited by obesity, contributing to the development of diabetes.

Adrenal cortex. The outer layer of the adrenal gland from which aldosterone is released.

Adrenal gland. A gland resting atop each

kidney that secretes corticosteroids and epinephrine, aldosterone to regulate salt retention by the kidneys, and small amounts of testosterone and estrogen.

Adrenal medulla. The inner core of the adrenal gland, from which corticosteroids and epinephrine are released.

Adrenal-stimulating hormone. Adrenocorticotropic hormone, released by the anterior pituitary to instruct the adrenal glands to release corticosteroids, epinephrine, and aldosterone.

Adrenaline. Epinephrine. Released from the adrenal glands on stimulation from sympathetic nerves.

Adrenocorticotropic hormone (ACTH). Adrenal-stimulating hormone.

Aerobic bacteria. Bacteria that only grow in the presence of oxygen and that cannot grow in the absence of oxygen.

Afterbirth. The placenta, which detaches from the uterine wall several minutes after delivery of the baby.

AIDS. Acquired immune deficiency syndrome. A slow and often fatal disabling of the immune system by HIV virus.

Albumin. The most common protein in the bloodstream, it provides receptor sites to transport heme, drugs, and hormones in the bloodstream and helps to absorb water into the vascular tree.

Alcohol. A chemical toxic to all cells of the body when used in excess, and particularly toxic to the liver and brain.

Aldosterone. A hormone released by the adrenal gland to instruct the kidney to retain water.

Alert. Being awake enough to be aware of one's surroundings.

Ali, Muhammad. The prize fighter who developed Parkinson's disease because of repeated head trauma.

Alveoli. Tiny sacs at the ends of bronchioles where oxygen and carbon dioxide are exchanged between inhaled air and the body's bloodstream.

Alzheimer's disease. A slowly advancing dementia caused by neuron-clogging protein accumulation in the brain for unknown reasons.

Amanita. A poisonous mushroom.

Amenorrhea. No menstrual periods.

Amino acids, essential. Eight amino acids the body cannot synthesize from scratch and that must therefore be eaten.

Amniotic fluid. The fluid in which a fetus is suspended as it develops inside the uterus.

Amphetamine. A strongly epinephrine-like drug that also stimulates the pleasure center, resulting in addiction.

Anabolic steroid. A hormone that builds up muscles.

Anal fissure. A painful crack in the skin that connects to the anal opening.

Analgesic. A drug that stops pain.

Anaphylaxis. A sudden, life-threatening intravascular immunologic response to an antigen, causing massive leakage of fluid from small blood vessels throughout the body.

Androstenedione. A precursor molecule to testosterone and estrogen.

Anencephaly. A condition in which a baby is born with no brain tissue other than a brainstem.

Anerobic bacteria. Bacteria that grow only in the absence of oxygen, and not in the presence of oxygen.

Anesthesia, epidural. Placement of anesthetics into the epidural space through a needle or catheter.

Aneurysm. Dilation of an artery, any artery in the body.

Aneurysm, fusiform. Circumferential arterial dilation, resembling a snake after eating a large rat.

Aneurysm, saccular. A focal weakening and ballooning out of part of an arterial wall.

Angina. Chest pain behind the sternum coming from the heart from lack of oxygen.

Angioplasty. The opening of a blocked artery by slipping a deflated balloon into the obstruction and blowing up the balloon.

Angiotensin II. A harmful hormone synthesized in the bloodstream in response to low blood flow to the kidneys; stimulates arteries to constrict and thicken their walls, and the adrenal glands to release aldosterone, causing the kidneys to retain salt.

Ankle. The bony protrusions of the tibia (inside ankle) and fibula bone (outside ankle).

Ankle sprain. Tearing of a ligament or tendon. A strain is milder than a sprain. It is merely the stretching of a ligament or tendon.

Anorexia nervosa. The severe curtailment of all food intake, usually in a teenage girl or young woman, because of a morbid and distorted belief that her body is too fat.

Antacids. Drugs that temporarily relieve heartburn by mopping up acid in the stomach.

Anterior. In front of.

Antibiotics. Drugs that kill or inhibit the growth of bacteria, fungi, or viruses.

Antibodies. Large proteins that attach to foreign antigens to neutralize them and then present them to white blood cells for future reference.

Anticoagulation, oral. Pills that block the synthesis of one or more of the clotting factors.

Antidiuretic hormone. Vasopressin. The hormone released by the posterior pituitary to instruct the kidneys to retain water.

Antigen. Any substance considered foreign by the immunologic system.

Antigen–antibody complex. The combination of an antibody attached to its target antigen, floating in the bloodstream.

Anxiety. A state of fear before the specific threat is identified.

Aorta. The main artery carrying oxygenated blood from the left ventricle.

Aortic valve. The valve at the exit hole of the left ventricle.

Aphasia. An impairment of the expression of language, not simply slurred speech or sloppy handwriting, consisting of uncorrectable spelling and grammatical mistakes in written and spoken language.

Appendicitis. Inflammation in the appendix, almost always due to a bacterial infection.

Appendix. A hollow finger of intestine dangling from the cecum, filled with clusters of white blood cells sniffing the intestinal slurry entering the colon.

Aqueous fluid. A clear fluid that keeps the anterior chamber distended behind the cornea and in front of the iris and lens.

Arachnoid. A thin membrane overlying the surface of the brain under which cerebrospinal fluid flows.

Arrhythmia. An irregular, or dangerously fast or slow, heartbeat.

Arteries. Blood vessels that carry blood away from the heart.

Arteriole. Small artery.

Arteriovenous malformation. A congenital absence of capillaries in an isolated area of the vascular tree allowing high-pressure arteries to dilate up low-pressure veins, often resulting in hemorrhage by middle life.

Arteritis. Inflammation of arteries.

Artery, axillary. The artery in the upper arm palpable under the biceps muscle.

Arthralgias. Joint pains.

Arthritis. Inflammation in a joint.

Arthritis, old age. Joint pain and inflammation due to wear and tear.

Arthritis, rheumatoid. An autoimmune attack on joints, resulting in disabling joint deformities.

Ascites. Fluid accumulation in the abdominal cavity.

Aseptic necrosis. Death of tissue that remains sterile.

Aseptic. Not infected.

Aspiration. The inadvertent and dangerous inhalation of food or drink into the trachea.

Aspirin. A chemical that blocks inflammation and, by preventing platelets from adhering to one another, reduces the likelihood of arterial blood clots.

Asthma. Difficulty breathing due to narrowed and congested bronchioles.

Astigmatism. Blurred vision due to an elongated cornea.

Atherosclerosis. The clogging of arteries by the buildup of cholesterol, triglycerides, blood clot, and calcium.

Athetosis. Writhing movements of the trunk and limbs, twisting them into distorted postures.

Athletic heart. A heart so strong that it can pump more blood in three strokes than a nonathlete can pump with four strokes.

Atlas. The first cervical vertebra, so named because it, like Atlas, holds the world on its shoulders.

Atrial fibrillation. A quivering of the atria as they are bombarded by electrical impulses 300 times a minute.

Atrial septal defect. A hole in the atrial septum, normal during fetal development, abnormal if it persists after birth.

Atrium. A holding chamber of the heart that fills with blood while the ventricle is busy contracting, and that quickly dumps the blood into the ventricle when the ventricle is finished contracting.

Atrophy. Shrinkage or wasting away.

Atropine. A drug that blocks the effect of the neurotransmitter acetylcholine released from parasympathetic nerves.

Autism. A mysterious disturbance of brain development, characterized by withdrawn, uncommunicative behavior, fixation on objects, hypersensitivity to sounds, and often but not always, intellectual impairment.

Autoimmune disease. The result of immune surveillance turning on itself and attacking its own body's tissues.

Autonomic nervous system. All the nerves in the brain, spinal cord, and peripheral nervous system devoted to regulating the involuntary affairs of the body, such as pupil reaction to light, sweating, heart rate, blood pressure, gut movement, erections, and more.

Axilla. Arm pit.

Axis. The second cervical vertebra.

Axon. The long, outgoing arm of a nerve cell bearing electrical signals for the next nerve cell or muscle.

Bacterium. A tiny single-celled organism whose DNA is floating free in the cytoplasm, unlike larger cells, where the DNA is gathered inside a nuclear membrane (the nucleus). Bacteria are usually identified by the color they take on when stained with a Gram stain: Gram positive if the bacterium stains blue, Gram negative if it stains pink.

Ballism. Repetitive flinging movements of

a limb, voluntarily controllable for only a few minutes.

Banting, Frederick. Along with Best, Collip, and Macleod, one of the discoverers of insulin.

Barbiturates. In 1864, Baeyer synthesized barbiturates from urea and named them after someone named Barbara (Barbara + urea).

Basal ganglia. Clusters of nerve cell bodies in the upper brainstem and base of the cerebral hemispheres devoted to controlling the amount and speed of movement, not strength.

Basement membrane. The platform on which inner ear hair cells vibrate in response to mechanical stimulation by the stapes.

Belladonna plant. A source of atropine.

Bell's palsy. Weakness of one side of the face due to compression of the facial nerve traveling through the skull's facial canal en route to the facial muscles.

Benign tumor. A growth that, like malignant tumors, continues to grow, but that does so by simply enlarging, not infiltrating the host tissue or metastasizing to distant organs.

Berger, Hans. The inventor of the electroencephalogram.

Beriberi. Neurologic damage to peripheral nerves (in the arms and legs) due to thiamine (vitamin B1) deficiency.

Best, Charles. Along with Banting, Collip, and Macleod, one of the discoverers of insulin.

Bile. A greenish slurry made by the liver from old hemoglobin and cholesterol, stored in the gall bladder, and released into the duodenum to break up fat globules for easier digestion.

Bilirubin. A metabolic breakdown product of heme, forming an important component of bile.

Biofeedback. A method to develop voluntary control over the autonomic nervous system.

Biopsy. A sampling of tissue for testing, culturing, or examination under the microscope.

Birth control pills. Potent estrogen- and progesterone-mimicking drugs that inhibit follicle-stimulating hormone release from the pituitary by fooling the pituitary into thinking there's a pregnancy afoot.

Blackhead. See ACNE.

Bleb. A delicate bubble.

Blind spot. A small blind area best detected at arm's length about 6 inches to the side of central vision, corresponding to the optic disc, which is devoid of all rods and cones.

Blood clotting. The formation of a fibrin net by a complicated series of protein interactions within the bloodstream.

Blood manufacture. Takes place in the bone marrow.

Blood pressure. The pressure generated in arteries with each heartbeat.

Blood pressure cuff. An inflatable bladder wrapped around the upper arm to temporarily compress the axillary artery for blood pressure measurement.

Blood pressure, diastolic. The blood pressure at the end of systolic contraction.

Blood pressure, systolic. The blood pressure at the peak of systolic contraction.

Blood type. The immunologic signature for all red blood cells in any one person, based on the presence or absence of A and B antigens attached to the red blood cell surface.

Blood–brain barrier. The sealed gap between endothelial cells lining the capillaries of the brain.

Blue baby. A baby with blood that's poorly oxygenated.

Blue balls. Painful testicles due to stagnant circulation from a sustained erection.

Blue bloods. The upper class.

Bone marrow. Where red blood cells, white blood cells, and platelets are made.

Bones and joints system. The bones, joints, and attached cartilage used to support and house the body.

Botox. A dilute solution of injectable botulinus toxin for selectively paralyzing specific muscles.

Botulism. Muscle paralysis from a toxin released by *Clostridium botulinum*.

Brain dead. When the brain is dead, but the heart is still beating. Patients in this state never recover, because the death of brain tissue is permanent.

Brainstem. Located between the bottom of the cerebral hemispheres and the top of the spinal cord, the brainstem is the oldest part of the brain, controlling ancient functions shared by all vertebrates: consciousness, sleep, eye movements, pupillary reaction, eye closure, facial sensation, facial movement, hearing, swallowing, rotation of the head, tongue movement, articulation of sounds, blood pressure, pulse rate, and respirations.

Breastbone. The sternum, onto which the ribs attach with the help of a small piece of intervening cartilage.

Broca, Paul. The discoverer of one of the speech centers in the brain, now called Broca's area.

Broca's aphasia. Impaired speech due to injury to Broca's area; extremely halting, sometimes nonexistent, leaving nothing but the main nouns of a sentence.

Broca's area. The quarter-sized area in the left (almost always) frontal lobe that controls the fluency of speech.

Bronchial tubes. Cartilaginous branches of the trachea that conduct air into the lungs.

Bronchioles. The small branches of the bronchial tree.

Bronchitis, chronic. Chronic inflammation in the bronchial tubes, usually manifesting as a chronic cough and phlegm production.

Bruit. The sound of blood tumbling in an artery or vein with each heartbeat, usually due to some obstruction in the blood vessel, or else excessive blood flow.

Buffalo hump. The large pad of fat that accumulates over the upper back in people who take excessive corticosteroids.

Bulimia. Binge eating followed by induced vomiting and use of laxatives and diuretics.

Bundle of His. Two electrical excitable bundles of muscle (one for each ventricle) that transmit the electrical signals from the atrioventricular node throughout both ventricles.

Bunion. A bony deformity of the great toe due usually to wearing tight high-heel shoes.

Bursa. A pillow of fluid over which tendons ride as they pull bones this way and that.

Caesarian birth. Delivery of a baby by cutting through the abdominal and uterine walls.

Callus. A painless thickening of skin from continual rubbing or pressure.

Cancer. A growth that never stops growing and that spreads by infiltrating strands of tumor cells into the host tissue and also by metastasizing to distant parts of the body.

Capillaries. Tiny, thin-walled blood vessels through which oxygen, glucose, and other goodies are released into the body's tissues, and by which waste is gathered up to be brought to the lungs, liver, and kidneys for disposal.

Carbohydrates. Rings of carbon to which are attached molecules of hydrogen and oxygen.

Carbon dioxide. A waste by-product produced during the mitochondrial breakdown of glucose to make 36 ATP.

Carcinogen. An agent that causes cancer.

Cardiac arrest. Abrupt failure of the heart to pump blood, usually due to ventricular fibrillation or rapid ventricular tachy-cardia, and sometimes to pericardial tam-ponade or a large pulmonary embolus.

Cardiac resuscitation. An electrical shock delivered to get all the cells in the heart to agree on an electrical starting point, so that coordinated electrical impulses can resume again from the sinoatrial and atrioventricular nodes.

Cardiac system. The heart, which pumps blood in a circuit around the body.

Caries. Tooth decay.

Carotid sinus. A nubbin of tissue along the carotid artery that alerts the brain to any rise in blood pressure.

Carotid sinus reflex. Vagal slowing of the heart in response to hypertensive stimu-lation of the carotid sinus.

Carpal tunnel syndrome. Compression of the median nerve crossing the wrist through the carpal tunnel.

Cartilage. Gristle. A firm but flexible tissue comprising the ear, tip of the nose, intervertebral discs, bony coverings in joints, and trachea.

CAT scan. Computerized Axial Tomography. An X-ray generated slab of the human body.

Catabolize. To break down into simple molecules.

Cataplexy. Sudden limpness of the trunk or legs, sometimes the whole body, when a person is suddenly struck by something evoking a strong emotion, such as surprise, anger, or hilarity.

Cataract. Obscuration of central vision due to opacification of the lens or cornea.

Cauda equina. The bushy tail of nerve roots in the lumbar spinal canal, extending from the bottom of the spinal cord in the lower thoracic spine, down to the nerves' exit holes in the lumbar and sacral spine.

Cecum. A blind pouch forming the first part of the large intestine.

Cell body. The brains of a nerve cell where the decision is made whether or not to fire the axon.

Cellulose. The structural polysaccharide of plants.

Cementum. A thin covering of the tooth below the gum line that helps to hold a tooth in its socket.

Central nervous system. All the nerves that begin and end in the brain or spinal cord.

Cerebellum. An ancient structure behind the brainstem controlling balance and coordination.

Cerebral cortex. The corrugated rind of gray matter over the surface of the cerebral hemispheres.

Cerebral edema. Extra water within the substance of the brain.

Cerebral hemisphere. Located above the brainstem, the right and left cerebral hemispheres together make up the brain.

Cerebral palsy. A brain injury sustained around the time of birth.

Cerebrospinal fluid. A clear-as-water fluid made in the cerebral ventricles and circulating out over the surface of the brain to be absorbed, carrying brain waste with it.

Cervix. The opening to the uterus at the far end of the vagina.

Chemotherapy. The treatment of cancer with medications.

Chest tube. A sterile tube inserted into the pleural space to drain out air, fluid, or pus.

Chicken pox. A systemic viral illness caused by herpes zoster virus, presenting with widespread vesicles (tiny sacs of fluid on the skin) that crust over and itch.

Chlamydia. A treatable sexually transmitted bacterium that infects the genital system of men or women.

Cholecystokinin. A hormone released by the intestines that curbs our appetite by inhibiting the hypothalamus from releasing NPY and stimulating the hypothalamus to release melanocortin.

Cholelithiasis. The presence of gallstones.

Cholesterol. A fat used throughout the body for cellular structure, hormones, and bile and that accumulates along arterial walls as atherosclerosis.

Chorda tendineae. The tendons by which the papillary muscles insert on the undersurface of the mitral valve to prevent it from bulging backward into the left atrium during systole. See MUSCLES, PAPILLARY.

Chorea. Brief flickers of muscles or muscle groups distributed randomly about the body (unlike tics, which always affect the same muscles).

Chorionic gonadotropin. A hormone secreted for several months by the fertilized egg to keep the ovary producing high levels of estrogen and progesterone for a lush uterine endometrium, until the placenta can begin producing its own supply of estrogen and progesterone.

Chromosome. A chain of genes, with extra genes included to control gene activity.

Chronic. Longer than six months.

Chylomicrons. Droplets of triglycerides absorbed through the intestinal wall into lymphatic lacteals.

Ciliary muscles. Two small muscles attached to the lens that, by contracting, cause the lens to round up for close-up vision.

Cingulate gyrus. A section of cerebral cortex that forms part of the limbic system.

Circumcision. Surgical removal of the foreskin, a flap of skin covering the glans of the penis.

Cirrhosis. Severe scarring of the liver, enough to render it useless.

Citrate. A chemical that binds calcium and thereby prevents blood from clotting.

Claudication. Pain emanating from muscles from lack of oxygen.

Clavicle. See COLLAR BONE.

Clitoris. The female version of the male glans.

Clot busters. Drugs that break apart blood clots.

Cocaine. An epinephrine-like drug that, by stimulating the pleasure center, is also very addictive.

Coccyx. Tail bone.

Cochlea. A rolled up conch of fluid in the inner ear containing a basement membrane that converts sound waves into electrical signals to be interpreted by the brain.

Collagen. A structural protein that helps cement teeth in their sockets, gives structure to the skin and soft tissues of the body, and forms much of the underlying framework of scar tissue.

Collar bone. The clavicle, a bone stretching from the upper sternum to the shoulder joint that helps stabilize the shoulder joint.

Collip, James. Along with Banting, Best, and Macleod, one of the discoverers of insulin.

Colon. Large intestine.

Colony-stimulating factor. A protein that stimulates the production of white blood cells.

Colostomy. A surgical hole in the colon brought to the skin surface.

Common bile duct. The joining of the hepatic and cystic ducts, carrying bile into the duodenum.

Complement proteins. Special immunologic proteins in the blood that punch a hole in bacteria and other foreign cells.

Condom. A thin latex shield placed over the penis or cervix to block sperm from entering the cervix.

Cones. Retinal cells sensitive to color, used for day vision.

Congenital. From birth, but not of genetic origin.

Conjunctiva. The white of the eye.

Conjunctivitis. Inflammation in the white of the eye.

Conscious. Being awake enough to initiate voluntary movement.

Consumption. Tuberculosis.

Contusion. A bruise, the black and blue representing the breakdown products of small amounts of blood released into the soft tissues.

Convulsion. A grand mal seizure in which the patient falls unconscious to the ground and shakes all over.

Corn. A painful inward-growing thickening of the skin due to continual rubbing or pressure.

Cornea. The clear front part of the eye, very sensitive to touch or irritating chemicals.

Coronal plane. The side-to-side plane of the body.

Coronary arteries. The arteries feeding blood to the heart muscle.

Coronary bypass surgery. A procedure that by connecting one end of a donor vessel upstream, and the other end downstream, of a site of coronary artery obstruction is able to detour blood around the site of obstruction.

Corticosteroids. Hormones produced by the adrenal glands with strong anti-inflammatory properties.

Corticotropin releasing factor. The hypothalamic messenger transported down to the pituitary gland to stimulate the pituitary to release adrenocorticotropic hormone.

Cortisone. The anti-inflammatory stress hormone released by the adrenal gland.

Crabs. Lice.

Cramp, muscle. Involuntary contraction of a muscle.

C-reactive protein. A protein released during an inflammatory attack, hence a sign of ongoing inflammation somewhere in the body.

Creatine. By attaching high-energy phosphate molecules to creatine in muscle, creatine-phosphate is able to rapidly replace the high-energy phosphate bonds broken off adenosine triphosphate (ATP) during vigorous exercise, thereby enhancing endurance.

Crede. Balling up the fist in the lower abdomen and leaning over to put pressure on a weak bladder to help it empty itself. More than 100 years ago, Dr. Carl Crede, who developed this method, also discovered the usefulness of dabbing dilute silver nitrate into newborns' eyes to prevent the horror of gonorrhea eye infections.

Cribriform plate. The perforated bony plate through which the brain's delicate olfactory hair cells poke into the upper chambers of the nose.

Crocodile tears. Tears evoked by seeing or tasting food, due to misdirected regrowth of axons after Bell's palsy.

Cruciate ligaments. Two ligaments within the knee joint holding the femur to the tibia.

Cyanosis. Blue, from lack of oxygen.

Cylcooxygenase (COX). The enzyme that regulates the production of prostaglandins, unique fatty acids that help control the inflammatory attack and help coat the stomach wall to protect it from strong hydrochloric acid.

Cyst. A sac of fluid.

Cystic duct. The tube connecting the gall bladder to the hepatic duct to form the common bile duct.

Cystic fibrosis. A genetic disease in which excessive amounts of thick mucus continually secreted by the walls of the bronchial tubes become repeatedly infected.

Dam, Henrik. The discoverer of vitamin K.

Dark meat. Meat containing dark-red myoglobin to bind oxygen for long-duration, low-intensity muscular activity by slowly metabolizing glucose and fat into lots of ATP.

Decibel. A measure of the loudness of sound. The human ear is capable of detecting changes of one decibel.

Decompression illness. Joint pains and mental changes due to nitrogen bubbles forming in the bloodstream from too rapid an ascent during scuba diving.

Decongestants. Drugs that shrink the nasal and sinus mucosa.

Deep venous thrombosis. A blood clot in the deep venous system, usually of the leg.

Defecation. Making number two.

Defribrillator. The machine that delivers a massive electrical jolt to the heart in order to reset the heart's electrical rhythm. See CARDIAC RESUSCITATION.

Dehydration. Excessive loss of water.

Delusion. Any idea believed by only one person in the world and judged by experts to be impossible.

Dendrite. The bushy tail of a nerve cell that receives signals from other nerve cells, or from any number of sensory inputs, such as touch, pin prick, hot, cold, and so on.

Dentin. The soft layer beneath the enamel of a tooth.

Deoygenated. Without oxygen.

Depth of field. The nearest and farthest distance from the retina where objects still remain in focus.

Dermatome. A strip of skin supplied by one sensory nerve root.

Diabetes. The failure of insulin to lower blood sugar, because there is no insulin around or because the cells are ignoring insulin, and all the consequences that follow.

Diaphragm. The broad, thin muscle at the bottom of the chest that, when contracting on inspiration, pulls air into the lungs.

Differential diagnosis. The list of possible explanations (synonymous with etiologies) for a patient's symptoms and signs.

Differential diagnosis, anatomic. The list of possible sites where the patient's symptoms and signs could be coming from.

Differential diagnosis, etiologic. The list of possible diseases that could be causing the patient's symptoms and signs.

Digestion. The process of absorbing food

and drink from the intestinal tract.

Disc herniation. Protrusion of a disc material beyond the confines of the disc space.

Dissection, arterial. Bleeding into the wall of an artery.

Distal. Far away from the center of the body.

Diuretic. A water pill.

Diverticulosis. Small outpouchings of the colonic wall, providing sites for small, often painful, infections.

Diving chamber. A sealed chamber into which air is pumped at high pressure to force oxygen into ischemic tissues, or else to force nitrogen bubbles back into solution in patients suffering decompression illness.

Diving reflex. Sudden, involuntary slowing of the heart on diving, or just dunking the face, into cold water; a means of conserving oxygen under water.

DNA. Deoxyribonucleic acid. A coded set of instructions for assembling amino acids into proteins. Four carbohydrates—cytosine, adenine, guanine, and thymine—are strung together in a specific order. Each link of three carbohydrates codes for one amino acid.

Dopamine. One of the brain's neurotransmitters.

Double-jointed. Having a lax joint.

Drug addiction. Behavior totally devoted to the sole goal of obtaining more of a drug.

Duchenne muscular dystrophy. An X-linked muscular dystrophy that affects nearly all muscles, beginning in childhood with weakness in the legs.

Ductus arteriosus. A short artery connecting the pulmonary artery to the aorta during fetal development to divert blood around the still underdeveloped lungs;

generally closed by one week of age.

Duodenum. The short section of small intestine just beyond the stomach.

Dura. A tough membrane covering the brain.

Dyslexia. Reading difficulty due to improper deciphering of written symbols into meaningful words.

E. coli. *Escherichia coli.* The most abundant bacterium in the colon.

Ear system. The system of bones and nerves buried within the temporal bone that converts sound waves and head movement into electrical signals, and sends them to the brain for analysis.

Eardrum (tympanic membrane). Membrane situated deep inside the external auditory canal that converts sound waves into the mechanical movement of tiny bones in the middle ear.

Ecstasy. A serotonin-raising party drug that eventually burns up serotonin neurons in the brain.

Edema. Excess fluid.

Eijkman, Christiaan. The first person to show that something in the husks of rice could cure beriberi.

Ejaculation. The expulsion of sperm from the urethra.

Elastic fibers. Fibers in the skin and soft tissue that spring stretched tissue back to its original shape.

Electrocardiogram (EKG). A recording of the heart's ongoing electrical activity.

Electroencephalogram (EEG). A recording of the brain's ongoing electrical activity.

Electrolysis. A method for removing hair follicles using electricity or heat.

Embolus. A blood clot that breaks away from an arterial or venous wall and travels in the bloodstream, eventually lodging in a smaller vessel downstream.

Emphysema. The destruction of alveolar walls, reducing the oxygen-absorbing capacity of the lungs.

Emulsify. To break up into tiny droplets.

Enamel (of a tooth). The hard outer surface of a tooth.

Encephalitis. Inflammation of the substance of the brain.

Endocrine system. The pituitary, thyroid, parathyroid, islets of Langerhans, adrenal glands, and gonads (testes and ovaries), plus other organs that secrete hormones into the bloodstream to control the function of one or more distant organs.

Endolymphatic sac. Where fluid in the semicircular canals of the inner ear normally drains out.

Endometrium, uterus. The inner lining of the uterus, where the placenta implants and derives nutrients for the developing fetus.

Endorphin. A pituitary protein released with enkephalin to inhibit pain and provide a feeling of euphoria.

Endothelial cells. Flat, broad cells that line the interior walls of arteries and veins.

Endotracheal tube. A plastic tube inserted into the trachea to carry air into the lungs from a mechanical ventilator or a hand-pumped rubber bag called an Ambu bag.

Enkephalin. A pituitary protein released with endorphin to inhibit pain and provide a feeling of euphoria.

Enteric nervous system. Billions of nerves within the gut wall that, along with (or under the direction of) the autonomic nervous system, regulate gut movement (peristalsis) and probably other gut functions as well.

Enzyme. A protein that chemically alters other molecules.

Ephedrine. A drug with epinephrine-like actions.

Epidermis. Medical term for skin.

Epidural hematoma. An arterial or, less commonly, a venous blood clot outside the dura, typically occurring in the temporal region when a temporal bone fracture tears a small artery. The rapidly accumulating arterial blood under high pressure presses against the temporal lobe, causing early fatal brain herniation.

Epidural space. The space outside the dura, between the dura and skull bone.

Epiglottis. A cartilaginous flap that closes over the trachea during swallowing.

Epinephrine. The body's stress hormone released by the adrenal gland, mimicking the action of sympathetic nerves.

Erection. A flooding of the penis with blood, making it turgid.

Ergot drugs. Drugs that stimulate the smooth muscle in arterial walls and uterus to contract, derived from the ergot family of fungi.

Erythropoietin. The hormone secreted by the kidneys to stimulate the bone marrow to make new red blood cells.

Esophagus. The intestinal conduit from the mouth to the stomach.

Estrogen. The hormone that makes a woman look and do like a woman.

Etiology. The cause of a patient's illness.

Eustacian tube. The channel connecting the middle ear with the pharynx to equalize pressure on both sides of the tympanic membrane, thereby avoiding the risk of rupturing the membrane.

Exercise, aerobic. Exercise accompanied by sufficient oxygen delivery to muscles to forestall excess lactic acid accumulation.

Exercise, anerobic. Exercise without enough oxygen for mitochondria to metabolize the muscle's accumulating pyruvate into ATP, forcing the cytoplasm instead to convert pyruvate to lactic acid.

Exercise, isometric. Pulling or pushing of an immovable object, thus generating anerobic metabolism.

External auditory canal. The hole in the ear channeling sounds to the tympanic membrane.

Extrapyramidal fibers. Bundles of motor nerves in the brain carrying instructions from the basal ganglia.

Eye, anterior chamber. The space behind the cornea and in front of the iris and lens.

Eye, floaters. Bits of cellular debris in the vitreous humor.

Eye system. Two jelly-filled globes that convert electromagnetic radiation into electrical signals and send the signals to the brain for analysis.

Fallopian tube. A funnel-shaped tube extending from the upper uterus that each month catches an egg released from the ovary and directs the egg into the uterus.

Fat. Lipid. Water-insoluble ch. ins of carbon atoms, solid at room temperature.

Fatty acids. Long chains of carbon atoms chemically attached to hydrogen atoms.

Fatty acids, cis. A double-bonded fatty acid with the carbon chains on either side of the double bond kinked in the same direction, making it more difficult for the fatty acid to solidify.

Fatty acids, monounsaturated. A fatty acid with only one double bond.

Fatty acids, omega. Omega refers to the terminal carbon atom on a fatty acid, regardless of the number of double bonds, so omega fatty acids can be monounsaturated or polyunsaturated. Omega 3 indicates a double bond three carbons away from the omega carbon atom; omega 6 indicates a double bond six carbons away.

Fatty acids, polyunsaturated. A fatty acid with more than one double bond.

Fatty acids, saturated. Fatty acids with all the available carbon bonds occupied by hydrogen.

Fatty acids, trans. A double-bonded fatty acid with the carbon chains on either side of the double bond kinked in the opposite direction, making it easier to solidify than it is for a cis fatty acid.

Fatty acids, unsaturated. Fatty acids with some of the available carbon bonds doubled up—reinforced—with rigid double bonds, kinking the fatty acids and preventing them from stacking and solidifying at room temperature.

Femur. The thigh bone.

Fetus. A developing baby in its mother's uterus.

Fibrin. The final protein of the clotting mechanism, forming a protein net to trap proteins, red blood cells, and platelets into a gelatinous blood clot.

Fibula. A long, thin bone extending from just below the outside part of the knee to the ankle, and forming the outside ankle.

Fistula. An abnormal connection between two hollow organs or one hollow organ and the skin surface.

Fleming, Alexander. The discoverer of penicillin.

Flight of ideas. The complete disconnection of one thought with the next thought.

Floating ribs. Ribs that wrap only partway around the chest, without attaching to the sternum.

Florey, Howard. The developer of methods to manufacture penicillin in bulk.

Foam cells. White blood cells chock full of cholesterol gobbled up within arterial walls.

Folate. A vitamin used throughout the body, often working in tandem with vitamin B12.

Folie a deux. A pair of psychotics who believe the same delusion.

Follicle. Hair shaft.

Follicle-stimulating hormone. The hormone released by the anterior pituitary to instruct the ovaries each month to ready one egg for release into a fallopian tube.

Fontanelle. The soft spot on a baby's head corresponding to the gap between skull bones. It eventually disappears as the bones grow and fuse together.

Frontal lobe. The cerebral hemisphere from the motor strip forward.

Frostbite. Death of tissue from excessive cold.

Frozen shoulder. Rotator cuff syndrome. Stiffness of the shoulder due to adhesions or inflammation in the glenoid capsule.

Fungus. Non–chlorophyll-containing molds, yeasts, and mushrooms. A mold lengthens by budding newborn cells from its tips, forming long, delicate branching filaments (fuzzy mold on stale bread is a good example). A yeast multiplies by releasing individual buds.

Funk, Casimir. The first person to isolate thiamine, the cure for beriberi.

Funny bone. The ulnar nerve passing behind the elbow that, when accidentally struck, sends an electric tingling sensation down the ulnar nerve into the little and ring fingers.

GABA. A neurotransmitter.

Gage, Phineas. The unlucky victim of a pole being thrust through his frontal lobes, resulting in a dramatic change in his behavior, now called "frontal lobe behavior."

Gallbladder. A storage depot for bile, located under the liver.

Gallstones. Solidified bile.

Ganglia. Any cluster of nerve cell bodies.

Ganglion cell. A nerve cell carrying retinal signals through the optic nerve to the brain to be assembled into a visual image.

Ganglion. A firm cyst of fluid, typically developing over the back of the hand or wrist.

Gangrene. Infection of tissue that's lost its blood supply, hence beyond the reach of white blood cells.

Gas gangrene. Gas production by anerobic bacteria infecting gangrenous tissue.

Gastritis. Inflammation in the stomach.

Gastrocnemius. The large calf muscle that allows you to step on your toes or push the gas pedal.

Gastrointestinal system. The mouth, salivary glands, esophagus, stomach, liver, gall bladder, pancreas, duodenum, small intestine, and colon.

Gene. A snippet of DNA carrying chemical instructions to assemble one protein.

Genital system. All the apparatus necessary to reproduce, including in men, the testes, vas deferens, penis, prostate, and other semen-producing glands and, in women, the ovaries, fallopian tubes, uterus, and vagina.

Genital warts. Very contagious, rough growths on the genitals and anus due to infection by papilloma virus, predisposing some patients in later life to cancer of the cervix.

Ghrelin. A hormone released by the stomach that stimulates the hypothalamus to release NPY.

Gland. An organ that secretes hormones into the bloodstream.

Glans. The head of the penis.

Glaucoma. Elevated pressure within the globe of the eye, compressing and eventually damaging the optic nerve, leading to blindness.

Glenoid cavity. The shallow cup of the scapula (wing bone) into which the head of the humerus inserts to form the shoulder joint.

Glomeruli. The sieves of the kidney, through which the liquid part of blood is filtered and then selectively reabsorbed downstream in the kidney tubules, leaving behind urine to dribble into the ureters.

Glomerulonephritis. An autoimmune attack on glomeruli triggered by group A beta hemolytic streptococcal bacteria.

Glucagon. A hormone released by the pancreas to stimulate the liver to release glucose into the bloodstream.

Glucose. A six-carbon atom configured into a circular chain to which are attached molecules of hydrogen and oxygen. Distinguished from galactose and other simple sugars by the way the atoms are attached to each other.

Glycogen. Long, branching strings of glucose molecules stored in the liver and muscle for rapid release during times of high-energy need.

Goiter. Enlargement of the thyroid gland.

Goldberg, Joseph. The discoverer of niacin deficiency as the cause of pellagra, who went through hell to convince a skeptical establishment that poverty lay at the root of pellagra.

Golgi tendon organ. A tiny sensor in a muscle's tendon that gauges how tense a muscle is.

Gonorrhea. A sexually transmitted bacterium that infects the genital system or any mucosal surface.

Gout. Painful inflammation of a joint, usually in the great toe, caused by deposition of uric acid crystals from excessive uric acid in the blood.

Graft versus host reaction. An attack by a bone-marrow donor's white blood cells on the host's tissues.

Gray matter. The areas of the brain where cell bodies congregate.

Greater trochanter. The bony protrusion of the femur mistakenly thought by laypeople to be the hip joint.

Growth hormone. The anterior pituitary hormone that stimulates growth of bone and soft tissue.

Growth plate. The area near the ends of a bone from which new bone is added to lengthen the bone.

Guillain Barre syndrome. An immunologic attack on the myelin of peripheral nerves resulting in rapid widespread paralysis. Recovery generally takes place over a period of weeks, months, and even years.

Gynecomastia. Breast enlargement.

Haber, Fritz. The developer of a process to chemically extract nitrogen from the air for use in fertilizers and explosives.

Hallucination. An awake image with no basis in reality.

Hallucinations, hypnagogic. Vivid awake dreams during descent into sleep.

Hallucinations, hypnopompic. Vivid awake dreams on awakening in the morning.

Hard palate. The bony roof of the mouth.

Harvey, William. The first person to prove that the heart pumps blood around a circuit.

Hashimoto's thyroiditis. Unexplained inflammation of the thyroid gland, often resulting in either too much thyroid hormone release or not enough.

Heart attack. Coronary infarct. Death of heart tissue due to lack of blood flow.

Heart enlargement. What the heart does when it fails—as a way of improving its ability to pump.

Heart failure. A tiring of heart muscle, so that the heart can no longer pump enough blood to meet the body's needs.

Heart valves. Flaps of cartilage at the entry and exit holes of the right and left ventricles to keep blood flowing in a forward direction.

Heartburn. Painful inflammation of the lower esophagus behind the breast bone, mostly due to reflux of hydrochloric acid through an incompetent lower esophageal sphincter muscle.

Heat stroke. Hypotension and delirium due to excessive heat and dehydration.

Heimlich maneuver. Forcefully compressing the abdomen to rapidly elevate the diaphragm and force expiration.

Helicobacter pylori. A bacterium that causes gastric (stomach) and duodenal ulcers.

Hematocrit. The percent of blood made up of red blood cells.

Hematologic system. Anything to do with the blood—red blood cells, white blood cells, platelets, clotting factors, plasma proteins, and the spleen.

Hematoma. A blood clot outside an artery or vein.

Heme. A small, iron-containing molecule cradled by globulin that's broken down by the liver to form bilirubin and then bile.

Hemiparesis. Weakness of the arm and leg on one side of the body.

Hemiplegia. Paralysis of the arm and leg on one side of the body.

Hemoglobin. A protein nestling a small heme molecule, in the center of which lies a molecule of iron that binds oxygen. Hemoglobin is spring-loaded to release oxygen in oxygen-starved peripheral tissues.

Hemoglobinuria. Blood in the urine.

Hemophilia. An X-linked defect in the synthesis of factor VIII, one of the clotting factors.

Hemorrhoids. Dilated veins at the anus and terminal rectum, often painful, often bleeding small amounts of bright red blood; caused by damming up of venous blood into the rectum.

Heparin. A chemical that coats the clotting factors, preventing blood from clotting.

Hepatic duct. The tube carrying bile downward from the liver.

Hepatitis. Inflammation of the liver.

Hernia. Synonymous with herniation. Protrusion of a structure through any opening or gap.

Hernia, hiatal. Protrusion of the stomach upward through the diaphragm, allowing stomach acid to wash up into the esophagus as painful acid reflux.

Heroin. A superstrong version of morphine.

Herpes. Herpes type I is a virus that causes cold sores on the mouth and lips, and a serious encephalitis. Herpes type II causes recurrent infections of nerves supplying skin around the genitals.

Herschel, William. The discoverer of infrared radiation.

Hiccup. Sudden involuntary contraction of the diaphragm, causing a sudden rush of air into the trachea that is abruptly terminated by sudden closure of the epiglottis.

High blood pressure. Hypertension.

Hippocampus. The brain's new memory structure in the temporal lobe.

Histamine. One of a number of chemicals that dilate blood vessels and cause them to leak fluid.

HIV. Human immunodeficiency virus, the virus that causes AIDS.

Hives. Blebs of fluid collecting under the skin, usually due to the release of histamine for any number of reasons.

Hofmann, Albert. The first person to synthesize LSD-25 and recognize its psychedelic properties.

Hopkins, Frederick. Early on, realized that there was something in the diet necessary for normal growth and development.

Horizontal plane. The plane parallel to the ground.

Hormone. A chemical secreted into the bloodstream to affect the function of a distant organ.

Horner's syndrome. The combination of a small pupil, ptosis (slight drooping of the eyelid), and loss of sweating over the face due to interruption of the sympathetic nerves en route to the face.

Humerus. The bone of the upper arm.

Hydrocephalus. Dilation of the cerebral ventricles, due to a damming up of spinal fluid behind an obstruction to spinal fluid flow. Also due to compensatory enlargement as the brain atrophies in a disease such as Alzheimer's.

Hydrochloric acid (HCl). A strong acid released by the stomach to denature proteins.

Hymen. A thin membrane covering the entrance to the vagina, permanently obliterated once sexual activity begins.

Hyperglycemia. High blood glucose.

Hyperopia. Farsightedness.

Hypertension. High blood pressure.

Hyperthyroid. Overactive thyroid gland.

Hyperventilation syndrome. Overbreathing due to high anxiety.

Hypoglycemia. Low blood sugar.

Hypotension. Low blood pressure.

Hypothalamus. A small but critical area of the brain, just above the brainstem (and hence phylogenetically quite old), devoted to monitoring and responding to basic bodily functions related to hunger, thirst, temperature, salt, sleep, and emotions. The hypothalamus also instructs the pituitary to release its hormones and stimulates the autonomic nervous system to respond to emotions.

Hypothyroid. Low thyroid function.

Ileum, terminal. The end of the ileum, just before it plugs into the cecum of the large intestine.

Illusion. A distortion of a true image.

Immunologic system. The collection of white blood cells, lymphatics, and lymph nodes clustered and scattered about the body guarding against anything foreign.

Incus. The middle bone of the middle ear.

Infection. An invasion of one or more organ systems by an infectious agent, usually, but not always, eliciting an inflammatory response.

Inferior vena cava. The main vein carrying deoxygenated blood up from the abdomen and legs to the right ventricle.

Inflammation. An attack by white blood cells resulting in redness, warmth, tenderness, and swelling.

Ingrown toenail. Painful growth of a toenail into adjacent skin.

Inner ear. The innermost part of the ear, where sound waves, having been amplified in the middle ear, are converted into electrical signals for transmission to the brain.

Insulin. A hormone released by the pancreas to lower blood sugar by escorting glucose into cells; also informs the brain of the body's carbohydrate status.

Intercostal muscles. The muscles between the ribs that expand and contract the rib cage during each breath.

Interferon. A protein that mobilizes cells to resist a viral attack.

Interleukins. Chemicals that help organize an inflammatory attack.

Interstitial cell–stimulating hormone. In men, the anterior pituitary hormone that stimulates the testes to make testosterone. In women, it is called luteinizing hormone and instructs the ovaries to make estrogen and to release one egg.

Interstitial space. The space between cells.

Intervertebral discs. Cartilaginous slabs between adjacent vertebral bodies to cushion them and provide mobility for the spine.

Intestine, incarcerated. A trapped loop of herniated intestine at risk of having its blood supply cut off.

Intracranial pressure, increased. Excessive pressure inside the skull due to excess blood, water, or tissue in the skull.

Intrinsic factor. A protein secreted by the wall of the stomach that attaches to vitamin B12, permitting it to be absorbed in the terminal ileum.

Intubation. The process of introducing an endotracheal tube into the trachea and securing it by blowing up a soft, inflatable cuff encircling the shaft of the endotracheal tube.

Intussusception. Telescoping of a tubular structure.

Iodine. A mineral component of thyroid hormone.

Iris. The colored part of the eye, made up of a muscle that constricts in response to light and dilates in response to darkness.

Iron atom. Held by a heme molecule in hemoglobin and myoglobin, iron binds oxygen.

Iron deficiency anemia. Low red blood cell count because of impaired hemoglobin production due to lack of available iron.

Irritable bowel syndrome. Anxiety- and stress-induced urgency to have a bowel movement.

Islets of Langerhans. Thousands of clusters of cells, buried throughout the pancreas, that secrete insulin in response to hyperglycemia.

Jakob Creutzfeldt disease. A rapidly fatal prion disease of the brain.

Jasper, Herbert. The physiologist who, with Wilder Penfield, first mapped out the motor strip.

Jaundice. Yellowing of the skin due to bile in the bloodstream.

Jenner, Edward. The first person to make vaccination a legitimate way to prevent certain diseases.

Jet lag. Feeling like you've been up all night, but are too tired to sleep, after flying across several time zones; thought to be due to a disruption of our inner time clock located in the hypothalamic suprachiasmatic nucleus.

Joint position sense. The ability to tell where our limbs and digits are in space.

Judgment. The process by which a person chooses the best answer among several possible answers to a problem.

Kekule, Friedrich. The chemist who in his sleep figured out the structure of benzene (a ring of carbon atoms).

Keloid. A thick scar that extends beyond the edges of a cut.

Keratin. The protein, derived from dead skin cells, that makes up a hair shaft.

Ketones. Two-carbon fragments snipped off long chains of fatty acids during periods of starvation to supply the body with a source of energy.

Kidney stone. A chip, often as tiny as a grain of sand, usually made of calcium, very painful when it lodges in the ureter. Large ones have to be fished out through the urethra, or surgically removed, or shattered with lithotripsy to prevent infection or dangerous back pressure on the kidney.

Kneecap. Patella.

Knee jerks. Reflex contraction of the quadriceps muscle when its tendon below the kneecap is suddenly stretched.

Kuru. A prion disease passed from one generation to the next in Papua New Guinea by the eating of the brains of diseased relatives who have died with the disease.

Kyphosis. Excessive outcurving of the thoracic spine, common in osteoporosis.

Labor. Painful contractions of a pregnant woman's uterus trying to expel the baby.

Labyrinth. Semicircular canals in the inner ear that detect twisting movements of the head.

Lacteals. The intestinal lymphatics that absorb chylomicrons, so named because chylomicrons inside the lacteals are white, resembling milk.

Lactic acid. Equivalent to about half a glucose molecule, lactic acid accumulates during heavy exercise (which you feel as burning muscles) and is rapidly reassembled into glucose by the liver.

Lactose intolerance. Inability to break down lactose in the gut for ready absorption, allowing lactose to reach the colon, to the delight of gas-forming bacteria.

Large intestine. The last section of the intestines, shaped like an inverted U, where the final step of digestion, by loads of bacteria, takes place, and where the final drops of water are wrung out of the intestinal slurry to form stool. Synonymous with colon.

Laryngoscope. A lighted instrument with a long blade inserted into the back of the throat to guide an endotracheal tube into the trachea.

Lasik surgery. A surgical procedure to change the shape of the cornea and obviate the need for glasses.

Lateral collateral ligament. The ligament along the outside of the knee holding the femur to the tibia.

Lateral. Away from the midline.

Learning disability. A delay in the development of one or more learning skills.

Legumes. Plants capable of snatching nitrogen from the air to make amino acids.

Lens. Situated behind the iris, helps the cornea focus images on the macula.

Leprosy. A chronic, low-grade, mildly contagious infection of nerves and soft tissues resulting in terrible disfigurement of the face, hands, and feet.

Leptin. A hormone released by fat cells telling the brain the status of our fat stores. The more leptin, the less our appetite.

Lesion. Any abnormality visible to the naked eye or under a microscope, in other words, not chemical.

Leukemia. A cancerous growth of white blood cells.

Leukotrienes. One of many chemicals released during inflammation to help attract more white blood cells to the battle.

Lice. Crabs. Tiny insects that live in warm, moist hair.

Ligaments. Bands of very tough tissue binding bone to bone.

Lightheadedness. The sensation one feels prior to fainting.

Limbic system. The collection of brain structures devoted to creating emotions, including the cingulate gyrus, hippocampus amygdala, mamillary bodies, anterior thalamus, nucleus accumbens, and other structures.

Lipase. The pancreatic enzyme that breaks apart fatty acids.

Lipid. Fat.

Lipoproteins. Proteins that carry lipids in the bloodstream.

Lipoproteins, high-density. Lipoproteins that carry cholesterol from arterial walls to the liver.

Lipoproteins, low-density. Lipoproteins that carry cholesterol to arterial walls.

Lister, Joseph. The person who introduced antiseptics into the armamentarium of doctors.

Lithotripsy. The delivery of a shock-wave to shatter large kidney stones.

Liver. The large organ in the right upper quadrant of the abdomen up under the rib cage that synthesizes most of the proteins in the bloodstream, detoxifies chemicals circulating in the bloodstream, stores glycogen to counteract periods of hypoglycemia, and houses white blood cells looking for foreign antigens in the bloodstream and absorbed food.

Locked in. Total paralysis of all muscles except those that move the eyes and the diaphragm due to severe damage to the brainstem below the reticular activating system (allowing the patient to remain conscious and alert), but above the respiratory control centers in the lower brainstem, allowing the patient to continue breathing.

Lockjaw. Continuous contractions of the masseter and temporalis (and other) muscles due to the toxin of *Clostridium tetani*.

Loewi, Otto. The first person to prove that axons release neurotransmitters.

Loosening of associations. When thoughts start to lose their connections to the next thought.

Lordosis. A normal incurving of the spine. Excessive lordosis of the lumbar spine is called swayback.

Lower motor neuron. The horizontal nerve extending from the brainstem or spinal cord out to the muscle.

Lumbar puncture. The insertion of a needle into cerebrospinal fluid in the lumbar subarachnoid space, where there is no spinal cord to be injured by the needle.

Lumen. Hollow center.

Luteinizing hormone. The female version of interstitial cell-stimulating hormone.

Lymph nodes. Glands. Nubbins of lymphoid tissue tucked away in the skin and deep body cavities.

Lymphatics. A collection of microscopic canals throughout the body (except for the brain) designed to collect proteins and fluid leaking from tiny capillaries and transport them to the nearest lymph node for analysis, before dumping them back into the bloodstream.

Lymphedema. Swelling of tissues because of the obstruction of lymph flow.

Lymphoid tissue. Collections of white blood cells in the bone marrow, lymph nodes, bloodstream, tonsils, adenoids, appendix, lining of the intestines, liver, and spleen.

Lysergic acid-25 (LSD). A serotonin-acting drug with extremely strong effects on normal thinking, capable of rendering someone temporarily psychotic.

Macewen, William. One of the world's first great neurosurgeons, and the first to recommend intubation of a patient during surgery to deliver continuous anesthesia.

Macleod, John. Along with Banting, Best, and Collip, one of the discoverers of insulin.

Macula. The center of the retina made up of pure cones where the retinal image is most focused.

Mad cow disease. A fatal disease of cattle caused by prions.

Malignant. Cancerous.

Malleolus. Ankle. The medial malleolus is the inside ankle; the lateral malleolus, the outside ankle.

Malleus. The first of the three bones in the middle ear, gently pressed up against the inside of the tympanic membrane.

Mast cells. Histamine-containing white blood cells lining the bronchial tubes and gut.

Mastoiditis. An infection in the mastoid bone, the part of the skull behind the ear.

McKay, Frederick. The dentist who discovered the benefit of fluoride for preventing dental caries.

McLean, Jay. The discoverer of heparin.

Measles. A potentially fatal viral illness presenting with red papules (slightly raised dots on the skin), fever, and upper respiratory symptoms.

Medial collateral ligament. The ligament along the inside of the knee holding the femur to the tibia.

Medial meniscus. A slab of cartilage along the inside half of the knee joint.

Median nerve. The nerve passing through the forearm and hand to supply nearly half the muscles that move the hand and fingers, often compressed where it passes through the carpal tunnel in the wrist.

Melanin. A chemical in the skin that absorbs ultraviolet rays and gives skin its brown color.

Melanocortin. A hypothalamic hormone that tells our brain we're full.

Melanoma. A highly malignant form of skin cancer that metastasizes early and often.

Melatonin. A hormone released primarily at night by the pineal gland whose function is still unclear.

Meniere's disease. Vertigo, progressive hearing loss, and tinnitus due to a buildup of pressure in the inner ear from an obstructed endolymphatic sac.

Meninges. A two-part membrane gently overlying the surface of the brain, the inner part consisting of a very delicate pia mater membrane carrying blood vessels feeding blood to the brain, the outer part being an arachnoid membrane. Cerebrospinal fluid circulates between the pia mater and arachnoid membranes.

Meningitis. Inflammation of the meninges.

Meningitis, chemical. Inflammation of the meninges due to something other than an infectious agent, for example, blood, irritating chemicals released from a burst cyst in the brain, or drugs injected into the subarachnoid space as a treatment for tumors or infection.

Menopause. Permanent failure of the ovaries to synthesize estrogen or release their eggs.

Menstrual cycle. The five or so days during which the uterus sheds its endometrium if it is not implanted by a fertilized egg.

Mental retardation. A delay in intellectual development of the brain.

Messenger molecules. Molecules inside cells that initiate a cascade of chemical activity when receptors on the cell surface are stimulated by hormones and other chemicals.

Metabolize. To chemically transform one molecule into another molecule.

Metastasize. To spread via the bloodstream or lymph to distant locations of the body.

Middle ear. Connected to the pharynx through the eustacian tube, contains three tiny bones that conduct sound vibrations from the tympanic membrane to the cochlea in the inner ear.

Middle meningeal artery. The artery running along the inside of the temporal bone, vulnerable to being lacerated by a temporal bone fracture and then bleeding dangerously into the epidural space.

Migraine headaches. Recurrent headaches that improve with migraine medication, whose mechanism appears to involve vascular dilation of arteries in the scalp.

Milkmaid's complexion. A smooth complexion from having avoided smallpox by contracting cowpox first.

Minot, George. Along with George Whipple and William Murphy, discovered that raw liver could cure vitamin B12 deficiency.

Misdirection. Seen following damage to the facial motor nerve, when misguided regrowth of some of the axons into the wrong muscles results in simultaneous contraction of unexpected muscles, for example, closure of the eye when smiling. Similarly, following laceration of parasympathetic nerves, tearing when salivating (crocodile tears).

Mitochondrion. A tiny powerhouse with its own DNA and enzymatic machinery to convert pyruvate and fatty acids into gobs of ATP, present in every cell in the body except red blood cells.

Mitral valve. The valve between the left atrium and left ventricle, regulating blood flow into the left ventricle.

Mitral valve prolapse. Benign bulging of the mitral valve backward into the left atrium during ventricular contraction.

Molds. A type of fungus that grows as filaments.

Mole, atypical. A mole on the skin unusual enough to raise a suspicion of a precancerous or cancerous lesion.

Mole. A pigmented area of skin.

Mononuclear white blood cells. White blood cells that follow polymorphonuclear white blood cells to clean up the debris of an inflammatory attack and catalog the foreign antigens for future battles.

Morphine. A narcotic analgesic whose side effect is suppression of the respiratory center.

Motor strip. The origin of the pyramidal tract, a strip of nerve cell bodies in the cerebral cortex of the frontal lobe organized into an image of the human body, with important areas such as the lips and fingers getting more cell bodies than less complex areas such as the chest.

Mountain sickness. Leakage of fluid into the brain from blood vessels exposed to insufficient oxygen.

Movement disorders. Chronic illnesses that prevent a person from being completely still.

MRI. A highly detailed, non–X-ray image of slabs of the human body.

Mucosa. The soft, moist, pink lining of the sinuses, eyelids, nose, mouth, esophagus, gut, bladder, urethra, vagina, and many other hollow structures.

Mucus. The sticky fluid that drips out the nose and coats the membranes of the nose, mouth, trachea, and bronchial tubes, in fact, all mucosal surfaces.

Multiple myeloma. A cancerous proliferation of a single antibody-producing white blood cell.

Multiple sclerosis. A neurologic disease intermittently damaging the myelin insulation around axons of the brain and spinal cord, manifesting as bouts of neurologic disability that eventually accumulate into more serious neurologic disability.

Mumps. A systemic viral illness that particularly affects the salivary glands, pancreas, and testicles.

Murmur. The sound of blood tumbling over some obstruction or abnormal hole in the heart.

Murmur, functional. A murmur in the heart due to forceful ejection of blood from a superhealthy heart.

Murphy, William. Along with George Minot and George Whipple, discovered that raw liver could cure vitamin B12 deficiency.

Muscle, biceps. The muscle that bends the elbow when one "makes a muscle."

Muscle, brachioradialis. The muscle that bends the elbow with the thumb pointing upward.

Muscle cells, smooth. Muscle cells that contract slowly and weakly, but are capable of holding a single contraction for a long time.

Muscle, cremasteric. The muscle that lifts a testicle when it's cold outside.

Muscle, deltoid. The muscle, forming the rounded contour of the shoulder, that lifts the arm.

Muscle, gastrocnemius. The calf muscle that pulls the heel upward when we are standing on our toes or stepping on the gas.

Muscle, gluteus maximus. The large muscle of the butt that pulls the leg back (extends the hip).

Muscle, masseter. The jaw-closing muscle at the angle of the jaw.

Muscle, pectoralis. The broad muscle over the upper chest that pulls the arms together.

Muscle, psoas. The muscle located deep in the abdomen that raises the knee.

Muscle, quadriceps. The large muscle above the knee that straightens the leg.

Muscle, sternocleidomastoid. The long muscle on either side of the neck that rotates the head in the opposite direction.

Muscle, temporalis. The muscle that bulges in the temple when the jaw is clenched, and that is used to close the jaw.

Muscle, tibialis anterior. The large muscle over the front of the lower leg that lifts up the foot. Without it, we walk with a footdrop.

Muscle, triceps. The muscle behind the upper arm that straightens the elbow.

Muscles, hamstring. The muscles behind the thigh that bend the knee.

Muscles, papillary. Small muscles stretching from the left ventricle to the undersurface of the mitral valve that contract during ventricular contraction to keep the mitral valve from bulging backward into the left atrium and thereby leaking. See CHORDA TENDINEAE.

Muscular dystrophy. A slow deterioration of muscle due to genetic abnormalities of proteins and enzymes within the muscle. Different muscular dystrophies affect different muscles.

Mycobacterium. A wax-coated bacterium impermeable, and therefore invisible, to the Gram stain. The Ziehl-Neelsen stain penetrates the waxy coat and adheres so tightly that even acids cannot remove the stain, making mycobacteria "acid fast." The most notorious mycobacterium is tuberculosis.

Myelin. The fatty insulation around axons that prevents short-circuiting between adjacent axons and helps speed electrical transmission.

Myoglobin. The protein in muscle that snatches oxygen from hemoglobin; it also gives muscle its dark red color.

Myopia. Nearsightedness.

Narcolepsy. A disturbance of sleep characterized by irresistible urges to fall asleep given the slightest chance. Episodes often occur in embarrassing situations. Narcolepsy is commonly associated with sleep paralysis, cataplexy, and hypnagogic or hypnopompic hallucinations.

Natriuretic hormone. A hormone released by the atrium of the heart instructing the kidneys not to retain salt.

Necrosis. Death of tissue.

Nerve, facial. The cranial nerve originating in the brainstem that supplies the muscles of the face.

Nerve root. Nerves exiting and entering the spinal cord; the part of the nerve between the spinal cord and plexus.

Neurologic system. The brain, spinal cord, peripheral nerves, and muscles.

Neuromuscular junction. The gap between a nerve axon and the muscle it is innervating, where the axon's neurotransmitters are released to stimulate the muscle to contract.

Neurotransmitter. A chemical released from the tip of an axon signaling the dendrites of another nerve cell to fire its axon, or signaling a muscle to contract.

Nicotine. One of the active ingredients in tobacco smoke, constricts arteries and stimulates the pleasure center.

Night terrors. Sudden terrifying inconsolable nightmarish awakenings in a sleeping child incapable of being fully awakened, and who forgets the episode by the morning. Night terrors occur during stage 4 sleep, unlike true dreams, which occur during stage 1 REM sleep.

Nitric oxide. A chemical released from arterial walls that causes them to relax.

Node, atrioventricular. The pacemaker for the ventricles.

Node, sinoatrial. The pacemaker for the atria.

Norepinephrine. A neurotransmitter.

NPY. A hypothalamic hormone that tells our brains we're hungry.

Nucleus accumbens. The pleasure center at the base of the frontal lobes.

Occipital lobe. The back of the brain, where vision is formed.

Occipital notch. The bony protrusion at the back of the skull.

Oils. Lipids that are liquid at room temperature.

Olfaction. Smell.

Ondine's curse. The failure of automatic breathing, leaving only voluntary breathing, and thus requiring ventilatory support when asleep to breathe.

Ophthalmic artery. The artery supplying the retina.

Ophthalmoscope. The instrument doctors use to look into the eye.

Optic chiasm. The neurologic structure behind the eyes where nerve fibers carrying signals from the inside half of each retina cross to the opposite side, enabling each occipital lobe to receive a stereoscopic view of the opposite half of the visual world.

Optic disc. The optic nerve plugging into the back of the eye, seen end-on through an ophthalmoscope.

Optic nerve. Plugged into the back of the eye, the optic nerve carries retina signals to the brain.

Organ. A structure made up of various tissues that performs a vital function for the body, for example, the heart, brain, and lungs.

Organ system. A collection of organs that work together to perform a set of important bodily functions, for example, the gastrointestinal system, made up of the mouth, salivary glands, esophagus, liver, gall bladder, pancreas, stomach, and small and large intestines.

Oscillopsia. Jiggling of the visual word when the head moves.

Osteoporosis. Thinning of adult bones.

Otoscope. A lighted instrument for looking into the external auditory canal at the tympanic membrane.

Oval window. The entryway to the inner ear, where mechanical vibrations of the middle ear bones are transmitted to nerves within the inner ear.

Ovaries. The storehouse for a woman's eggs and the major source of estrogen in a woman.

Ovulation. The release of an egg from an ovary.

Oxygen. A molecule that mops up hydrogen atoms being released by mitrochondria busy making the body's energy molecule, ATP.

Oxytocin. The hormone released by the posterior pituitary to stimulate the uterus to contract when it's time to deliver.

P wave. The part of the EKG tracing that represents depolarization of the atria, which initiates atrial contraction.

Pacemaker, cardiac. A wire threaded into the heart to take over the electrical pacemaking of the heart in the event of a dangerous arrhythmia.

Pain, colicky. A wave of pain precipitated by contraction of a hollow organ such as the intestines, ureter, or gall bladder against an obstruction.

Palpate. Feel.

Pancreas. An organ lying up against the back wall of the midabdomen that secretes three different enzymes into the duodenum to digest fats, carbohydrates, and proteins. It also houses the islets of Langerhans, the makers of insulin.

Pancreatic duct. The tube carrying pancreatic enzymes into the duodenum,

joining the common bile duct just before inserting into the duodenum.

Pancreatitis. Inflammation of the pancreas.

Papilledema. Swelling of the optic disc due to increased intracranial pressure.

Paraplegia. Paralysis of both legs.

Parasite. Any organism, ranging from unicellular amebae to complex tapeworms, that lives off the earnings of others.

Parasympathetic nerves. Autonomic nerves that rule during times of relaxation to slow the heart, lower the blood pressure, release saliva into the mouth, move food along the gut, empty the bladder, and during romantic moments, enhance blood flow to the genitals.

Parathormone. The hormone released from the parathyroid glands to raise the calcium level by extracting calcium from bones, improving calcium absorption from the intestines, and reducing calcium excretion from the kidneys.

Parathyroid glands. Four small glands buried in the thyroid gland that release parathormone to maintain adequate calcium in the bloodstream.

Pare, Ambrose. The first person to recognize that pus was not helpful to a wound.

Parietal lobe. The section of cerebral hemisphere between the frontal and occipital lobes.

Parkinson's disease. A disease characterized by a paucity and slowing of movements, a shuffling and imbalanced gait, and a tremor at rest that lessens or disappears when the person reaches for something.

Paronychia. A painful infection at the edge of a fingernail or toenail.

Pasteur, Louis. The first person to realize that microorganisms were the cause of wine spoilage and infectious diseases, the first to develop a vaccine for rabies and anthrax, the first to prove that life could not develop spontaneously but required a parent, the first to protect foods from spoiling by heating them to kill dangerous bacteria—quite simply, an absolutely brilliant mind who, accepting nothing that could not be proven scientifically, was able to greatly advance scientific knowledge with the most primitive resources.

Pasteurization. The process of heating food to kill harmful bacteria.

Patella. Kneecap.

Pathophysiology. Or, pathologic physiology, the mechanism by which an etiologic agent causes a disease process.

Pellagra. Dementia, dermatitis, and diarrhea due to niacin deficiency. Niacin is critical for normal mitochondrial function.

Pelvis. Three bones—the ilium, ischium, and pubis—fused together and paired up with another set on the other side, connected to the sacral bone in the back to form a pelvic bowl.

Penfield, Wilder. The neurosurgeon who, with Herbert Jasper, first mapped out the motor strip.

Penicillin. An antibiotic that kills certain bacteria by interfering with bacterial cell wall synthesis.

Penis. The shaft of inflatable venous channels surrounding the urethra.

Pepsin. The enzyme released into the stomach to snip apart proteins for easier digestion.

Pericardium. The sac surrounding the heart.

Peripheral nervous system. Any nerve that begins in either the brain and spinal cord and ends up in a peripheral tissue.

Peristalsis. The way the gut moves to propel food along.

PET scan. Positron emission tomography. A test that directly measures an organ's cellular activity by monitoring the activity of radioactive chemicals taken up and used by the organ's cells.

Peyer's patches. Thousands of clusters of lymph tissue lining the gut wall, checking food being absorbed for foreign antigens.

Pharynx. The back of the throat. The part of the pharynx above the soft palate is the nasopharynx.

Phoneme. A sound bit.

Photophobia. Glare from lights.

Pimple. See ACNE.

Pinched nerve. See RADICULOPATHY.

Pineal gland. The gland in the center of the brain that triggers the onset of puberty.

Pinna. The outside part of the ear that collects sounds from the air.

Pituitary. The pea-sized organ dangling from the undersurface of the brain behind the bridge of the nose, nicknamed the master gland because its hormones help control so many organs of the body.

Pituitary gland, anterior. The source for FAT PIG: Follicle stimulating hormone, Adrenal-stimulating hormone, Thyroid-stimulating hormone, Prolactin, Interstitial cell–stimulating hormone (in men; luteinizing hormone in women), and Growth hormone.

Pituitary gland, posterior. The source of oxytocin, the hormone that simulates a pregnant uterus to contract and the breasts to release (not synthesize) milk, and of the hormone vasopressin (antidiuretic hormone), which stimulates the kidneys to retain water.

Placebo effect. An improvement in symptoms from nothing more than believing the treatment will work.

Placenta. The organ that allows a

developing fetus to receive nutrients from its mother by bathing fetal blood vessels in the mother's blood within the placenta.

Plaque, demyelination. A patch of myelin stripped off its axons.

Plaque, dental. Tenacious gunk that collects at the base of teeth and rots out the gums and teeth.

Plasma. What's left over after red blood cells, white blood cells, and platelets are removed.

Platelets. Tiny membranous pellets floating in the bloodstream ready to plug small holes that develop in the vascular tree.

Pleasure center. Nucleus acumbens, a nerve center deep in the frontal lobe that animals will, if allowed to, continue to stimulate until they drop dead from lack of food and water.

Pleura. The membrane covering the surface of the lung and lining the inside of the chest wall.

Pleural space. The space between the pleura overlying the surface of the lung and the pleura lining the inside of the chest wall.

Pneumonia. Any infection of the lungs.

Pneumothorax. Air in the pleural space causing a lung to partially collapse.

Polygraph. Lie detector, based on the detection of lying-induced changes in the sympathetic nervous system.

Polymorphonuclear white blood cells. White blood cells that initiate the attack on a foreign antigen.

Polyneuropathy. Weakness, pain, and numbness usually in the hands and feet and due to a widespread disturbance of all peripheral nerves in the body.

Polysaccharides. Long chains of sugar molecules forming mucus, starch, cellulose, and glycogen.

Posterior. Behind.

Postpartum. The period immediately following birth.

Prednisone. A commonly prescribed corticosteroid.

Preeclampsia. Dangerous hypertension during pregnancy, cured by delivering the baby.

Prefrontal lobotomies. An old method, now considered barbaric, to control otherwise uncontrollable schizophrenics, criminals, and retarded patients, consisting of slicing through wide swaths of axons in the frontal lobes, leaving the patient apathetic and dull.

Pregnancy, ectopic. Pregnancy in which the fetus develops outside the uterus, usually in one fallopian tube.

Pregnancy, tubal. Pregnancy in which a fetus develops inside one fallopian tube.

Premature atrial contractions. Atrial contractions that preempt the normal signal from the sinoatrial node.

Premature ventricular contractions. Ventricular contractions triggered by aberrant electrical signals preempting the usual atrioventricular signal.

Presbyopia. The development of farsightedness with advancing age, usually beginning around age 40.

Pressure, left atrial. The first indication of a failing heart is rising left atrial pressure as blood backs up behind the left ventricle into the left atrium. Left atrial pressure has to be indirectly measured with a tube guided up a large vein, through the right ventricle, and wedged into a small arteriole in the lungs.

Pressure points. Spots where nerves crossing bones can be pinched to incapacitate a person.

Pressure, right atrial. Failure of the right

ventricle raises pressure in the right atrium, which you can see as dilated neck veins because there are no valves at the entrance of the right atrium. The rising pressure in the right atrium is transmitted backward into the neck veins.

Prions. Infectious proteins that unfold and induce other proteins to do so, too, leading to neuronal damage.

Progesterone. A hormone released by the ovary, and later by the placenta, stimulating endometrial thickening to nourish a placenta.

Prolactin. The hormone released by the anterior pituitary to instruct the breasts to make milk and the ovaries to inhibit ovulation.

Prolapse. Sagging of a structure through a natural hole in the body due to gravity and loss of structural integrity in the surrounding supporting tissue.

Prone. Lying face down.

Prostaglandins. Complex fatty acids, some of which help direct an inflammatory response and others of which coat the stomach and protect it from stomach acids; so named because they were first discovered as a product of the prostate gland that contracts smooth muscle in the uterus and thereby helps sperm reach the fallopian tubes.

Prosthesis. Artificial body part.

Protein. A chain of amino acids.

Protein denaturation. Unraveling of a protein.

Protozoa. Single-celled organisms that move about by ingenious adaptations. Spirochetes, for example, being spiral shaped, move by spinning like a corkscrew.

Proximal. Close to the center of the body.

Psychosis. An illness characterized by delusions of one sort or another.

Psychosis, functional. A psychosis due to some unidentifiable cause.

Psychosis, organic. A psychosis due to an identifiable cause.

Puberty. The beginning in the early teenage years of increased estrogen and testosterone release, probably triggered by the pineal gland in response to unknown signals.

Pulmonary artery. The main artery carrying deoxygenated blood from the right ventricle to the lungs.

Pulmonary edema. Excess fluid in the lungs, audible through a stethoscope as snapping open (crackling) of the alveoli with each inspiration.

Pulmonary embolus. A venous embolus that travels through the right atrium and right ventricle and lodges in a small pulmonary arteriole if you're lucky, in the main pulmonary artery if you're not.

Pulmonary vein. The main vein carrying oxygenated blood from the lungs to the left ventricle.

Pulmonic valve. The valve at the exit of the right ventricle.

Pulp (of a tooth). The center of a tooth, housing its blood vessels and nerves.

Pulse, irregular. Arrhythmia.

Punch drunk. Dementia due to repeated head trauma.

Pupil. The central black part of the eye, representing a hole through which light enters the eye.

Purkinje fibers. Electronically excitable heart muscle that carries electronic signals from the bundle of His into the left and right ventricles.

Pus. The gooey yellow remnants of an inflammatory attack, containing dead bacteria (if that's what caused the inflammation), proteins, white blood cells, and destroyed tissue.

Pyelonephritis. Infection of the kidney; produces a chandelier sign when the back is thumped. (A chandelier sign is anything done to a patient that sends the patient leaping onto the chandelier in pain.)

Pyloric sphincter. A muscle controlling when food may exit the stomach into the duodenum.

Pyramidal tract. The bundle of upper motor neurons carrying movement instructions from the brain to the brainstem and spinal cord, where the instructions are handed off to the lower motor neurons; so named because of the pyramidal tract's triangular shape in cross-section.

Pyridoxine. Vitamin B6.

Pyruvic acid. After glucose is broken down to pyruvate, making two ATP along the way, pyruvate is either shunted in the presence of oxygen into mitochondria to make 36 more ATP, or it is left in the cytoplasm without oxygen to be converted to lactic acid without further ATP production.

PYY. A hormone released by the intestines and colon that stimulates the hypothalamus to release melanocortin, shutting off our appetite.

QRS complex. The part of the EKG tracing representing depolarization of the ventricles.

Quadriplegia. Paralysis of all four limbs.

Rabies. A virus that enters peripheral nerves at the site of animal bites and works its way to the brain, where it causes a devastating fatal encephalitis.

Radial nerve. The nerve supplying muscles that lift the hand.

Radiation. High-frequency (high-energy) electromagnetic radiation that kills fast-growing cells, such as cancer cells and hair cells.

Radiculopathy. Compression of a nerve root, usually by a herniated disc or piece of overgrown bone (osteophyte).

Radiculopathy, cervical. Compression of a cervical nerve root.

Radiculopathy, lumbar. Compression of a lumbar nerve root.

Radiculopathy, sacral. Compression of a sacral nerve root.

Radius. The forearm bone that flip-flops over the ulnar to turn the palm up or down.

Rancid. Referring to the oxidation of fats, releasing foul-smelling free-fatty acids.

Rapid eye movement (REM) sleep. The period of sleep when eye movements are actively watching a dream.

Rat poison. Main ingredient is warfarin, which causes fatal internal bleeding.

Raynaud's disease. Spontaneous spasm of arteries in the fingers (usually), leaving them white, blue, and cold.

Reactive hypoglycemia. Excessive fall in blood glucose after a carbohydrate meal.

Reasoning. The process by which a person arrives at the single correct answer to a problem.

Rectum. The last, straight part of the colon, right before the anal opening.

Red blood cells. Nonnucleated, nonmitochondrial cells in the bloodstream that carry hemoglobin, making up 40% of an average person's blood. Being nonnucleated and nonmitochondrial, red blood cells survive only about three months.

Reentry signal. An electrical signal in the heart that doubles back to sneak in a premature impulse to the sinoatrial or atrioventricular node.

Referred pain. Pain from an injury in one part of the body mistakenly felt in another part of the body because of a shared nerve root supply.

Refraction. The bending of light as it travels into another medium.

Regurgitant (insufficient). Failure to close properly.

Relaxin. A protein released by the placenta that relaxes ligaments, allowing the pelvis to expand, to accommodate the enlarging fetus and facilitate movement of the baby's head through the pelvis.

Releasing hormones. Hormones secreted by the hypothalamus to instruct the pituitary to release its hormones.

Renin. A hormone released by the kidneys in response to low renal artery pressure, converting angiotensinogen in the bloodstream to angiotensin I, which is then converted by angiotensin converting enzyme (ACE) to angiotensin II. Angiotensin II raises the blood pressure by stimulating arteries to constrict, by thickening their walls, and by stimulating the adrenal glands to release aldosterone, thereby causing the kidneys to retain salt.

Resistin. A protein that tells cells to resist insulin.

Respiration, accessory muscles of. Muscles in the neck that, during a big breath, lift and expand the upper rib cage.

Respiratory center. A collection of nerve cells in the lower brainstem (medulla) controlling the rate and depth of relaxed breathing.

Respiratory system. The system devoted to sniffing and breathing the air, generating voice sounds, and helping to regulate the acidity of the blood—consisting of the nose, pharynx, larynx, trachea, bronchi, and lungs.

Reticular activating system. An extensive meshwork of nerve cells in the upper brainstem that controls consciousness.

Reye's syndrome. Unexplained liver disturbance and brain swelling in a child, triggered in some cases by taking aspirin for a viral illness.

Rh factor. An antigen attached to the surface of red blood cells.

Rheumatoid arthritis. An autoimmune disease of the joints, often causing serious and disabling joint damage.

Rhodopsin. The chemical in rods that makes them so exquisitely sensitive to light.

Rickets. The failure of growing bones to calcify because of vitamin D deficiency.

Rigor mortis. Stiffening of a body after death, due to inability of the corpse's muscles to relax by recapturing the calcium that's naturally released into the muscles after death.

Rigors. Coarse shivering of the whole body.

Rods. Retinal cells extremely sensitive to light, used for night vision.

Root canal. Replacement of the dental pulp with a tight sealant.

Rotator cuff. The glenoid capsule, a cartilaginous seat for the head of the humerus to attach to the scapula.

Roux, Emile. The unsung hero in Pasteur's lab who developed the rabies vaccine.

Saccule. Along with the utricle, detects the position of the stationary head in space and the movement of the head forward, backward, up, and down when the neck is rigid.

Sacral bone. The triangular-shaped flat bone at the bottom of the spinal column, out of which depart the five sacral nerve roots to the legs and pelvis.

Sagittal plane. The front-to-back plane of the body.

Sanatorium. A large housing/health facility located far from the community to isolate patients thought to be dangerous to themselves or others—those suffering from schizophrenia, mental retardation, tuberculosis, and leprosy. Now largely outmoded.

Scapula. The shoulder blade.

Scar tissue. Tough but virtually functionless tissue deposited in the wake of inflammation.

Sciatic nerve. The largest nerve in the leg, cascading from the buttock down the back of the leg, supplying the hamstrings and all the muscles below the knee.

Sciatica. Irritation of the sciatic nerve.

Scoliosis. A side-to-side curvature of the spine.

Scrotum. The sac holding the testicles.

Scurvy. A disease caused by insufficient levels of ascorbic acid (vitamin C) that impairs the synthesis of collagen and causes collagen to weaken, resulting in tiny capillary hemorrhages, loosening of teeth, and joint pains. Almost exclusively a disease of primates, as all other mammals (except the guinea pig) can synthesize their own vitamin C.

Sebum. A thick lubricating oil secreted by sebaceous glands onto growing hair follicles.

Semicircular canals. See LABYRINTHS.

Seminal vesicles. A pair of glands behind the bladder that secrete vital nutrients into semen to keep sperm active.

Sepsis. A bacterial or fungal infection that's gained entry to the bloodstream.

Septic shock. Life-threatening low blood pressure due to the release of toxic proteins in the bloodstream by bacteria or by the white blood cells attacking them.

Septum. A baffle separating two chambers.

Serotonin. A widely distributed neurotransmitter with many roles in the brain and spinal cord, among them mood stabi-

lization—elevating a person's serotonin levels improves depression.

Serum. Plasma without its clotting proteins.

Sexually transmitted diseases. An infectious disease transmitted by sexual contact. Examples include syphilis, gonorrhea, HIV, trichomonas, herpes virus, hepatitis B, chlamydia, venereal warts, and lice.

Shock. A state in which blood pressure is so low that vital organs begin to malfunction.

Shoulder blade. The scapula, the shoulder and wing bone, to which most of the shoulder muscles attach.

Shoulder dislocation. Displacement of the head of the humerus from the glenoid cavity.

Shoulder separation. A dislocation of the clavicle from its attachment to the scapular bone.

Shunt. A detour or bypass.

Shunt, intraventricular. A tube inserted into a hydrocephalic ventricle to relieve high spinal fluid pressure (which causes the ventricles to dilate in the first place). Also used to deliver chemotherapy into the cerebrospinal fluid.

Sick sinus syndrome. Dropped signals from the sinoatrial node, usually due to ischemia of the sinoatrial node.

Sickle cell anemia. Condition due to a genetically defective hemoglobin that causes red blood cells to collapse into a sickle shape, in turn causing blood to sludge.

Sigmoid colon. The short S-shaped section of colon leading to the rectum.

Sign. An objective, observable abnormality on physical exam, that is, something the doctor finds on physical exam.

Sinuses. Hollow chambers in the skull bone.

Sinusitis. Inflammation within the sinuses, usually due to infection.

Skin. The thick covering of the body containing, beneath its waterproof surface of dried-out compacted cells, a dense scaffolding of elastic tissue, blood vessels, lymph, hair follicles, sweat glands, and nerves.

Sleep apnea. A sudden interruption of breathing while sleeping, either because the tongue and blubbery soft tissues of the pharynx sag into the airway, or because the brainstem breathing center mysteriously turns off, followed within a minute or so by a brief awakening as the brain becomes alarmed at the resulting hypoxia. The interrupted sleep manifests the next day with excessive daytime sleepiness.

Sleep paralysis. Spells of terrifying paralysis on descending into or arising from sleep, thought to be fragments of REM sleep.

Slipped disc. A poorly chosen term for a herniated disc, because it mistakenly gives the impression that the disc can be slipped back into place—it can't, but the herniated disc can be made less symptomatic by exercises, medications, surgery, and many other claimed therapies.

Soft palate. The floppy part of the roof of the mouth.

Soft spot. See FONTANELLE.

Somatostatin. The hormone that inhibits the release of growth hormone from the pituitary.

Spasticity. Stiffness of a joint due to damage to the upper motor neuron.

SPECT scan. Single photon emission computed tomography. A test that measures an organ's blood flow by monitoring the activity of intravenously injected radioactive chemicals.

Speculum. A flat blade used by doctors to keep soft tissue out of the field of view during an examination.

Speech, circumstantial. Speech that takes forever to get to the point, because the speaker insists on including parenthetical comments and lots of tiny details.

Sphincter muscle, esophageal. A muscle at the juncture of the esophagus and stomach that prevents stomach acid from washing up into the esophagus, a painful condition called acid reflux.

Sphincter. Any muscle that closes a hole.

Spina bifida. A maldevelopment of the brain causing hydrocephalus and herniation of the spinal cord out the skin of the back (leaving the kids paraplegic). Left untreated, the hydrocephalus grows to enormous dimensions and the spinal cord, being exposed, becomes infected.

Spinal column. The stack of vertebral bodies and attached spinous processes forming the backbone and, behind the vertebral bodies, the vertical elevator shaft for the spinal cord.

Spinal cord. The part of the central nervous system beginning at the bottom of the brainstem (the medulla), carrying signals to and from the brain and peripheral tissues.

Spinal fluid. Cerebrospinal fluid.

Spinal tap. Lumbar puncture.

Spiral groove. A groove in the back of the humerus bone where the radial nerve, wrapping around the humerus, is vulnerable to being compressed and damaged.

Spleen. A soft, palm-sized organ tucked up behind the rib cage in the upper left quadrant of the abdomen whose function is to remove dead red blood cells from the blood and to help monitor the blood for foreign antigens.

Spores, botulinus. The hibernating form of botulinus bacteria, resistant to drying out.

St. Anthony's Fire. Ischemic infarction of the arms due to intense vasoconstriction from eating food contaminated with ergot fungi.

Stapes. By vibrating its foot against the oval window, the stapes mechanically stimulates the inner ear.

Statins. Drugs that block the synthesis of intracellular cholesterol, to which cells respond by absorbing cholesterol from the bloodstream and lowering the blood cholesterol.

Status epilepticus. A state of continuous seizure activity.

Stem cells. Cells capable of developing into one or more of the body's tissues.

Stenosis. Narrowing.

Sterile. Free of bacteria.

Sterility. Inability to reproduce.

Sternum. The breastbone.

Steroids. A class of chemicals that share a complex chemical skeleton (viewable in most organic chemistry and biochemistry books). Examples include cortisol, aldosterone, estrogen, testosterone, and all their relatives.

Stethoscope. That Y-shaped instrument a doctor inserts in his or her ears to listen to a patient's heart and lungs.

Stool, black. A sign of free iron in the stool, indicative of iron pills in the diet or of hemorrhage into the stomach or upper intestines, with subsequent digestion of blood and freeing of the iron.

Strabismus. A turning of one eye so that the two eyes are no longer yoked. Commonly referred to as "lazy eye."

Strep throat. A throat infection caused by the bacterium streptococcus.

Streptomycin. The first antibiotic to effectively treat tuberculosis.

Stroke. Sudden death of a section of brain due to an interruption of its blood supply.

Subacute. Lasting weeks or months.

Subacute bacterial endocarditis. An infection of a heart valve lasting days and weeks, sometimes presenting with flu-like symptoms of low-grade fever and fatigue.

Subarachnoid hemorrhage. An arterial, or occasionally venous, hemorrhage into the cerebrospinal fluid circulating underneath the thin arachnoid that rests atop the surface of the brain.

Subclavian vein. A major vein in the upper chest draining venous blood from the arm.

Subdural hematoma. A venous blood clot within the subdural space.

Sudden Infant Death Syndrome (SIDS). Sudden, unexplained death of a sleeping infant; incidence is reduced by placing infants on their back to sleep and avoiding soft bedding into which the infant can burrow its face.

Superficial temporal artery. The visible and palpable artery in the temples.

Superinfection. An infection by antibiotic-resistant bacteria after antibiotics have wiped out the previous antibiotic-sensitive bacterial flora.

Supine. Lying flat on the back.

Suprachiasmatic nucleus. The hypothalamic nucleus helping to control the daily rhythms of our body.

Surface tension. The inward pull of molecules at a liquid's surface due to the way electrically charged molecules at the surface align themselves.

Surfactants. Agents that break up surface tension.

Sutures. The seam where two skull bones fuse together, visible on a shaved head.

Sympathetic nerves. Autonomic nerves that prepare the body for fight or flight by raising the blood pressure, increasing the pulse rate, dilating the bronchial tubes, diverting blood to the vital internal organs, dilating the pupils, raising the hairs on the back of the neck, slowing the gut, stimulating the adrenal glands, and on and on.

Symphysis pubis. The bony joint of the pelvis palpable just above the groin.

Symptom. A subjective complaint; something a patient complains about.

Synapse. The gap between the axon of one neuron and the dendrites or cell body of another neuron, where the neurotransmitter is released.

Synovial fluid. Lubricating fluid secreted into joints.

Syphilis. A slow but deadly disease of the whole body caused by a spirochete and transmitted by blood or other body fluids.

Systemic lupus erythematosus (lupus). An autoimmune disease that primarily attacks arteries and joints, causing widespread inflammation in the body.

T wave. The part of the EKG tracing that represents repolarization of the ventricles.

Tachycardia. Rapid heart rate.

Tailbone. Coccyx, a small vestigial bone attached to the bottom of the sacrum.

Tamponade. Compression, usually by fluid.

Tangential speech. Speech that repeatedly takes off in a new direction from one small point in the conversation.

Tapetum lucidum. A reflective membrane behind the retina in nocturnal animals to enhance nighttime vision.

Tear duct. The tunnel at the inner corner of the eye that conducts tears into the upper nasal chamber.

Temporal arteritis. An illness causing inflammation in the walls of arteries, especially those in the head; generally seen in elderly people; often obliterates the blood supply to the optic nerves, resulting in sudden blindness in one or both eyes; stoppable with corticosteroids.

Temporal lobe. The part of the cerebral hemisphere situated to the side of the frontal lobe.

Temporomandibular joint. Where the jaw attaches to the skull in front of the ear.

Tendon, achilles. The large cord behind the ankle connecting the gastrocnemius muscle to the heel.

Tendons. Round cords that attach muscles to the bones they move.

Tension pneumothorax. The accumulation of air in the pleural space under high pressure—high enough to shove the heart to the opposite side of the chest and prevent it from pumping blood.

Testes. Testicles. The site for the synthesis and storage of sperm, and the major site of testosterone production in men.

Testicle, undescended. A testicle that fails to descend from its embryonic origin in the abdomen into the scrotal sac; must be retrieved because of the high risk of it later turning cancerous.

Testicular torsion. Painful twisting of the testicle.

Testosterone. The hormone that makes a man look and behave like a man.

Tetanus. Widespread continuous muscle contractions caused by the toxin of *Clostridium tetani*.

Thoracic duct. The main lymphatic duct returning lymph up through the chest into the venous circulation.

Thromboembolism. An embolus that has broken free from a thrombus.

Thrombophlebitis. Inflammation of a deep venous thrombus.

Thrombose. To clot off.

Thrombus. A blood clot inside an artery or vein.

Thyroid. The bow-tie–shaped organ on either side of the trachea below the larynx controlling the speed of metabolic activity in the body.

Thyroid-stimulating hormone. The hormone released by the anterior pituitary to instruct the thyroid gland to release thyroxine.

Tibia. The main supporting bone of the lower leg, extending as a flat bone downward from the knee next to the large tibialis anterior muscle.

Tics. A brief repetitive flicker of a muscle or muscle group, such as blinking or head jerking, sometimes involving more complex movements.

Tinnitus. Ringing in the ear.

Tissue factor. Something that triggers the clotting factors to begin forming a blood clot.

Tissue. A collection of similar cells within an organ, for example, the liver, that help the organ to carry out its function.

Tonsils. Lymphoid tissue attached to the side walls of the pharynx.

Torsion. Twisting of a long tubular structure.

Tourette's syndrome. A childhood illness characterized by involuntary tics and vocalizations with no effect on intellect.

Trachea. The windpipe, which carries air from the nose and mouth into the lungs' bronchial tubes.

Tracheostomy. A hole cut into the trachea and brought to the skin surface, allowing air to be breathed directly into the lungs.

Tragus. The small triangular flap in front of the external ear canal.

Transcutaneous electrical nerve stimulators (TENS). An electrical device to stimulate large nerve fibers in a nerve and thereby relieve pain.

Transient ischemic attack (TIA). Any transient neurologic deficit due to ischemia; often due to a tiny embolus dislodging from a carotid artery thrombus, lodging downstream in a small cerebral artery, and then breaking apart minutes to hours later.

Tremor. Rhythmic shaking.

Triangle of death. The area across the middle front of the face where venous blood can carry facial bacteria directly into the brain.

Trichomonas. A parasite that infects the genital system of men and women.

Tricuspid valve. The valve at the entryway to the right ventricle.

Triglycerides. Three long-chain fatty acids hooked to a glycerol molecule.

Tuberculosis. A highly dangerous contagious disease of the lungs and deep body tissues caused by a mycobacterium that protects itself from most antibiotics by a waxy coat.

Tumor necrosis factor. A chemical released during inflammation to help direct an inflammatory attack.

Turbinates. Bony plates in the nasal chambers, covered by mucosa, that warm and moisten inhaled air.

Twins, fraternal. Twins with different genetic makeups.

Twins, identical. Twins with the same genetic makeup.

Tympanic membrane. Eardrum.

Typhoid fever. An illness spread by food and water contaminated with the bacterium salmonella, presenting with fever, abdominal pain, diarrhea, enlarged liver and spleen, and a slow heart rate (for the degree of fever) and often finding a long-term home in the gall bladder.

Ulna. The stationary bone of the forearm, palpable along the undersurface of the forearm.

Ulnar nerve. The funny bone nerve passing behind the elbow to supply about half the muscles that move the hand (the median nerve controls most of the other half, leaving the radial nerve simply to lift the hand).

Ultrasound. Images of the internal organs generated by sound waves bounced off them.

Umbilicus. An arterial and venous lifeline from the fetus to the placenta.

Umbrella, inferior vena cava. A cage that's slipped into the inferior vena cava to trap pulmonary-bound emboli from the legs and pelvis.

Upper motor neuron. The vertical nerve extending from the brain to the spinal cord (or brainstem) carrying motor instructions for the lower motor neuron.

Urea. The chemical used by the body to rid itself of the nitrogen discarded during the disassembly of amino acids.

Ureter. The tube carrying urine from the kidney to the bladder.

Urethra. The tube carrying urine from the bladder outside the body.

Uric acid. The chemical used by the body to rid itself of the nitrogen released from the breakdown of DNA.

Urination. Making number one.

Urologic system. While the kidneys, ureters, bladder, and urethra help clear the blood of undesirables by storing it in urine, the kidneys also regulate the level of calcium, sodium, potassium, acid, and a slew of other chemicals in the blood stream, help control the blood pressure, regulate the production of red blood cells by the bone marrow, and help synthesize vitamin D and angiotensin, earning the kidney its title as the second smartest organ in the body.

Utricle. See SACCULE.

Uvula. That fleshy tab dangling from the soft palate.

Vaccine. Part of an infectious agent purposely introduced into the body to prime the body's immune system in case the real infectious agent does try to enter the body.

Vagina. The hollow canal below the uterus through which a baby is delivered, bordered on one end by the cervix and the other by the outside world.

Vagus nerve. The parasympathetic nerve originating in the brainstem and wandering ("vagus" means wandering in Latin) through the chest and abdomen that, among other things, slows the heart, narrows the bronchial tubes, and moves the intestines.

Valsalva. Bearing down against a closed epiglottis.

Vas deferens. The tube carrying sperm from the testicles to the urethra.

Vascular system. The system of arteries, veins, and capillaries that carry blood to and from distant sites in the body.

Vasoconstrictor. Anything that causes an artery or vein to constrict.

Vasovagal reflex. Involuntary slowing of the heart in response to fear, anxiety, pain, or anything else that stimulates the vagus nerve to slow the heart.

Vasovagal syncope. Fainting due to sudden vagal nerve slowing of the heart, or pooling of blood in the legs without reflex tachycardia to maintain the blood pressure.

Vegetative. A conscious patient with roving eye movements unaware of his surroundings, unable to communicate any needs, and unable to coordinate his arms or legs for any useful activity; usually due to severe widespread damage to both cerebral hemispheres. Colloquially characterized by "the lights are on but nobody's home." Vegetative patients require long-term nursing care.

Veins. Blood vessels that carry blood to the heart.

Veins, varicose. Bulging, dilated veins visible on the skin surface.

Venereal warts. Genital warts.

Ventilator. A machine that pumps air into the lungs.

Ventricle, cerebral. Any of the hollow chambers within the brain where cerebrospinal fluid is made and out of which it circulates.

Ventricle, left. The thick-walled chamber on the left side of the heart that pumps oxygenated blood to the body.

Ventricle, right. The thin-walled, right-pumping chamber on the right side of the heart that pumps deoxygenated blood to the lungs.

Ventricular fibrillation. Chaotic quivering of the ventricles due to failure of the atrioventricular node and bundle of His to deliver a coordinated jolt of electricity to the ventricles.

Ventricular tachycardia. An arrhythmia of the heart in which the ventricles beat extremely rapidly, so rapid they often don't have time to fill with blood between beats.

Vertebrae, cervical. The bones of the spinal column in the neck.

Vertebral body. A cube of bone, seven of which form the cervical spine, twelve of which form the thoracic spine, and five of which form the lumbar spine.

Vertigo. The sensation that either you or the external world is moving when, in fact, both are stationary.

Viagra. A drug that raises nitric oxide levels in the penis, relaxing its blood vessels and allowing more blood into the penis.

Virus. A packet of DNA or RNA that reproduces by injecting its DNA or RNA into a host cell and substituting its reproductive commands for the host's.

Visual scintillations. Sparkles and jagged lines visible to the patient during an attack of migraine.

Vitamin A. The chemical converted into rhodopsin in rods.

Vitamin B12. A complex cobalt-containing chemical necessary for normal neurologic and hematologic function; requires intrinsic factor from the stomach to be absorbed downstream in the terminal ileum.

Vitamin C. Ascorbic acid.

Vitamin D. A hormone synthesized in the skin to help the parathyroid glands control the level of calcium in the blood.

Vitamin K. A vitamin necessary for synthesis of some of the clotting proteins.

Vitamins. Chemicals necessary for certain enzymes to do their job.

Vitreous humor. A clear jelly that keeps the eyeball distended.

Vocal cords. Two elastic bands of tissue that, when pulled taut by tiny muscles in the larynx (voice box), are made to vibrate by exhaled air, carrying the newly created sounds into the pharynx and mouth to be formed into words.

Warfarin. A chemical that inhibits the synthesis of one or more of the clotting proteins by interfering with vitamin K metabolism.

Warning leak. Sentinel hemorrhage. A leak of blood from an aneurysm or arteri-

ovenous malformation into the subarachnoid spinal fluid, causing flu-like
symptoms of headache, neck pain
radiating down the back, neck stiffness,
nausea and vomiting, and feeling out of
sorts. A small subarachnoid hemorrhage
such as this needs immediate medical
attention, as it is a warning of an
upcoming larger subarachnoid hemorrhage.

Waxman, Henry. The discoverer of streptomycin, the first antibiotic to effectively
treat tuberculosis.

Wernicke, Carl. The discoverer of the
speech center in the left posterior
temporal lobe that bears his name.

Wernicke's aphasia. Impaired speech due
to injury to Wernicke's area, characterized
by the inability to understand spoken or
written language and by the use of
nonsense words in speech and writing
because of the inability to assemble
phonemes into proper words.

Wernicke's area. The quarter-sized area in
the left posterior temporal lobe that
deciphers sounds and symbols into
language and assembles sound bits into
words.

Wheezing. High-pitched whistling sounds
due to narrowed bronchioles.

Whiplash. A whipsawing of the neck,
typically suffered in accidents when the
unsuspecting victim is caught off guard
and fails to hold his neck rigid.

Whipple, George. Along with George
Minot and William Murphy, discovered
that raw liver could cure vitamin B12
deficiency.

White matter. The areas of the brain
where axons traverse.

White meat. Muscle devoid of mitochondria, hence no fat and no dark red
myoglobin to bind oxygen; used for brief
periods of intense physical activity.

Whitehead. See ACNE.

Wrist drop. Inability to elevate the wrist,
usually due to a radial nerve injury.

X-linked diseases. Genetic diseases
carried on the long arm of the X chromosome, manifesting primarily in males.

Yeast. A type of fungus that reproduces by
budding.

INDEX

———∿∿∿∿∿∿∿———

ABOUT THE AUTHOR

Sheldon Margulies, M.D., is a board-certified practicing neurologist in Silver Spring, Maryland, and a member of the American Academy of Neurology. He graduated from the University of California at Berkeley in 1966, Stanford School of Medicine in 1971, completed an internal medicine residency at McGill University in 1973, and a neurology residency at the University of California San Francisco in 1976. He is also an inactive member of the Maryland Bar, having graduated from the University of Baltimore School of Law in 1988. Dr. Margulies currently holds the rank of clinical assistant professor in the Department of Neurology at the Uniformed Services University of the Health Sciences, having been a clinical assistant professor of neurology at Johns Hopkins University and assistant professor of neurology at the University of Maryland and University of Alabama.

Dr. Margulies is the author of *Everyday Doctoring: A New Approach to the Logic and Reasoning of Neurology and Medicine*, a textbook on medical and neurologic physical diagnosis, and coauthor of *Learning Law*, a textbook outlining legal reasoning. He has also published articles concerning the postconcussion syndrome and its causes; the medical evidence for and against the diagnosis of brain damage following mild head injuries; the Supreme Court's 1993 decision in *Daubert* concerning the trial court's role in excluding junk science from the courtroom; and the applicability of *Daubert* to the use of differential diagnosis and neuropsychological testing in proving claims of brain damage.

FURTHER READING

For further reading and specific references, please visit www. fascinatingbody.com, where you will also be able to ask Dr. Margulies questions, view the answers, and offer comments.